Nursing management
of diabetes mellitus

Nursing management of diabetes mellitus

Edited by

Diana W. Guthrie, R.N., M.S.P.H., F.A.A.N.,C.

Department of Nursing, Wichita State University; University of Kansas School of Medicine—Wichita Branch, Wichita, Kansas

Richard A. Guthrie, M.D., F.A.A.P.

University of Kansas School of Medicine—Wichita Branch, Wichita, Kansas

The C. V. Mosby Company

Saint Louis   1977

Printed in the United States of America

Distributed in Great Britain by Henry Kimpton, London

The C. V. Mosby Company
11830 Westline Industrial Drive, St. Louis, Missouri 63141

Library of Congress Cataloging in Publication Data

Main entry under title:

Nursing management of diabetes mellitus.

    Bibliography: p.
    Includes index.
    1. Diabetes—Nursing.   I. Guthrie, Diana W.
II. Guthrie, Richard A.
RC660.N83   616.4′62′0024613   76-27828
ISBN 0-8016-1995-5

TS/VH/VH 9 8 7 6 5 4 3 2 1

Contributors

ELIZABETH L. BURKE, R.N.

Coordinator of Diabetic Education, Good Samaritan Hospital and Medical Center, Portland, Oregon

BETSY S. DESIMONE, M.S.W.

Medical Social Worker, Los Angeles County Hospital, Los Angeles, California

LIDDY DYE, R.N.

Diabetes Teaching Nurse, Los Angeles County Hospital, Los Angeles, California

DIANA W. GUTHRIE, R.N., M.S.P.H., F.A.A.N.,C.

Assistant Professor, Department of Nursing, Wichita State University; Diabetes Nurse Specialist, University of Kansas School of Medicine—Wichita Branch, Wichita, Kansas

RICHARD A. GUTHRIE, M.D., F.A.A.P.

Professor and Chairman of Pediatrics, University of Kansas School of Medicine—Wichita Branch, Wichita, Kansas

JUDY JORDAN, R.N.

Nurse Specialist in Diabetes, Gainsville Medical Group, Andrews and Associates, P.A., Gainsville, Florida

RITA NEMCHIK, R.N., M.S.

Diabetes Nurse Educator, G. Duncan Research Foundation, Philadelphia, Pennsylvania

DONNA NICKERSON, R.N., M.N.

Nurse Specialist in Diabetes, Gainsville, Florida

COLLEEN SHEETS, R.N., B.S.N.

Diabetes Nurse Educator, G. Duncan Research Foundation, Philadelphia, Pennsylvania

MARIA SMITH, R.N., M.S.N.

Clinician in Diabetes; Former Assistant Professor of Nursing, University of Rochester, School of Medicine and Dentistry, Rochester, New York

VIRGINIA STUCKY, R.D., M.A.

Nutritionist, Wichita, Kansas

Preface

Diabetes mellitus is being increasingly recognized as a prevalent disorder, and much written information concerning the care and management of patients with this disease is quickly becoming outdated as more recent advances are made. This book is written for student nurses, registered nurses, nurse specialists, and other health professionals, as a tool for expanding and updating their knowledge in the care of those afflicted with diabetes.

Initial education of health professionals requires the advantage of up-to-date material as well as contact with varying schools of thought. Medical opinions vary with regard to the cause, cure, prevention, management, and control of diabetes mellitus and other associated problems. Continuing education sources need to become available so that this field of information and controversy may constantly be updated for the professional. The goal of this book is to present current information and ongoing resources so that health professionals, working together with involved consumers of health care, may develop and maintain optimal care.

In presenting a variety of thought predominant in the study of diabetes, we have cooperated with a number of nurses and dieticians who recommend various methods of both nursing and medical management. Our contributors are leaders in the field of management, representing such areas as office nursing management and consulting as well as specializing in a medical center setting or working in various aspects of primary and secondary care. Their individual areas of interest involve psychologic adjustment, better injection techniques and educational systems, treatment of atrophy, the child as well as the older adult with diabetes, and diet plans and resources available to the diabetic person as well as to the professional.

We trust that the professional or future professional will find this book a useful resource. The references included with each chapter provide a source of supportive information for continued study of areas of more specific interest. We hope that the glossary will clarify the terms used in the text and that the short directory of resources and services will be useful in guiding diabetic patients to better services.

The contributors to this book have been enthusiastic in their endeavor to share their experience and knowledge with others. We wish to thank them for their input, cooperation, and response to ideas and thoughts. We congratulate them on their excellent presentations and their cooperation in meeting deadlines.

Appreciation is expressed to Sandra Norris for the fine job she has done in typing the manuscript and to Dee Goodwin from the Media Resources Center of Wichita State University who handled the illustrations.

All of us join together in wishing that diabetes will soon be cured—and, even better, prevented—so that one day this book will become a part of history. Until that time, we hope that this book will in some way assist those who are afflicted with this chronic problem and, in so doing, give those individuals knowledge and motivation as they and their families participate meaningfully in their care.

Diana W. Guthrie

Richard A. Guthrie

Contents

Appendices

Introduction

Diabetes mellitus is a metabolic disease of unknown cause resulting from a deficiency of the pancreatic hormone insulin and, as recent evidence indicates, an irregularity in the release of glucagon. The disease has been known for centuries, and although research has elucidated many of the mysteries and has designed life-saving treatments, the cause and the prevention remain elusive. The word *diabetes* is from the Greek word meaning to siphon and refers to the most obvious sign of the disease—the marked loss of water by urination, polyuria. The word *mellitus* is derived from the Latin word for sweet and thus differentiates diabetes mellitus (sweet urine disease) from diabetes insipidus (bland urine disease), which is a disease of the posterior pituitary gland.

Diabetes mellitus was first described in an ancient Egyptian papyrus dating from the second millennium B.C. An Egyptian priest had observed that the urine of people afflicted by a disease of weight loss and excessive urination attracted insects, particularly bees and ants. Over the centuries, various other authors described a similar phenomenon without completely characterizing the disease or naming it.

It was the Greeks who characterized the excessive urination and the siphoning effect, or "the melting of the body through the loins" (weight loss and polyuria). A few centuries later, the Romans added the name mellitus, presumably because some enterprising physician gave the urine the taste test, discovering for sure its sugar content.

There were few developments that advanced our understanding of diabetes over the next millennium and a half. In more modern times, various diets were tried, some of them quite horrible. The rancid fat diet, popular in France in the 18th and 19th centuries, is one such example. It is questionable whether such diets extended the life span, but for the unfortunate victims, life certainly must have seemed longer.

Scientific progress in our knowledge of diabetes began in the 18th century with the development of the microscope and Langerhans' descriptions of the beta cell containing islets in the pancreas. Subsequent pathologists such as Virchow (1821-1902) and others then described the lesions of the pancreas, leading Minkowsky (1858-1931) to hypothesize that the pancreas was somehow involved in diabetes. Minkowsky then performed pancreatectomy in animals and produced diabetes. This experiment led to the speculation that the pancreas contained an internal secretion whose deficiency was responsible for the disease. Many experienced investigators searched in vain for the internal secretion of the pancreas. All efforts were thwarted because the enzymes of the exocrine pancreas digested the beta cells.

In the dramatic summer of 1921, Dr. Fredrick Banting devised a way of ridding the body of the exocrine pancreas while preserving functioning beta cells. Charles Best, a young graduate student working with Dr. Banting that summer, developed the alcohol techniques for extracting the hormone from the remaining pancreatic tissue and for measuring blood glucose. In August 1921, after several failures, an extract of pancreas produced a dramatic drop

1

in blood glucose in a diabetic dog, thus the internal secretion of the pancreas had been isolated. This secretion, named insulin, was soon purified and concentrated, and a new era dawned for the unfortunate victims of diabetes. Insulin has since been refined and further concentrated and has been modified to extend the duration of action, but no further dramatic breakthroughs have been made in the field.

In the 1950's, the oral hypoglycemic agents were developed, but these have been a mixed blessing. Recent research has finally begun to enlighten our understanding of the basic pathophysiology that leads to beta cell failure, and the outlook for a cure in the near future is brighter than before but is still some time away.

Berson and Yalow's development of the radioimmunoassay technique for measuring insulin levels, in the early 1960's, has introduced new techniques of research that may ultimately lead to the final answers. Use of electron microscopes for the morphologic study of the ultrastructure of the beta cells is another important technique leading us to an understanding of the mechanisms of insulin secretion. Most recently, Unger's discovery, that diabetes is a disease that involves a variation in glucagon as well as a deficiency of insulin, has also opened up exciting new vistas in diabetes research. These developments are discussed more thoroughly in Chapter 19 but are listed here to bring the history of diabetes development up to the modern era.

This book is concerned with the education of the diabetic patients and what the nurse and dietitian should know to properly educate them. A brief discussion of some of the controversies in diabetes is indicated here to put the diabetic education program in proper perspective.

With the discovery of insulin in 1921, a certain complacency settled over the diabetic world—diabetes was cured. After a few years, however, it became evident that insulin treatment was not the final answer. Insulin would extend the life span, but

within a few years, the diabetic person began to go blind and die from vascular disease. Thus began the most important of the many controversies concerning diabetes and one that continues to the present time. This controversy may be briefly stated as follows: Is the vascular disease, which causes most of the morbidity and mortality, a genetic component of the disease, that is, a concomitant of the diabetes and unrelated to control? Or—Is the vascular disease a complication of diabetes, somehow related to insulin deficiency and/or to hyperglycemia, and thus preventable by control? If the first position is correct, diabetes control is of little importance because the vascular disease is inevitable and unpreventable. Little effort should be made to achieve control, and diabetes education is unnecessary. If the latter position is correct, every effort should be made to effect control. Education of the diabetic patient, the public, and the health professional will be needed to accomplish this goal.

It is the bias of the editors of this book that control of diabetes is important in the prevention of both acute and chronic complications and that education of the diabetic patient is a vital part of the control program. The authors of this book have been selected with this thesis in mind; each chapter is intended to bring the student nurse, the staff nurse, the diabetes educator, and other health professionals the latest information we feel should be transmitted to diabetic individuals and their families to assist them in achieving control. It is our belief that people with diabetes should understand their disease so well that they can make adjustments themselves in their control program. The physician and the health care team, as their consultants, should assist these individuals when necessary in their control program.

Knowledge and motivation are needed if such a self-care program is to be effective. Motivation must come from within the patient, but self-motivation is facilitated by knowledge. Rarely will individuals do what they ought to do unless they understand why they are being asked to do it. Thus emotional support and an educational program are clearly needed to assist diabetic individuals in attaining both the motivational force necessary to control the diabetes and the information they need to carry out the prescribed program. Diabetes can be difficult to control under the best of circumstances, but in the presence of emotional disturbance, home instability, or lack of a will to try, it is impossible.

This book is divided into five sections. Section one presents the definition of the disease in some detail. Chapter 1 lists facts and statistics that have been updated to December 1975. Methods and criteria for diagnosis are reviewed in Chapter 2, and the process of intermediary metabolism and its derangement in diabetes are discussed in Chapter 3.

Section two considers the management, both medical and nursing, of the child and the adult with diabetes. In Chapter 4, childhood diabetes is presented in its relationship to the parent, the preschooler, the elementary school child, and the adolescent. The major emphasis in Chapter 5 is the older adult because individuals in this age group often develop many problems associated and nonassociated with diabetes. In all management, the psychosocial adjustment of the patient becomes most evident; Chapter 6 discusses the positive, supportive role of the health professionals in a variety of settings for a variety of needs.

Section three is concerned with acute and chronic care. Acute care is both preventive and crisis in nature. In Chapter 7 each of these aspects is balanced with information about medical management. Chronic complications are presented in a straightforward manner in Chapter 8. Chapters 9 and 10 discuss various medications, including their time action and the problems associated with their physical or mechanical administration. All methods of urine testing are presented in Chapter 11, including information to be placed on the individual's record. Hygiene, which involves the total person, and foot care receive special emphasis in Chapter 12.

Chapter 13 in Section three includes a variety of approaches in the dietary management of diabetic patients. Among the variety of approaches is the "point system" fathered by Dr. Rollin T. Woodyatt, who became involved with diabetes in the early years when insulin was discovered. His method of calculating and teaching diet involves the use of points and colored symbols related to carbohydrate, protein, and fat intake and represents a simplicity in the choice of the three food groups. The exchange program of the American Diabetes and American Dietetic Associations is the most commonly used method of diet calculation and patient education. It was currently updated by both associations working cooperatively. The exchange system often places foods of diverse content into the same category; for instance, peanut butter would be placed in the meat list, with some notice of its fat content. The point system developed by Woodyatt and perfected by Stucky, who authors Chapter 13, overcomes many of these problems. Each food is assigned carbohydrate points for its carbohydrate content, fat points for its fat content, and protein points for its protein content. Thus each food can be classified more precisely and diets calculated more closely to the needs of each individual. The point system like the exchange system is not perfect but does represent an alternative method of meal planning, which should be carefully considered by the health care team. The pros and cons of each of these programs are discussed.

Special problems is the major emphasis of Section four. Although other specific problems concerning diabetes are not covered in this section, the ones of more common occurrence—pregnancy, infant of the diabetic mother, and surgery—are discussed in Chapters 14, 15, and 16.

Section five portrays the resources available to the nurse and other professionals for patient education. Chapters 17 and 18 discuss methods available and assessment of education, which are tools to assist health professionals in their contacts with the involved patient and family. This section ends on a positive note, with an updating of research in Chapter 19. Its major emphasis, the importance of cure and prevention, is directed toward motivating the individual to optimal care.

Appendices A through F, presented for fingertip use, list practical information, including a suggested course outline, MET levels of activities, calorie-exercise expenditures, and a revised exchange list. The glossary, Appendix A, defines as many associated terms as possible. The resources and services are listed in Appendix B for the convenience of professionals and their clients as well. Many of the services are found in each state and often in the major cities of that state.

The health care team must involve people trained to handle the emotional as well as the medical aspects of diabetes. The team must be alert to prevent or handle the problems as they arise. Diabetes is not the problem. The problem is the individual with diabetes. Diabetes is a disease that affects every organ and every organ system of the body; moreover, it affects and is affected by the emotions.

Control of diabetes requires a team effort, involving the cooperation of the individual with diabetes, the physician, nurses, dietitians, podiatrists, physical therapists, social workers, psychologists, and other allied health personnel. This book is dedicated to the proposition that diabetes can and should be controlled through the teamwork of the health care professionals and the person with diabetes.

SECTION ONE

Definition

1

Diabetes mellitus: facts and statistics

Maria Smith

PREVALENCE AND INCIDENCE

In June 1975 the Committee on Statistics of the American Diabetes Association[1] reported that there are 6,000,000 people in the United States with known diabetes. Of these, 1.25 million are receiving insulin, 1.25 million are treated by oral agents, and 3.5 million control the disease by diet alone. At least 2,000,000 more people have diabetes and do not know it. By methods of projection statistics, it is estimated that an equal number of people will develop diabetes within their lifetime. From these figures, it is evident that there are at least 10 to 12 million known and potential diabetic persons in the United States (Table 1-1). In other words, 1 out of every 20 people will develop diabetes in their lifetime. At present 1 out of 4 families have a history of diabetes.

Some other important facts are: (1) diabetes has become the leading cause of new cases of blindness; (2) $1/2$ of all heart attacks, $3/4$ of all strokes, and $4/5$ of all gangrene are caused by diabetes[2]; (3) 160,000 people with diabetes are confined to their home; (4) 37% of diabetics, a total of 40,000 persons, die from their disease each year (this figure does not include those deaths from cardiovascular disease in which diabetes is the underlying cause of death); (5) the incidence of diabetes increases with age—the majority of known diabetic persons are at least 45 years of age; (6) the sex ratio is nearly equal, as stated in the 1965 report of the National Center for Health Statistics.[3]

The recent official report of the National Diabetes Commission, submitted to Congress on December 10, 1975, lists diabetes officially as the third leading cause of death, with between 300,000 and 350,000 deaths attributable to diabetes each year. However, with up-to-date studies of vital statistics, an important discovery is noted. On death certificates, the final cause rather than the underlying, or contributory, cause of death is counted for statistical evalua-

Table 1-1. Diabetes incidence

	USA*		Kansas*	
Known diabetes		6,000,000		66,338
Insulin dependent	1,250,000		13,821	
Oral drugs	1,250,000		13,821	
Diet	3,500,000		38,696	
Unknown and potential estimate		6,000,000		66,338
TOTALS		12,000,000		132,676

*According to the 1970 census, the population of the USA is 203,235,298 and that of Kansas, 2,247,000. Projected information provided by the Research and Analysis Section, Division of Registration and Health, Statistics Services, Kansas Department of Health and Environment.

tion. The 1970 statistics are very revealing if tabulated by the underlying cause of the vascular disease that finally resulted in death. The 1970 totals would be calculated as follows:

Diabetes—fifth leading cause of death	40,000
Heart attacks—530,000 deaths $\frac{1}{2}$ caused by diabetes	265,000
Strokes—211,000 deaths $\frac{3}{4}$ caused by diabetes	158,000
Total deaths in which diabetes was either the direct or contributory cause	463,000

According to this accounting method, diabetes may be considered the leading cause of death by disease.[2] Fatal diseases would compare as follows:

Diabetes (both as direct and contributory cause of death)	463,000
Cancer	300,000
Heart disease (total caused by heart disease minus those due to diabetes)	265,000

The life expectancy of the general population is increasing, and there appears to be a corresponding increase in the total number of persons with diabetes. In its 1975 report (mentioned above), the National Commission on Diabetes also states that diabetes affects 10 million Americans, or 5% of the population. There is an increased risk in the development of diabetes with every 20% of excess weight. The incidence of diabetes appears to be increasing at the rate of 6% per year.[4]

Children constitute 5% to 10% of the insulin-dependent population. In the 1930's, Priscilla White[5] reported the prevalence of diabetes to be 1 in 2500 children. A recent study in Michigan reported that the prevalence of diabetes is 1 in 625 school-age children.[6] Diabetes is less common in children under school age. However, even if this younger group were added, a higher prevalence of diabetes in children would still be found today. In fact, these data, if correct, would indicate a doubling of the incidence of diabetes in children in the past 40 years.

Better disease reporting and statistical errors in both studies may account for some of the differences. However, environmental factors increasing the incidence of diabetes must be looked for and prevented when possible.

The prevalence of diabetes is also increasing dramatically in older individuals, who are the most frequent victims of the disease. The increased incidence of diabetes in black women has been extremely dramatic. It is estimated that 20% more nonwhites than whites develop diabetes.[5]

A number of causes account for the increased numbers of people having diabetes. Diagnostic testing and reporting are more refined today, and early detection of the disease is more common. Diabetic youth are living near-normal lives with insulin therapy, and their children are apt to inherit the diabetic gene. Also, people are living longer and developing diabetes in later life. Obesity is a significant problem and has been correlated as a "stress factor" in those persons predisposed to diabetes.[7] Some researchers have concluded that the incidence of diabetes has increased within recent years in those groups of people who consume large amounts of refined sugar.[8-10] The hormonal factors associated with pregnancy can be diabetogenic, resulting in abnormal glucose tolerance curves in pregnant women prone to diabetes and women taking birth control pills. In addition, environmental and personal stresses may be "trigger factors," causing an individual to change from a prediabetic stage to a symptomatic stage of diabetes.

There are slightly more women than men with diabetes and a marked increase in diabetes in older individuals (50% of diabetics develop their disease after 45 years of age). There is no geographical effect on the incidence or prevalence of diabetes in the United States, though there is in the world. The incidence of diabetes in various countries is closely correlated with affluency and the incidence of obesity.[7] Not all persons with a positive family history of diabetes develop the disease. Genetic characteristics,[11] stress factors,[7] and environmental conditions[12] probably determine susceptibility.

CLASSIFICATION

Diabetes mellitus may occur as a primary disease of unknown cause or as a secondary disease resulting from pancreatic disorders or other hormonal problems causing tissue resistance to the effects of insulin.

Primary diabetes mellitus

Ketosis-prone (juvenile) diabetes. Ketosis-prone diabetes commonly occurs during childhood or adolescence, although exceptions are frequently reported. The onset of the disease is usually sudden and dramatic, and the patient frequently experiences many symptoms and may have symptoms of ketoacidosis. During the first months after diagnosis, a "remission" frequently occurs, and normal or near normal amounts of insulin are released in response to a glucose stimulus. Hypertrophy of the beta cells may occur, followed by insulin deficiency, atrophy of beta cells, and hyalinization of the pancreatic islets. Ketosis-prone individuals require insulin, are unstable, and may develop complications, especially the microvascular complications, at a more rapid rate than the ketosis-resistant group.

Ketosis-resistant (adult) diabetes. Ketosis-resistant diabetes typically occurs in people 40 years or older, who are obese and less inclined to have gross fluctuations in blood glucose levels. Individuals with resistant diabetes secrete some insulin (hence the resistance to ketosis); however, their response to a glucose stimulus is often slow and subnormal. They often exhibit a late second peak of insulin release. Chronic complications, especially the macrovascular complications of diabetes, are more frequently seen in the ketosis-resistant than the ketosis-prone group.

Secondary diabetes mellitus

Secondary diabetes refers to insulin deficiency resulting from the loss of pancreatic tissue (as in cancer, surgical removal of the pancreas, and chronic pancreatitis) and to diabetes resulting from an excess of certain hormones (corticosteroids, growth hormone, catecholamines, and glucagon) that raise blood glucose levels and cause an increased resistance to or a decreased effect of insulin. Diabetes is also often an adjunct to pregnancy and may be precipitated by the use of birth control pills. Hormonal diabetes is often reversible when the stress factors (hormones) are removed.

CHARACTERISTIC STAGES

An individual may naturally progress from the prediabetic to the overt stage of diabetes (Table 1-2). However, it is also possible to see a reversal from the chemical or overt stage of the disease to the prediabetic or chemical diabetic stage when stress factors are withdrawn.

If diabetes is inherited as a recessive

Table 1-2. Characteristics of the stages of diabetes mellitus

	Signs and symptoms	Diagnostic testing
Prediabetes (a genetic potential for diabetes)	None	Normal
Chemical	None	Normal fasting blood glucose level; abnormal glucose tolerance test; abnormal serum insulin level
Overt	Actively symptomatic	Elevated fasting blood glucose level; grossly abnormal glucose tolerance test; decreased serum insulin level

trait, as geneticists[11] believe is true of most cases, the probability of developing diabetes should be 100% if both parents have diabetes or if the person has an identical twin with diabetes. If one parent or grandparent on one side of the family and an aunt and uncle on the other side have diabetes, then the statistical probability of having diabetes is 80%. If one parent is diabetic and a grandparent on the nondiabetic parental side also has diabetes the probability of diabetes in the offspring should be 60%. (See Table 14-2.) The actual incidence of diabetes in susceptible families usually falls below the expected statistical probability, indicating that environmental factors affect the expression of the diabetic gene.

ECONOMIC IMPACT

The cost of medical treatment of diabetes was reported by the Committee on Statistics of the American Diabetes Association at the 1975 annual meeting.[1] In 1974, more than 227 million dollars were spent by those having diabetes for direct medical care costs. In addition to the direct medical care costs, there is an additional economic loss from missed work days and disability, both temporary and permanent. The economic loss from diabetes is unknown, but even excluding the loss to society of productivity from early death, the loss is estimated to be in excess of 5 billion dollars per year, an incredible loss. All in all, by numbers and cost, diabetes is a startling disease that needs major recognition and financing in order to be controlled.

There needs to be a combination of education and research in order to maintain optimal management and, most importantly, to discover a prevention and cure for this devastating disease.

REFERENCES

1. American Diabetes Association, Inc., Report of Committee on Statistics, New York, June 1975.
2. Scoville, A. B.: Report to American Diabetes Association, June 1974.
3. National Center for Health Statistics: Characteristics of persons with diabetes, U.S., July 1964-June 1965, Washington, D.C., USPHS Pub. 1000, No. 40, Oct. 1967.
4. Report of the National Commission on Diabetes, vol. 3, part 2, December 1975, U.S. Government Printing Office, pp. 93-354.
5. Pincus, G., and White, P.: On the inheritance of diabetes mellitus, Am. J. Med. Sci., **186:**1, 1933.
6. Gorwitz, K., Howen, G., and Thompson, T.: The prevalence of diabetes in Michigan school age children. Diabetes, **25:**128, Feb. 1976.
7. West, K. M.: Culture, history and adiposity or Should Santa Claus reduce? Obesity and Bariatric Medicine **3:**48, 1974.
8. Cohen, A. M., and others: Change of diet of Yemenite Jews in relation to diabetes and ischaemic heart disease, Lancet **2:**1399, 1961.
9. Yudkin, J.: Sweet and dangerous, New York, 1973, Bantana Book Co.
10. Campbell, G. D.: Diabetes in Asians and Africans in and around Durban, S. Afr. Med. J. **37:**1195, 1963.
11. Steinberg, A. G.: Heredity and diabetes, Eugen. Q. **2:**26, 1955.
12. Tattersall, R. B., and Fajans, S. S.: A difference between the inheritance of classical juvenile onset and maturity onset type of diabetes of young people, Diabetes **24:**44, 1975.

BIBLIOGRAPHY

Cahill, G.: Physiology of insulin in man, Diabetes **20:**10, 1971.
Ellenberg, M., and Rifkin, H., editors: Diabetes mellitus theory and practice, New York, 1970, McGraw-Hill Book Co.
Levine, R.: Diabetes mellitus, Ciba Clin. Symp. **15:**4, 1963.
Smith, M. , and Burday, S. Z.: Nursing the patient with diabetes mellitus, Rochester, N.Y., 1970, Rochester Regional Medical Program.
Spencer, R.: Patient care in endocrine problems, Philadelphia, 1973, W. B. Saunders Co.
Williams, R. H.: Textbook of endocrinology, Philadelphia, 1968, W. B. Saunders Co.

2

Diagnosis of diabetes mellitus

Maria Smith

Diabetes mellitus may be extremely easy to diagnose or extremely difficult. In the ketosis-prone individual, the onset of diabetes is usually fulminate. Signs and symptoms are present, and the fasting blood glucose level is usually elevated. On the other hand, diabetes in the ketosis-resistant person may be symptomless and at times difficult to diagnose. The earlier and milder forms of the disease are often difficult to diagnose, especially because the norms and criteria for diagnosis have not as yet been completely standardized.

WHO SHOULD BE TESTED FOR DIABETES?

In adults, testing for the presence of diabetes should be carried out when there is glycosuria, a history of diabetes in the past, a strongly positive family history of diabetes, a history of fetal loss or large babies (babies over 9 pounds at birth), symptoms of hypoglycemia, presence of obesity, evidence of neuropathy, retinopathy, premature coronary artery disease or early peripheral atherosclerosis, evidence of lipid abnormalities (such as hypercholesterolemia or hypertriglyceridemia), or individuals in older age groups.[1]

In children, testing should be carried out when there is a strong family history of diabetes, obesity, or symptoms of hypoglycemia or glycosuria.[2]

RECOMMENDED TESTS

A variety of tests are available for screening for diabetes; they are discussed here in the order of their effectiveness from least to most effective.

Urine testing for glucose values

Testing of the urine for levels of glucose or reducing substances is one of the commonest and least effective methods of screening for diabetes. The urine glucose test has the advantage of being inexpensive, quick, and painless. However, it has the disadvantage of being insensitive. The urine test will be positive for glucose only after the blood glucose values have become sufficiently elevated to allow glucose to spill into the urine, usually a blood glucose value of 180 mg/dl (deciliter) or more. Thus, the urine test will be positive, especially in adults, only in advanced stages of the disease and is of no value for detection of the early stages of the disease. For this reason, urine testing should be abandoned for mass screening and should be reserved for quick screening in the office of individuals who are symptomatic or strongly suspected of being diabetic. A positive urine glucose test is usually significant (except in renal glycosuria), but a negative urine test does not rule out diabetes.

Blood testing for glucose values

Random blood sampling. Random sampling, that is, the taking of blood samples at any convenient time, is performed without standardization. Such values are difficult to interpret because there are no norms with which to compare them. Again, if the values are grossly abnormal, they may be

11

meaningful, but normal or mildly abnormal values are meaningless without standardization of dietary intake and sampling times and without the establishment of careful experimentation of the normal values. Random blood sampling is being used extensively by public health departments and diabetes associations for mass screening because of its simplicity, relative inexpensiveness, and convenience to the population being screened, but it is of limited sensitivity.

Fasting blood glucose test. The fasting blood glucose test (commonly referred to as FBS, fasting blood sugar) is probably the most frequently used laboratory test for diabetes. The FBS values are almost always elevated in the person with overt diabetes, especially in the child; thus the FBS is a good confirmatory test for diabetes in these symptomatic individuals. It is however, a poor diagnostic tool for the ketosis-resistant adult because FBS values usually remain constant throughout life even though the ability to handle a glucose load declines. The FBS is also a poor tool for screening of children for the earlier stages of diabetes because, by definition, individuals with chemical diabetes have normal FBS values. It can be said that a person is diabetic if the FBS value (using true glucose values) is greater than 130 mg/dl. This commonly used test will miss about 85% of the diabetic population.

Two-hour postprandial blood glucose test (2-hour PPG). The 2-hour PPG is a more sensitive test than the FBS because it does measure glucose after some degree of stress (for example, a meal). This test should not be considered totally diagnostic for diabetes, however, because it is influenced by a variety of factors: (1) The elderly often have a mildly elevated glucose level 1 or 2 hours after a meal, but the total curve never goes high enough to be truly diagnostic of diabetes. (2) Starvation may produce an abnormal glucose curve with a peak at 2 hours. (3) Food intake is usually not standardized; thus, the values are variable and difficult to interpret.

The 2-hour PPG can be diagnostic if a standard glucose load (1.75 gm of glucose per kg body weight) is administered with the meal and a reading of 180 mg/dl or greater is obtained in a person for whom there is no other cause for impaired carbohydrate intolerance.[3]

Oral glucose tolerance test (OGTT). The most sensitive method for detecting diabetes mellitus is some modification of the OGTT. Properly standardized and performed, the OGTT will detect early chemical and mild overt diabetes with great accuracy. There are many pitfalls, however, to accurate glucose tolerance testing. The individual to be tested should receive a high carbohydrate diet for 3 days before the test. For adults, the diet should contain 80 gm of protein, 300 gm of carbohydrate, and the rest fat. For children, the diet should contain 60% to 65% of the proper calories for age and size as carbohydrate. A high carbohydrate intake standardizes the glycogen reserves and sensitizes the beta cell to the glucose stimulus. Artificial diabetes can be created by starvation or carbohydrate deprivation. After an overnight fast of 10 to 12 hours, the adult is given 100 gm of glucose in a palatable base. For the child, the fasting period should be standardized to 10 hours: a snack is given at 10 PM and the test is started at 8 AM the following day. Failure to standardize the fasting period in children will result in an abnormal baseline (fasting) value. The child is given 1.75 gm of glucose per kilogram ideal body weight for height, which is administered as a 30% solution in a palatable, carbonated base. The glucose solution should be consumed within 5 minutes. Samples of blood and urine are obtained while the person is fasting, and then 30, 60, 120, and 180 minutes after oral glucose is administered. Some investigators also obtain a 90-minute sample and some extend the test to 4, 5, and even 6 hours. Most investigators have found the 3- or 4-hour test best for the diagnosis of diabetes, and the 5- or 6-hour test best for confirming reactive hypoglycemia. Medications should not be given during the

Table 2-1. Fajans-Conn criteria*

	Glucose values (mg per 100 ml)	
Sampling times	**Whole blood**	**Plasma or serum**
Fasting	—	—
Hours after glucose administered		
1 hour	160	185
1½ hours	140	160
2 hours	120	140
3 hours	—	—

*Glucose load 1.75 gm per kg ideal body weight as 25% solution in otherwise healthy and ambulatory individuals under age 50.

test, and smoking should not be allowed. Simple, light activity is desirable.

There are various criteria for the interpretation of the OGTT. The most widely used and best accepted criteria are those of Fajans and Conn[4] (Table 2-1). Values *above* the norms established by Fajans and Conn are interpreted as diabetes. Mildly elevated values after glucose is administered with a normal blood glucose value at the initial time (fasting) is chemical diabetes. Elevated values after glucose is administered with an elevated blood glucose value at the initial time (fasting) is overt diabetes. Fajans and Conn's values are for venous plasma. Values for whole blood are 15% lower than for plasma, and values for capillary or arterial blood will be slightly higher than venous blood values. In addition, values considered "normal" will vary with the chemical methods used by the laboratory for determining blood glucose values. Most laboratories use a method that measures levels of some other reducing substance in the blood besides glucose, and these values will be slightly higher than true glucose values as measured by the glucose oxidase method. Most good laboratories today use automated methods that measure nearly true glucose values. Appropriate corrections must be made for these modifications in technique.

Glucose tolerance changes with age. Normal values are slightly lower than the Fajans and Conn norms in small children,

slightly higher in older children, and considerably higher in children during the preadolescent growth spurt and early adolescence.[5] The glucose curve is flattened and prolonged during pregnancy and elevated with aging. Some authors[6] add to the Fajans and Conn criteria 10 mg per decade of age after age 50 to correct for the "normal" decline in glucose tolerance with age. Appropriate age-related norms must always be used. It is inappropriate to use Fajans and Conn's norms for interpretations of glucose tolerance in children. The best standardized norms for children are the norms of Pickens and Burkeholder.[7] These norms are for capillary whole blood and must be appropriately adjusted if venous plasma is used.

Various drugs will affect the outcome of the OGTT. The following drugs elevate the blood glucose levels: glucocorticoids, which stimulate gluconeogenesis; thiazide diuretics, which diminish total body potassium levels and aggravate existing diabetes; birth control pills containing mestranol, which impairs glucose metabolism; and nicotinic acid, which may damage liver cells. The following drugs decrease blood glucose levels: salicylates, whose mechanism is unknown; alcohol, which inhibits the release of glucose by the liver; monoamine oxidase inhibitors (MAOI), which are "mood elevators" that stimulate insulin release; and propranolol, which suppresses epinephrine and thus suppresses glycogenolysis by the liver.

Other tests. Other diagnostic tests for carbohydrate tolerance are the cortisone primed oral glucose tolerance test, the intravenous glucose tolerance test, and the tolbutamide tolerance test. Of these tests the cortisone primed OGTT is most useful. This test is more sensitive than the standard OGTT because it adds cortisone to glucose as an additional stress to the insulin-producing mechanism. It will diagnose chemical diabetes in the earliest stages. The test has, however, not been standardized for children.

The intravenous glucose tolerance test is

a useful tool for studying chemical diabetes, especially for studying the insulin reserve; however, it is not as sensitive as the OGTT for diagnosis. The tolbutamide tolerance test is useful in studying the responsiveness of the individual in the early stages of diabetes to the sulfonylurea compounds but likewise is not as sensitive as the standard OGTT for diagnosis.

Testing for serum insulin values

Since the advent of the radioimmunoassay for insulin concentrations in the early 1960's, it has been possible to measure the insulin-secreting ability of the pancreas during glucose tolerance testing. Testing for insulin-secreting ability markedly increases the reliability of the OGTT. When the laboratory has the capability for measuring serum insulin values, this measurement should always be a part of the OGTT. Fajans and Conn[8] have published norms for serum insulin values for adults, and Jackson and Guthrie[9] have published norms for children.

SUMMARY

The OGTT is the most sensitive test for the diagnosis of diabetes mellitus, especially in the earlier and asymptomatic stages. Combined with serum insulin determinations, the properly standardized and interpreted OGTT is an extremely sensitive tool for the diagnosis and study of diabetes. Its only disadvantage to the patient is its expense and inconvenience. The sensitivity of the test overcomes these disadvantages. When symptoms suggestive of diabetes are present, the FBS or 2-hour PPG determination may be all that is needed for diagnosis. When these are negative or when diabetes is suspected in an asymptomatic individual, an OGTT combined with serum insulin values, where available, should be performed under rigidly controlled conditions and the results compared with carefully selected appropriate norms for age.

Caution must be taken not to overdiagnose diabetes because a false diagnosis has serious implications in employment, insurability, and emotional impact. On the other hand, all actual cases of diabetes should be diagnosed as early as possible so that appropriate treatment can be prescribed in order to prevent complications of the disease. The standard OGTT properly performed and rigidly controlled and interpreted should lead to neither false-positive nor false-negative tests but to a proper diagnosis of diabetes mellitus.

REFERENCES

1. Smith, M., and Burday, Z.: Nursing the patient with diabetes mellitus, Rochester, N.Y., 1972, Rochester Regional Medical Program, pp. 1-2.
2. Rosenbloom, A. L., Drash, A., and Guthrie, R. A.: Chemical diabetes mellitus in childhood: report of a conference, Diabetes **21**:45, 1972.
3. Ellenberg, M., and Rifkin, H.: Diabetes mellitus: theory and practice, New York, 1970, McGraw-Hill Book Co. p. 445.
4. Fajans, S., and Conn, J.: The early recognition of diabetes mellitus, Science **82**:208, 1959.
5. Burkeholder, J. N.; Pickens, J. M.; and Womack, W. N.: Oral glucose tolerance test in siblings of children with diabetes mellitus, Diabetes **16**:156, 1967.
6. O'Sullivan, J. B.: Oral glucose tolerance tests. In Hammi, G. J., and Danowski, T. S., editors: Diabetes mellitus: diagnosis and treatment, vol. 2, New York, 1967, American Diabetes Association, Inc., pp. 47-50.
7. Pickens, J. M.; Burkeholder, J. N.; and Womack, W. N.: Oral glucose tolerance test in normal children, Diabetes **16**:11, 1967.
8. Fajans, S., and Conn, J. W.: Prediabetes, subclinical diabetes and latent clinical diabetes: interpretation, diagnosis and treatment. *In* Leibel, B. S., and Wrenshall, G. A., editors: The nature and treatment of diabetes, Proceedings of the 5th Congress of the International Diabetes Federation, Excerpta Medica, Series 84, Amsterdam, 1965, pp. 641-656.
9. Jackson, R. L., and Guthrie, R. A.: The child with diabetes, Kalamazoo, Mich., 1975, The UpJohn Co., p. 19.

3

Intermediary metabolism

Maria Smith

An intensive interdependence between physician, nurse, and patient is essential for the proper control of diabetes mellitus; few chronic diseases demand such cooperation. The physician will diagnose and outline a plan of treatment, while the nurse implements the plan of care together with the diabetic person and the family. To best accomplish this task, the nurse must have an understanding of the mechanism of diabetes, including normal carbohydrate, protein, and fat metabolism, the physiologic role of insulin, and the consequences of insulin deprivation. These concepts are discussed in this chapter.

GLUCOSE-INSULIN RELATIONSHIP

Glucose is the primary fuel for all body tissues. The brain utilizes 25% of the total body glucose—an especially high demand. Because brain energy stores are very small, a constant supply of glucose must always be available to maintain adequate brain function. It is, therefore, imperative that the blood glucose level be maintained in the 60 to 120 mg/dl range to prevent central nervous system compromise.

Insulin is the primary hormone for regulating blood glucose levels and does so by controlling the rate at which blood glucose is taken up by muscle, fat, and liver cells. Each of these three types of cells utilizes glucose in a different way, as determined by specific enzyme systems. Many of the principles of diabetic management and control are based on the intricate interaction of insulin and other hormones with these three cellular processes.

Fat cell

The primary function of the fat cell is providing storage. It contains unique enzymes that convert glucose into triglycerides as well as enzymes that convert triglycerides to fatty acids, which are released and converted to ketones in the liver, when needed.

The conversion of glucose to triglycerides and the breakdown of triglycerides to free fatty acids take place continuously and simultaneously within the same fat cell, and both processes are regulated by insulin. High blood insulin levels stimulate the uptake of glucose by fat cells to form triglycerides; thus there is a net gain of storage fat. During low blood insulin levels, glucose uptake into the fat cell is poor; thus less triglyceride is formed. Triglyceride breakdown then exceeds formation, resulting in a net loss of the storage fat. Thus, by regulating glucose uptake into fat cells, insulin can influence net fat metabolism.

Insulin also inhibits the enzyme lipase, which breaks down storage fat into fatty acids and glycerol. When insulin is high and lipase is inhibited, there is also a net increase in storage fat. There is a net decrease in storage fat when insulin is low, because lipase becomes activated and fat is then broken down.

Muscle cell

The muscle cell has two primary functions: it converts glucose into energy needed for muscle function, and it serves as a reservoir for protein and glycogen. During starvation, the protein of the contractile apparatus itself can be made available in the form of amino acids, which can then be converted in the liver into glucose in order to maintain blood glucose at an adequate concentration for brain function.

In the muscle cell, as in the fat cell, insulin promotes the uptake of glucose. The muscle cell, however, has different enzymes that control two metabolic pathways for glucose. First, glucose can be converted into "contractile energy." Second, glucose can be converted to glycogen, a storage form of glucose that is more readily available than triglycerides in times of glucose insufficiency.

When blood glucose levels are normal, insulin also affects the enzymes of the muscle cell to maintain muscle mass by promoting the uptake of amino acids and preventing the breakdown of protein.

Liver cell

Liver glycogen is another storage form of glucose. As mentioned above, glycogen is more readily available for use than are triglycerides, which first have to be converted to free fatty acids and then converted to ketones. The liver monitors these conversions and also converts amino acids to glucose when necessary. The latter process is called gluconeogenesis (new glucose formation).

Although insulin is not required for the transport of glucose into the liver, insulin directly affects the liver to promote the uptake of glucose by reducing the rate of glycogenolysis (glycogen breakdown), increasing glycogen synthesis, and decreasing the rate of gluconeogenesis.[1]

Beta cell

Insulin is secreted by the beta cells of the pancreas, which continually monitor glucose levels. The beta cells function first as a sensor of blood glucose levels. The beta cells then secrete enough insulin to regulate the carbohydrate load, maintaining the blood glucose level within a very narrow range. A feedback system exists whereby a small amount of carbohydrate stimulates a small amount of insulin release. The liver responds to increased insulin secretion by suppressing glycogen release (glycogenolysis). The formation of

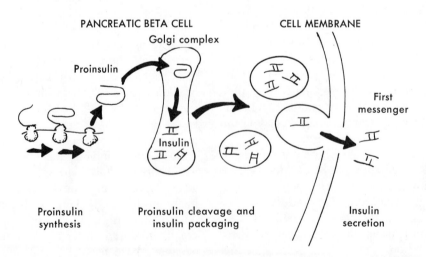

Fig. 3-1. Synthesis of first messenger.

new glucose (gluconeogenesis) is likewise suppressed. A large carbohydrate intake stimulates a greater insulin response, and the peripheral and liver cells take up glucose. When glucose levels are low, insulin release is suppressed and glycogenolysis and gluconeogenesis occur in order to feed glucose into the system and maintain the blood glucose levels.

Although the process of beta cell stimulation and insulin release is not entirely understood, it is recognized that glucose metabolism signals the synthesis of the pre-cursor of insulin called proinsulin. Proinsulin is transformed into insulin within the beta cell, and the insulin is then stored in granules and released in response to several stimuli (Fig. 3-1). Glucose is the most profound stimulus to insulin release. Other stimuli include amino acids, hormones (such as adrenocorticotropic hormone [ACTH], growth hormone, glucocorticoids, thyroxin, and estrogens), vagal stimulation, sulfonylureas, and ketones. Those substances diminishing insulin secretion are epinephrine, norepinephrine, insulin, bi-

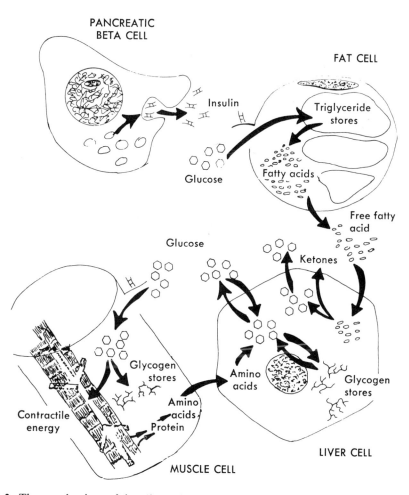

Fig. 3-2. The mechanism of insulin action in fat, muscle, and liver cells: In fat cells, insulin promotes the uptake of glucose and enhances triglyceride stores. In muscle cells, glucose enters via the membrane, made permeable by insulin, and is converted to glycogen stores or used for contractile energy. In liver cells, glucose is stored as are amino acids.

guanides, and thiazide diuretics; starvation and hypoxia also inhibit insulin secretion.

Pancreatic insulin is secreted directly into the portal circulation and is carried to the liver, the central organ of glucose homeostasis, where 50% of the insulin is degraded. The peripheral circulation then transports insulin to body cells and ultimately to the kidney, where 25% is degraded, and excretion occurs.

Other hormones

Epinephrine. Epinephrine is a hormone that has multiple effects to prepare the body for many different kinds of stress. Its effect on glucose is very rapid and can produce minute-to-minute changes in blood glucose levels. Stress stimulates epinephrine release, and the hormone then serves to mobilize glycogen to yield a higher blood glucose level. Epinephrine also suppresses insulin release to further enhance blood glucose levels.

Growth hormone. Growth hormone, together with insulin, promotes body growth. Its effect on blood glucose levels is a slow one. Growth hormone elevates blood glucose, making it available for the growth process. However, the physiologic role of growth hormone in glucose control is unknown. Though growth hormone elevates blood glucose levels and hypoglycemia will increase growth hormone levels, it is not known whether growth hormone plays any meaningful role in minute-to-minute regulation of blood glucose levels.

The second messenger

Insulin affects intracellular functioning, as outlined in Fig. 3-2. The intracellular effect of insulin is accomplished by "second messengers," which are activated by receptors on specific cell membranes that determine whether or not the cell responds to insulin. Specific enzymes then allow the cell to perform its functions in response to insulin. One enzymatic mechanism that all insulin-responsive cells have is the hexokinase system. When insulin stimulates these cells, the cell membrane is modified to allow the uptake of glucose. The hexokinase system is also stimulated to allow the cell to take up and metabolize glucose. The enzymatic system for lipogenesis (formation of fats) is specific to the fat cell, while the enzymatic system for conversion of glucose to energy is specific to the muscle cell. By a separate set of enzymes, the

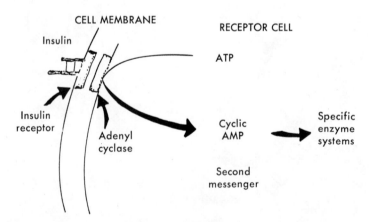

Fig. 3-3. Activation of second messengers: Insulin is synthesized from proinsulin within the beta cell of the pancreas. Second messengers, which are receptors on specific cells, determine cellular responsiveness to insulin. Specific enzyme systems then permit the cell to respond to insulin action.

fat cell can, of course, also convert glucose to energy for its own metabolic processes, which include conversion of glucose to fat, an energy-requiring process. All these specific functions are mediated by a second messenger called cyclic AMP (adenosine monophosphate). When insulin stimulates the responsive cell membrane receptor, cyclic AMP is activated through a long chain of chemical events. The cyclic AMP then activates the particular cell's metabolic processes that use the absorbed glucose (Fig. 3-3).

THE PROBLEM OF INSULIN DEFICIENCY

Thus far, normal homeostatic mechanisms have been discussed. Fig. 3-4 illustrates the abnormal state of insulin deprivation, as observed in individuals with

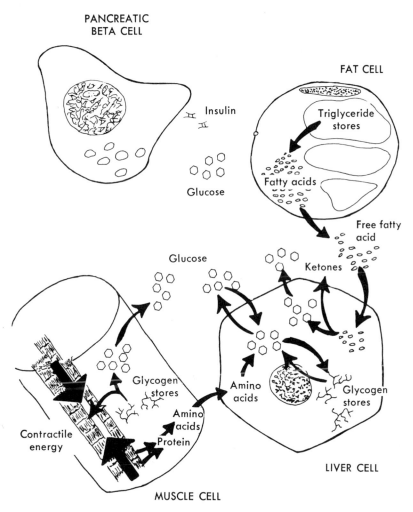

Fig. 3-4. Insulin deficiency: An immediate consequence of insulin deficiency is the lack of glucose uptake by cells. In fat cells, triglyceride stores are liberated in the absence of insulin, yielding free fatty acids, which are ultimately converted into ketones. In muscle cells, glycogen stores are activated and amino acids are converted into glucose in the liver to provide contractile energy.

unknown or uncontrolled diabetes. The degree of insulin lack will influence the extent of this process. If untreated, complete insulin deprivation, as often observed in the young child with diabetes, will terminate in ketoacidosis and coma. The diabetic adult with minimal insulin lack may not even experience symptoms of the disease.

Diabetes mellitus may be defined as an absolute or relative lack of insulin that results in aberrations of fat, protein, and carbohydrate metabolism. Absence of insulin production initially affects the uptake of glucose in muscle and fat cells. As glucose entry into cells diminishes, the body signals for fuel, and glycogen is released from the liver. The blood glucose level is thereby further elevated. As the glucose levels approach 180 mg/dl of blood,* the capacity of the renal tubules to reabsorb glucose (renal threshold) is exceeded, and glucose is excreted into the urine (glycosuria). Because glucose is an osmotic diuretic, water and salts are also excreted in large quantities, and cellular dehydration occurs. Prolonged, excessive diuresis (polyuria) combined with caloric loss causes polydipsia (increased thirst), polyphagia (increased hunger), and fatigue—the classic symptoms of diabetes mellitus.

In addition to the classic symptoms mentioned, others may also be present. Weight loss, commonly seen in the child with diabetes, is uncommon in the adult, who is often obese. Fluctuation in blood glucose levels with changes of osmotic pressures may change the shape of the lens of the eye, resulting in refractive changes manifested by blurred vision. Headache is often a major complaint, and its cause is unknown. Faintness, nervousness, and hunger, experienced chiefly by adults, occur 1 or 2 hours after a meal; these problems are caused by a delayed, extra insulin release. Weight gain, skin infection, and recurrent vulvovaginitis are fairly common complaints in the diabetic adult.

Individuals with stable maturity-onset diabetes are often asymptomatic, and the diagnosis is made incidentally by routine blood or urine laboratory tests. These adults frequently have chronic complications of diabetes, such as recurrent infection, atherosclerosis (caused by decreased clearance of fats from the blood, thus resulting in hyperlipidemia, or increased fat in the blood), peripheral vascular disease, neuropathy, and ocular complications.

The onset of diabetes may continue unchecked, especially in younger, ketosis-prone individuals. Cells attempt to respond to glucose deprivation initially by metabolizing protein, resulting in the liberation of amino acids in large quantities. Some of these amino acids are converted into urea in the liver and are excreted, which results in a negative nitrogen balance.

The fat cell attempts to provide fuel in the absence of insulin by mobilizing fat stores. The free fatty acids are initially utilized for energy production, but the majority reach the liver where three strong acids are formed: acetoacetic acid, beta-hydroxybutyric acid, and acetone. The keto-acids are ultimately excreted by the kidney along with sodium bicarbonate. The combination of ketoacid accumulation and bicarbonate excretion causes a fall in plasma pH, resulting in acidosis. The body attempts to correct the acidosis by the characteristic Kussmaul's respiration, which is deep, labored respiration caused by the body's effort to convert carbonic acid (H_2CO_2) to carbon dioxide and water and to excrete the carbon dioxide. In an unchecked state, acidosis, dehydration, and electrolyte inbalance ultimately affect brain function, and coma results. Death may occur if insulin deficiency remains untreated.

Total body potassium may be decreased because of cellular breakdown and excretion. Dehydration, however, may cause the serum potassium to be concentrated in less

---

*The renal threshold is lower in women during pregnancy and in children. It may be elevated in the elderly patient or in persons with a long history of diabetes.

body fluid, resulting in normal or elevated serum potassium levels. Sodium is lost along with water in the urine, and serum sodium is almost always severely depleted.

Insulin treatment reverses the catabolic state created by insulin deficiency. Blood glucose levels fall, fats cease to break down, ketones are no longer produced, serum bicarbonate and pH levels rise, and potassium shifts intracellularly as anabolism (tissue rebuilding) begins.

SUMMARY

Diabetes mellitus is a catabolic state caused by a deficiency of insulin. In the absence of insulin, normal body functions are inhibited and tissue breaks down, causing acidosis. Uncorrected, diabetic ketoacidosis can lead to coma and death. Diabetes mellitus is a serious metabolic derangement affecting almost every body organ and function. The abnormality should be detected as early as possible and corrected with adequate fluid, electrolyte, and insulin administration.

REFERENCE

1. Ellenberg, M., and Rifkin, H., editors: Diabetes mellitus: theory and practice, New York, 1970, McGraw-Hill Book Co., p. 137.

SECTION TWO

Management

4

The child

Diana W. and Richard A. Guthrie

This chapter summarizes the various aspects of diabetes management, adjustment, and exercise in the child. A number of the principles discussed may be applied to the adult as well, especially to the insulin-dependent adult. Consequently, material that could have been included elsewhere has been grouped here for simplicity.

All too often children and youth with diabetes are treated as miniature adults. Children grow and therefore have changing needs that require special consideration. Insulin-dependent, or ketosis-prone, diabetes usually occurs rather suddenly, especially when compared with the non-insulin-dependent, maturity-onset disease. Diabetes is usually more severe in young people, whose nutritional and insulin needs are changing as they grow to adulthood. Stabilization of exercise is virtually impossible. Emotional responses are quite variable, especially in the adolescent. All of these variables require careful consideration and individualization of management. Children with juvenile diabetes mellitus do finally develop into adults. When this occurs, fewer changes in the food and insulin requirements are needed.

The main goal of management of children with diabetes is to promote normal growth and development—mentally, spiritually, and physically—in order to prevent or delay possible complications associated with the disease. Life expectancy is increased if proper management of the disease is attained and maintained. The high degree of metabolic control needed to prevent or delay complications will involve all members of the health care team. Medical treatment, overall management, education regarding the how to's and why's, continuing communication and education, and treatment of intercurrent illness and injury become an integral part of maintaining control of the disease. Support of healthful eating practices and the aim for physiologic normality are principles appropriate for any individual; however, these principles are often lacking in the management of the child with diabetes. Although there are varied opinions regarding the outcome of such practices, the general health of individuals should be maintained for their best longitudinal development.

COMPLICATIONS OF INSULIN-DEPENDENT DIABETES

The complications of insulin-dependent diabetes mellitus can be divided into three groups: (1) short-term, or acute, (2) intermediate, and (3) long-term, or chronic, complications.

Short-term, or acute, complications

There are two important short-term complications of diabetes in children: *diabetic ketoacidosis* and *hypoglycemia.*

Diabetic ketoacidosis (DKA) may be the initial problem experienced by the undiagnosed diabetic child, or it may be an intercurrent problem at any time during the course of the disease. Except in the newly diagnosed diabetic individual, DKA is an avoidable complication and is most often observed in the poorly controlled diabetic child. If hyperglycemia is allowed on a continuing basis, then the margin of safety before ketosis develops is very small.

The commonest precipitating factor of DKA in the child is infection. Emotional stress and failure to take the prescribed amount of insulin are other common causes of DKA. Contrary to commonly held opinions, overeating will rarely cause the development of DKA. Children are commonly told that eating sweets, such as a candy bar, will make them "go into coma." The explanation of the pathogenesis of DKA in Chapter 7, however, readily reveals the fallacy of this scare tactic. Ketosis develops when fat breaks down because of a lack of insulin to stabilize the lipase enzymes or when other hormones, such as glucagon and epinephrine, are present in excess, causing lipolytic activity. An excessive carbohydrate intake will cause hyperglycemia but will not affect fat breakdown and thus will not in itself cause ketosis or ketoacidosis. Children should not be trained with such obviously false scare tactics. They will most assuredly test the statement and, finding it false, will doubt the credibility of anything else that has been said. The facts alone should be presented simply and straightforwardly.

DKA is a serious, potentially fatal, acute complication of diabetes and is avoidable. Education of the family and the child regarding the pathophysiology of DKA—its causes, its signs and symptoms, and the methods of prevention and treatment—is an important part of the training program by the health care team. Unfortunately, there are still many rehospitalizations and many unnecessary deaths each year from this complication. A high degree of metabolic control with normal or near-normal basal blood glucose levels, education of the family, and access to the health care team

through open communication would prevent many hospitalizations and deaths.

Hypoglycemia, or insulin reactions, is the second of the short-term, or acute, complications to be considered. Hypoglycemia is, for the most part, also avoidable. Occasional shaky spells before a regular meal or one that is a little late are probably unavoidable but are not serious. Serious or severe insulin reactions can be and should be avoided. Ironically, children with poorly controlled diabetes often have more and more severe insulin reactions than do children with well-controlled diabetes. Children on multiple doses of insulin per day have significantly fewer reactions than do those on a single injection per day, where 24-hour control is being attempted by a single large dose. The causes of hypoglycemia are overdoses of insulin, the improper distribution of insulin, and too little intake of food or too much exercise without a concurrent adjustment of the food intake. All of these problems are preventable with good management, proper education, and access to the health care team.

Management of DKA and hypoglycemia are further discussed on p. 35. Points of differentiation between these two important acute problems can be found in Table 4-1. Medical personnel and the families of the children should be able to differentiate the two. Delays in treating hypoglycemia to await laboratory confirmation can result in serious brain damage, especially in small children, and should never be allowed. If the diagnosis is doubtful, the child should be treated for hypoglycemia, because it is the most immediate threat to the child's continuing welfare.

Intermediate complications

The intermediate complications of insulin-dependent diabetes include *problems of growth and development, infection,* and *psychologic problems.*

The growth and development of diabetic children and their corresponding blood glucose levels have been observed in a number

Table 4-1. A comparison of diabetic ketoacidosis with hypoglycemia

	Ketoacidosis* (elevated blood glucose levels)	Hypoglycemia† (lowered blood glucose levels)
Causes	Too much food Too little insulin Stress: illness, surgery, injury, growth, or emotional stress	Too little food Too much insulin Too much exercise without extra food
Signs and symptoms Appearance	Flushed face Weight loss Tired Kussmaul's respiration Coma	Pale Staggering gait Delirious Seizures Coma Yawning Blanching around nose and lips (circumoral pallor)
Eyes	Double or blurred vision Soft eyeballs (caused by dehydration)	Crossed Dazed Dilated pupils
Emotional response	Irritable	Irritable Anxious Unexpected behavior change
Physical response	Fruity smelling breath Abdominal cramps Nausea and vomiting Diarrhea Polydipsia (thirst) Polyphagia (hunger) Polyuria (frequent urination) Headache	Trembly Weak Drowsy Cold, clammy sweat Light headed Headache Difficulty in talking Mouth and tongue numb
Circulation	Low blood pressure Weak and rapid pulse	Rapid heart rate Strong pulse
Urine specimen	Urine test positive for glucose and acetone	Urine test negative for glu- cose (at least by second voiding)

*Diabetic ketosis = elevated blood glucose levels, ketones in blood and urine. Diabetic ketoacidosis = elevated blood glucose levels, ketones in blood and urine, electrolyte imbalance, more acid pH.
†Hypoglycemia = insulin reaction or insulin shock.

of studies. Jackson and Kelly[1] found that those children who were poorly controlled did not grow well, while those in good control grew at a normal rate (Fig. 4-1). Even in identical twins, if there was a difference in the degree of hyperglycemia, there was a difference in rate of growth. Although the one variable was overt diabetes, the affected or hyperglycemic twin was shorter.[2] It now seems abundantly clear, from the Iowa studies of Jackson and Kelly and from a review of the data that we (Guthrie, Guthrie, and Jackson) collected over a 20-year period at the University of Missouri, that growth, an important intermediate problem in the diabetic child, is related to control. Poor control, or marked, persistent hyperglycemia, results in growth failure through mechanisms that are as yet undefined. Good control of the diabetes through careful management and education of the family will result in children who grow nor-

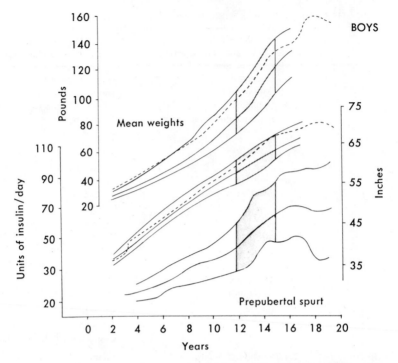

Fig. 4-1. Insulin requirements and growth in children with diabetes mellitus. (From Jackson, R. L.: The child with diabetes, Nutr. Today 6(2):9, 1971. Reproduced by permission of Nutrition Today ©.)

mally and follow developmental guidelines consistent with their genetics.

Infection is common in diabetics. Urinary tract infection, especially pyelonephritis, vulvovaginitis, skin infections, and greater susceptibility to systematic infection have been reported in greater frequency in diabetics. Tuberculosis was once the most common complication of diabetes. Recent data from both clinical observation and experiment reveal that the problem of more frequent infection in diabetics is almost certainly caused by poor control. Recent studies, for example, reveal that white blood cells from both normal and diabetic patients phagocytize bacteria less well in a high than a low glucose environment.[3] The author's experience has been that children with well-controlled diabetes are no more susceptible to infection than are nondiabetic children.

Psychologic problems in children with diabetes are many and varied and are often said to result from attempts at good control. Many people who care for children with diabetes believe that the discipline required to follow a diet, take multiple doses of insulin, and check urine will cause psychologic problems resulting in dependency relationships and rebellion. This theory presupposes something inherently bad about discipline, and admittedly child-rearing theory of the past 30 to 40 years has emphasized the need for leniency to prevent the "stifling of creativity." It is our opinion, however, that psychologic and child-rearing theory have been grossly misinterpreted. The encouraging of creativity has been confused with indulgence. Our observation over the past 20 years has lead us to believe that child-rearing practices have often been backwards. The practice since the Depression has been to indulge children and discipline adolescents. This practice has led to pampered immature children and rebellious adolescents. It is our belief that we should discipline children and teach them the rules of life, including the difficult and harsh ones, then when the children become adolescents, the restrictions can be relaxed as the children are able to make increasingly responsible, mature decisions and take responsibilities. Maturity is learning self-discipline, but children do not learn self-discipline without being first disciplined. It is our belief that the discipline required to promote diabetes control rather than being psychologically damaging may in fact have beneficial effects in promoting a mature, self-controlled, productive adult.

Recent studies by Simond[4] of a well-controlled diabetic population at the University of Missouri indicates that these assumptions may be true. Simond's data indicates that, at the very least, "tighter" diabetic control does no harm to the diabetic child. The study also shows, however, that disorganized families or families with preexisting problems often cannot attain a high level of diabetic control and that more understanding, education, and support may be needed from the health care team for these families.

Obviously, there are many individual differences, and all management and education must be individualized. Psychologic problems must be watched for and handled promptly by the health care team. When problems develop, they should be vigorously approached and appropriate professionals mobilized to help. For some of the minor psychologic problems, group sessions, such as properly handled diabetes association meetings for youths and camps for youths, can be very helpful.

Long-term, or chronic, complications

The long-term, or chronic, complications of insulin-dependent diabetes are primarily those that are caused by damage to the blood vessels and nerves, resulting in diabetic *microvascular* and *macrovascular*

diseases. Diseases of clinical significance are primarily *retinopathy* and *nephropathy* and are the primary causes of morbidity and mortality in children with diabetes. Macrovascular disease (a premature aging process with early heart attack, stroke, and loss of extremities) is more commonly observed in the diabetic adult but may be seen in children who survive the microvascular disease long enough for macrovascular disease to develop. *Neuropathy* may be observed in both the adult and child with diabetes but is more common in the adult with poorly controlled diabetes.

The scientific data supporting the concept that the vascular (particularly the microvascular) disease and the neuropathy are related to control are presented in Chapter 19. Suffice it to say at this point, that an increasing number of previously skeptical diabetologists have now come to accept this concept because of the weight of the accumulating data and have accelerated research on better methods of facilitating control. Though the facts are far from complete at the present time, there appears to be enough data to say that until all the answers are found, we must give the children with diabetes the benefit of the doubt and provide them with the highest degree of control possible while research continues. A recent statement by Dr. Roger Unger[5] of Dallas from his Banting Award address will illustrate this important concept:

1. Nature's efforts are seldom purposeless.
2. Nature, through the coordinated secretion of insulin and glucagon, makes a formidable, and in most humans a remarkably successful, effort to avoid hyperglycemia throughout life.
3. These humans virtually always escape microangiopathy, whereas those humans in whom nature fails in its efforts to avoid hyperglycemia usually develop microangiopathy.

The cooperative effort of the entire health care team, including children and their families, will be needed to provide the

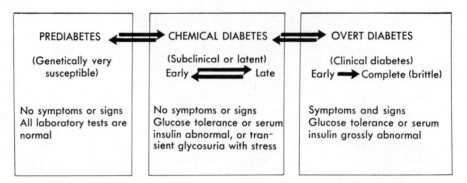

Fig. 4-2. Classification of diabetes. (From Jackson, R.L.: The child with diabetes, Nutr. Today **6**(2):8, 1971. Reproduced by permission of Nutrition Today ©.)

level of care needed to accomplish the goal of normoglycemia or near-normoglycemia on a continuing basis.

EARLY DIABETES MELLITUS

Abnormal glucose tolerance may exist in children for many years before the development of overt diabetes. The current concepts and terminology are outlined in Fig. 4-2.

Prediabetes

The prediabetic phase is a stage of genetic susceptibility in which there are no signs or symptoms and in which all tests are normal. It begins at conception in the genetic diabetic child and continues until chemistry becomes abnormal.

Chemical diabetes

Chemical diabetes in children may be of long or short duration before overt diabetes develops. Because of the shorter time it takes for diabetes to develop in children, most specialists recommend for detection of diabetes in children, a 3- to 5-hour OGTT with insulin assay, where possible, rather than involving children in detection drives. Detection drives do not diagnose a significant number of children with diabetes and thus do not warrant the cost and the time. Children who have a strong family history of diabetes or a sibling (brother or sister)

with diabetes are in the high-risk group, as are children who are obese or who have symptoms of hypoglycemia. These high-risk children should have frequent glucose tolerance testing in which standardized glucose tolerance methods and norms standardized for children are used (Fig. 4-3). Other children need not be tested unless symptoms develop. Two or more glucose tolerance tests with two or more blood glucose values beyond the 97th percentile of normal values for glucose tolerance in children and with the fasting specimen within normal limits is considered diagnostic for chemical diabetes by many specialists.[6] Overdiagnosis of chemical diabetes in children should be avoided because of the negative social implications of the disease (for example, difficulty in obtaining insurance and employment).

A number of children with chemical diabetes will have glycosuria during an intercurrent infection. An OGTT should be administered if there are positive results from following *glucose loading test:*

1. Empty bladder.
2. *Under 6:* Drink 4 oz orange juice or 2 oz grape juice with 1 tablespoon sugar. Twenty minutes later, drink 3 oz of regular cola.
   6 years and older: Drink 8 oz orange juice or 4 oz grape juice with 2 tablespoons of sugar. Twenty minutes later, drink 6 oz of cola.

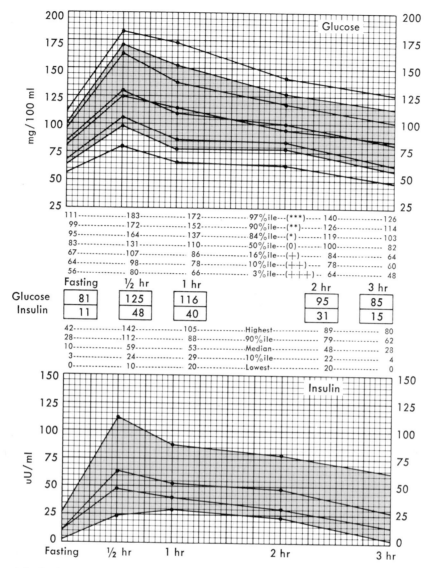

Fig. 4-3. Oral glucose tolerance test norms, include normal glucose and insulin levels for children (gray area).

3. Two to 3 hours later, empty bladder and test urine for glucose levels.

Studies continue to observe the progression of diabetes in the chemical stage and the methods by which the progression may be reversed or halted. These studies of the natural history of diabetes must, of necessity, be long-term observations; thus data accumulation is slow. They are important studies, however, as they may lead not only to better methods of treatment but also to an understanding of the metabolic alterations in the evolution of diabetes and to methods of prevention.

Management of chemical diabetes in children has been varied. If a child has significantly abnormal glucose tolerance and low serum insulin levels, even though diabetic ketoacidosis has not occurred, valuable time can be saved and more severe "damage" to beta cells prevented if insulin treatment is started. Some children have been started on diet alone or diet with oral hypoglycemic agents. The oral agents have been found to be ineffective for overtly ill children with diabetes and probably have limited, if any, value for children with chemical diabetes. Early administration of adequate insulin often leads to a more stable diabetes, perhaps prolonging the ability of some beta cells to produce insulin. Early administration of insulin usually results in smaller doses of insulin over the years and better overall control of the disease.[7]

The diet for the child with chemical diabetes should be no different from the diet of the child with overt diabetes. The 3 meal–3 snack dietary distribution should be emphasized because the pancreas can meet small frequent insulin requirements better than large infrequent loads. The composition of the diet is not nearly as important as the distribution, though concentrated sweets should certainly be avoided to reduce the stress on the beta cell. The 3 meal–3 snack meal distribution and the avoidance of concentrated sweets are especially important in the child with hypoglycemia. These children often have a delay in the secretion of insulin, with hypoglycemia between meals or late in the glucose tolerance test. Food between meals when the delayed insulin secretion is at its peak is important to prevent symptoms.

Concurrent with the administration of insulin and a balanced diet is the need for comprehensive and continuing education. The whole family should be given information so that they are able to make intelligent decisions, to develop an understanding of the disease, to assist in the control of the disease, and to adjust to the implications concerning the disease. The children should be educated when they are old enough to understand. Gradual participation in self-care must be balanced with loving support and discipline from the fam-

ily. The family should also be instructed on methods of communication with various members of the health team. Only with these three aspects (education, communication, and adequate management) can the child grow up to be a healthy, fully functioning adult.

OVERT DIABETES MELLITUS

In the majority of cases of juvenile diabetes mellitus, the child loses all, or almost all, beta cell function. The beta cells may actually become hyalinized to form scar tissue. In contrast, individuals with maturity-onset diabetes may maintain 40% or so of the beta cell population.[8] The child with insulin deficiency has decreased synthesis of glycogen, fats, and protein, as well as inhibition of glucose uptake at the periphery. DKA develops from a reversal of the normal glycolytic pathways, as well as from marked mobilization of fats from adipose tissue. Gluconeogenesis occurs despite hyperglycemia. When the rate of free fatty acid release exceeds the rate of free fatty acid utilization, excessive ketones are produced. Ketonuria occurs as soon as tissue capacity for use of ketones is exceeded by ketone production.

Weight loss is most noticeable in the child in the overt stage of diabetes if over 50% of the ingested foods are carbohydrates. Polyuria of 3 to 5 liters and polyphagia of 2800 to 3000 calories, with a glucose concentration of over 5% in the urine, could lead to a loss of over 250 gm of glucose, or 30% to 40% of the caloric consumption each day when insulin is deficient.

The onset of overt diabetes in the child is generally acute. Mothers notice fatigue, bed wetting, polyuria, polyphagia, polydipsia, and weight loss in their children, often more readily than a diabetic adult notices symptoms in himself. It is usual to have parents pinpoint, to the day, when the symptoms developed. The metabolic changes may rapidly lead to DKA. If acute infection or other stress does not occur, mild ketosis may interfere with the normal rate of growth. (This is usually reversed once the diagnosis is made and the catabolic state is corrected.)

As DKA occurs, skin turgor becomes poor, mucous membranes become dry, and eyes become sunken as dehydration progresses. An imbalance of electrolytes and ketonemia lead to nausea, vomiting, Kussmaul respirations, and often abdominal pain.

In the child, the differential diagnosis of DKA must be considered. Salicylate intoxication may produce hyperpnea, ketunuria, and a positive Clinitest. Salicylate intoxication may be ruled out by a negative or almost-negative Testape reading and a negative Acetest after the urine is boiled. Serum salicylate and glucose levels will provide definitive differentiation. Acute infections may cause ketonuria and a mildly positive

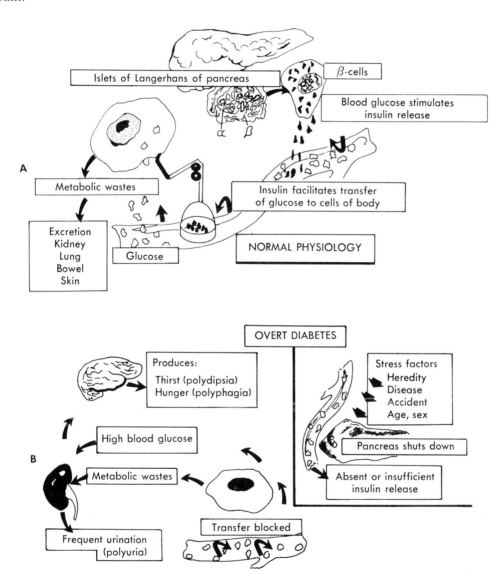

Fig. 4-4. A, Normal physiology. **B** to **E,** Diabetes cycle. **B,** Overt diabetes—glucose unable to be transferred into the muscle and fat cells.   *Continued.*

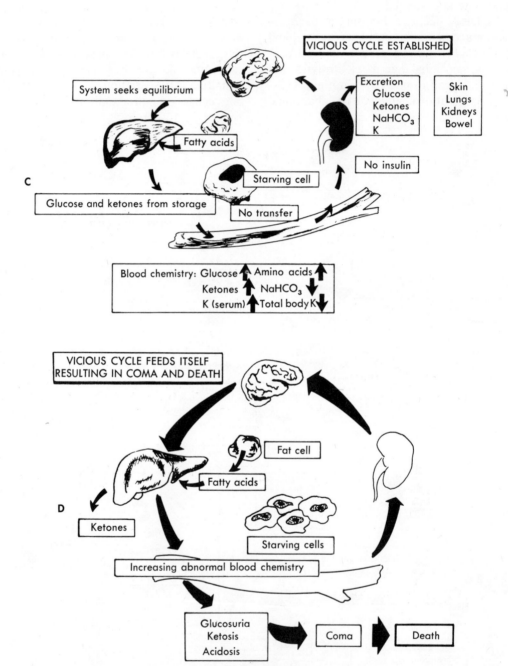

Fig. 4-4, cont'd. C, Vicious cycle established—levels of blood glucose, ketones, serum potassium, and amino acids elevated; NaHCO₃ and total body potassium levels lowered. **D,** Vicious cycle feeds itself—results in coma and death when an external source of insulin is lacking. **E,** Insulin intervention—the cycle is broken.

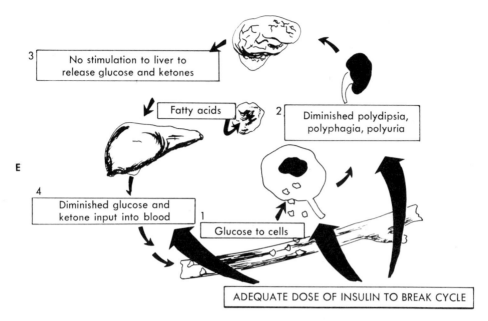

Fig. 4-4, cont'd. For legend see opposite page.

Clinitest but a negative Testape reading. Hyperalimentation, the administration of parenteral fluids to premature infants, hypokalemia, hypernatremia, acute pancreatitis, encephalitis or other central nervous system disorders, the administration of steriods, and severe burns or other trauma may caused hyperglycemia and in some cases glucosuria. Once the underlying conditions are reversed, normoglycemia usually follows.

Mellituria (sugar in the urine) may also be seen when an individual has a low renal threshold (blood glucose levels are normal), Fanconi's syndrome, or problems with other reducing substances such as galactose or fructose. Endocrine disorders, such as hyperthyroidism and Cushing's syndrome, may also result in glucose in the urine. Lead encephalopathy may produce glycosuria without hyperglycemia.

DIABETIC STATES

Once the diagnosis of diabetes is confirmed, insulin therapy is instituted. Insulin therapy for diabetes may vary depending on the level of deterioration of glucose tolerance, that is, whether the child has: (I) DKA, (II) diabetic ketosis, or (III) hyperglycemia.

Diabetic ketoacidosis (I)

DKA is the most acute state of glucose intolerance and includes dehydration and electrolyte imbalance. It is an acute emergency state that may also include hyperlipidemia, hyperkalemia or hypokalemia, and various degrees of central nervous system depression. Elevated temperature frequently accompanies dehydration in the child. Kussmaul respiration and fever may make the physician consider pneumonitis. The acetone smell to the breath and urine may become quite marked.

The following abnormal laboratory values are observed in children with DKA:

Elevated glucose levels in blood—usually >300 mg/ dl, often >500 mg/dl

Elevated glucose levels in urine—>2% (4+), often >5%

Elevated ketone concentration in blood and urine

Decreased plasma bicarbonate concentration—often to 10 mEq/liter or less

Low blood pH—<7.3, often to <7.1

Elevated blood urea nitrogen values—possibly >20 mg/dl

Table 4-2. Normal laboratory values for children*

	Birth	12 weeks	6 months	2 years	12 years
Red cells (millions/cu mm)	4.1-7.5	3.5-4.5	4.0-5.0	4.2-5.2	4.5-5.4
Hemoglobin (grams/100 cc)	14-24	10-13	10.5-14.5	12-15	13-15.5
White cells (average/cu mm)	17,000	10,500	10,500	9500	8000
Platelets (average/cu mm)	350,000	300,000	300,000	300,000	300,000
Hematocrit	54 ± 10	35	30-40	37	40

*Reproduced with permission from Silver, H. K., Kempe, C. H., and Bruyn, H. B.: Handbook of pediatrics, ed. 11, Los Altos, Calif., 1975, Lange, Medical Publications.

Table 4-3. Normal pulse rates*

Age	Beats per minute
First day	75-155
Under 3 years	100-200
3 to 8 years	70-150
Over 8 years	50-125
Adults	70

*Reproduced with permission from Silver, H. K., Kempe, C. H., and Bruyn, H. B.: Handbook of pediatrics. ed. 11, Los Altos, Calif., 1975, Lange Medical Publications.

Urine with increased numbers of red cells, white cells, and often casts
Elevated white cell count—often >15,000/cu mm
Increased or decreased serum potassium levels
Decreased total body potassium levels
Decreased serum sodium levels—<130 mEq/liter

Insulin. Children require large doses of insulin in DKA because they are relatively refractory to the action of insulin. The initial dose is usually administered ½ intravenously and ½ subcutaneously or intramuscularly, and subsequent doses are given subcutaneously or intramuscularly. A new method is being tested to administer the insulin in smaller doses in moderately diluted quantities in small-volume containers by continuous intravenous perfusion or in small frequently administered doses given intramuscularly. Small frequent doses of regular insulin or small doses administered by continuous intravenous infusion are preferable to large infrequent doses. Approximately 2 units of regular insulin per kilogram of body weight are given by the intravenous-subcutaneous route as the initial dose. The initial dose is followed in 3 to 4 hours by a dose of 0.5 to 1 unit of regular insulin per kilogram of body weight administered by the subcutaneous route. The second dose is followed by doses every 4 to 6 hours of 0.25 to 0.5 units per kilogram. Insulin will then be decreased as body needs decrease.

Fluids and food. When a child in the ketoacidotic state has low blood pressure, a "pump primer" solution, such as 360 ml of sodium chloride (0.9%) per square meter of body surface area, is given intravenously during the first 45 minutes. Plasma or plasma expanders, such as whole blood or dextran, might also be used rather than normal saline solution if the child is in shock. "Pump primers" may be continued until the child recovers from the "shock" state.

When a child in the ketoacidotic state has normal blood pressure, half-normal saline solution may be started until urine output is restored. Dextrose (5%) in a multielectrolyte solution is usually begun once the child is moderately rehydrated and acidosis has been corrected, usually a few hours after therapy is initiated.

Fluid and electrolyte therapy administered to the child with DKA should be no different from that given to any dehydrated, acidotic child, as outlined in standard pediatric texts. Glucose should be added early, even in the presence of hyperglycemia, because the total body glucose level is low and insulin therapy will readily deplete these stores. Early administration of glucose will prevent "overshoot" hypoglycemia. Potassium should be added early in therapy because the total body potassium level is decreased. As soon as urinary output is established, potassium in large amounts (usually 40 mEq/liter) should be added to the intravenous fluids. Once the child is stabilized and awake, oral fluids (usually clear liquids containing sugar) can be begun. Once the child is able to eat, the initial feedings may be given as four equal feedings or three feedings and a midnight snack.

Hypoglycemia should be prevented by careful monitoring of glucose levels in the blood and urine. On an hourly basis, the Clinitest and Acetest should be performed, and urine volume, and the vital signs, particularly the pulse rate, should be monitored. The pulse will become fast and pounding as epinephrine is released in response to hypoglycemia. Blood glucose levels may be monitored at the bedside as often as needed by means of the Dextrostix. This method is most accurate if read in a Reflectance or Eyetone meter.

When Dextrostix are used, the following techniques must be rigorously followed if blood glucose levels are to be meaningful:

1. Clean finger with alcohol
2. Wipe dry
3. Pierce finger
4. Touch "hanging" drop of blood to stick (cover entire rectangle)
5. Count exactly 60 seconds from moment blood touches stick with watch
6. Wash off drop of bood by small stream of water
7. Blot dry
8. Read against bottle or in reflectance meter

Carefully plot intake and output of fluids. Note any emesis and urinary flow and concentration. It is our opinion that every child with DKA should be in an intensive care unit or should have a private duty nurse so that all aspects of care can be carefully monitored. Electrocardiogram (ECG) monitoring can help in determining the need for potassium therapy. (See an explanation of normal ECG in a standard text.) Hypokalemia results in a prolonged Q-T interval with wide, low-amplitude T waves on the ECG. Hypokalemia may result in cardiac arrhythmias, gastric atony, ileus, leg cramps, weakness, and muscle paralysis. Hyperkalemia results in a shortened Q-T interval and high-peaked T waves. Hyperkalemia may result in tachycardia or bradycardia, oliguria, diarrhea, or numbness of the feet. Intercurrent infection should be carefully searched for and appropriate antibiotic therapy promptly initiated.

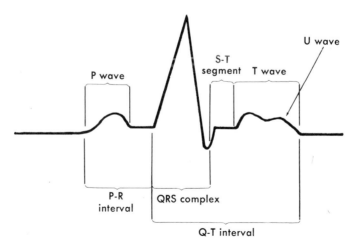

Fig. 4-5. U wave observed in hypokalemia. Potassium (K) levels are less than 4 mEq/liter.

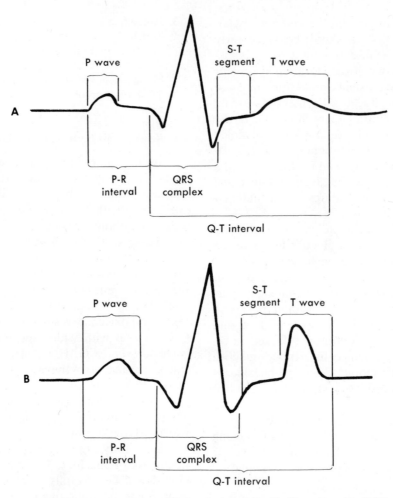

Fig. 4-6. A, Normal serum potassium (K) level, 4 to 5.5 mEq/liter. **B** to **E,** ECG patterns observed in patients with hyperkalemia. **B,** K level, 6 mEq/liter, with a peaked T wave and normal QRS complex and P-R interval. **C,** K level, 7 to 7.5 mEq/liter. **D,** K level, 8 mEq/liter. **E,** Sine (curved) wave is seen as terminal event. (From Conover, M. H., and Zalis, E. G.: Understanding electrocardiography, St. Louis, 1976, The C. V. Mosby Co., pp. 165-166.)

Diabetic ketosis (II)

In the ketotic state, the child has glucose in blood and urine, ketones in blood and urine, and possibly some dehydration. The pH, however, is normal and central nervous system depression has not yet occurred. This child may walk into the physician's office and be diagnosed by abnormal results from glucose and acetone tests.

Insulin. Insulin doses are ¼ to ½ the amount given in the ketoacidotic state, or 0.5 to 1 unit of regular insulin per kilogram of body weight as an initial dose. This total amount is then divided into four subsequent doses every 4 to 6 hours. Once the child is stabilized, doses may decrease to three or two per day (some physicians reduce to one) using mixtures of intermediate-acting and short-acting insulins.

Fluids and foods. A regular diet may be

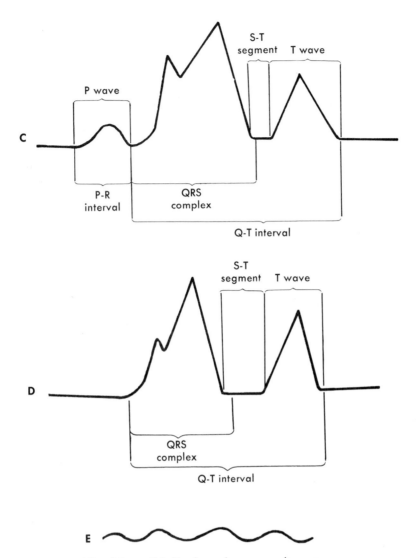

Fig. 4-6, cont'd. For legend see opposite page.

initiated early because the child is conscious and is usually not nauseated. Four feedings a day may be given, each feeding 20 to 30 minutes after the administration of regular insulin, until the child is stabilized. Once hyperglycemia is controlled and the blood is ketone free, a 3 meal–3 snack eating pattern may be instituted. Nursing care is less intense, but hypoglycemia must be prevented.

Hyperglycemia (III)

With hyperglycemia, glucose may be found in blood and urine but ketones are absent. The fasting blood glucose level is usually elevated so that an OGTT is usually not needed though occasionally may be needed if the FBS is borderline.

Insulin. Insulin requirements are usually 1/8 to 1/4 of that needed for the ketoacidotic state, or 0.25 to 0.5 units of regular insulin per kilogram of body weight as the initial dose and reduced as previously described. This may be given initially in four equal doses of regular insulin. By day 2 or 3, the insulin should be given on a percentage basis: 35%, ½ hour before breakfast; 22%, ½ hour before lunch; 28%, ½ hour before supper; and 15%, ½ hour before a midnight snack. The total daily dose of insulin (½ to 2 units/kg/dl) is adjusted each day by the previous day's fractional urines.

Fluids and foods. Four equal meals or three meals and a midnight snack may be ordered until insulin doses are decreased in number and intermediate-acting insulin is added. Then the 3 meal–3 snack pattern may be instituted.

STABILIZATION OF DIABETES MELLITUS

Whatever the initial state of the child, the subsequent management after initial stabilization is similar. The collection of urine (for testing glucose levels) on a fractional basis is the best overall guide to therapy. After the initial emptying of bladder of all urine, four fractional urines are collected daily at end of each of four time periods: 6 to 11 AM, 11 AM to 4 PM, 4 to 11 PM, and 11 PM to 6 AM. Urine volume and results of Clinitest and Acetest are measured and recorded on a daily flow sheet.

Injected insulin should aim at the promotion of a normal physiologic state. The goal of therapy is to promote normal growth and development and to prevent or delay vascular and neurologic complications. There are numerous methods of attaining this physiologic state. Whatever the method, it must give the child adequate, effective insulin levels 24 hours a day, and it must change as the child grows and needs increased intake for normal development.

The 3 meal–3 snack eating pattern with two doses of a mixture of intermediate-acting and regular insulin was devised over 40 years ago.[9] At that time, observation of over 200 normal children, who were allowed to eat whenever they felt hungry, resulted in a 3 meal–3 snack eating pattern. This same meal pattern was applied to children with diabetes, and insulin doses were administered in such a way that insulin levels would cause the child's blood glucose level to be within the normal range 2 hours after a meal without the child experiencing any significant hypoglycemia.

Numerous studies have noted that 87% of teenagers eat in a 3 meal–3 snack pattern, although the composition of the snacks may not be as nutritious as might be desired. Some states have instituted a midmorning nutrition break in the public schools, and teachers have observed a marked increase in effective teaching time. A Czechoslovakian study[9] revealed that obesity is better prevented by frequent meals and snacks than by larger, less frequent meals. Children are not able to hold as much food because of the small size of their stomachs; yet their caloric needs for activity and growth are larger than are the needs of adults. Adults have coffee breaks, which often include caloric intake. Why then restrict the child with greater needs and decreased stomach capacity to fewer meals and snacks than are taken by the adult? As children become adults, their lifestyles may warrant variations, but for the best absorption, nutritional level, and metabolism of food, the 3 meal–3 snack eating pattern is most desirable. Insulin is then adjusted to cover the needs of the food intake.

The goal of diabetic therapy should be to achieve normal or near-normal blood glucose levels around the clock. Because blood glucose levels cannot be measured frequently at home, urine glucose measurements are usually used. When the child is well, the goal is a urine as glucose-free as possible without the child's experiencing significant insulin reactions. This objective may only be achieved with adequate education. The parents as well as the child must learn to adjust insulin dosage and food intake to control glucose on an hour-to-hour basis. The child must also be able to partici-

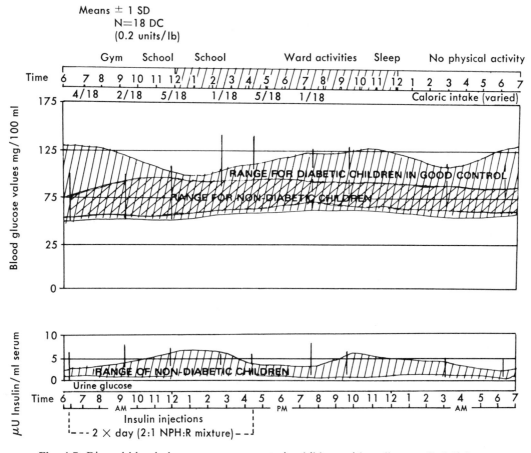

Fig. 4-7. Diurnal blood glucose measurements in children with well-controlled diabetes.

pate in play with his friends and be involved in normal childhood activities without fear of insulin reactions. As the family adjusts to the fact that the child has a chronic condition or as the child adjusts to the same fact, then methods must be devised to support continued understanding, good judgement, self-discipline, and motivation for optimum health.

PSYCHOLOGIC CARE

Ideally the child should be hospitalized for initial management in an environment that includes means for continuing education and provides ways of minimizing the physical activity differential when outside the hospital. Hospitalization not only

allows the team closer observation of the child in the acute state but allows time for:

1. Determining maintenance insulin requirements
2. Identifying and exploring psychosocial adjustments
3. Stabilizing child's nutritional status
4. Educating the parents and child
5. Making a metabolic recovery

Once the diagnosis is confirmed, the parents and older children need considerable emotional support. They need to have their questions answered honestly. They need knowledge to put "old wives' tales" into perspective. The first few days after the diagnosis is known, the parents as well as the older child need time to adjust mentally. The parents learn what parts the team members play in the care of their child. They see their child gradually change —from an acutely ill child to one who is recovering. The parents learn that each day their child is progressing toward stabilization so that eventually he may easily be controlled at home. They develop confidence in themselves as they are able to participate in their child's care under supervision of the hospital team.

The roles of the team members become increasingly clear to the family. They easily recognize the role of the physician. They learn that the nurse is a patient advocate and a more readily available source of information. They may find her using play therapy with the younger child to see how the youngster is adjusting to treatment and to learn something about care. They will find the nurse in the classroom along with the dietitian. If a dietitian is not available, the nurse may act as the dietary counselor. Questions regarding such activities as the child's school attendance, social activities, athletic events, and exercise are answered. A social worker is a resource person who coordinates team members for determining adjustment levels and for problem solving as the parents and child return to the community.

Diabetes does impose an emotional strain on the family. Their response may be to "make things easier" for the child. Their usual logic of discipline may be clouded by their sympathy for the child's condition. Proper control of the disease may only be attained by good emotional health on the part of the parents as well as the child. Development of self-discipline in any child is important. It is even of more importance in children with diabetes because it relates to their future health as an adult. Once the parents can admit that their child has a disease with no known cure and can recognize that their child may still be happy, healthy, and active, then they can more readily learn what is needed for adequate and finally for optimal care.

Younger children (and their parents) seem to adjust more easily. The parent who is overly sympathetic or reactive or overly protective has a tendency to smother the child and to cause the child to grow fearful or to develop feelings of inferiority. Children soon learn to use their diabetes to gain attention both positively and negatively. As the unwholesome attitude continues to grow, the child becomes more undisciplined and the physical status deteriorates.

On the other hand, if the family supports the growing child with empathy, understanding, and discipline, the child will become more self-confident and more self-disciplined. As the child develops into adolescence and young adulthood, self-management gradually dissolves into a pattern of daily care. More self-management assists the adolescent, in "breaking the apron strings." The parents develop confidence in their youth's independence, and the adolescent is well on the way to becoming a stable adult.

Perhaps one of the greatest difficulties for adolescents is letting others know they have diabetes—revealing to others that they are "different." This attitude is adjusted as the youth recognizes the needs of others and the opportunities for health education. Adolescents may have some rough moments, but support from the health team and from the parents helps them accept the reality of the situation.

Ideally, association with other children or youth with diabetes may be one of the best methods for individual adjustment. This association may be at meetings, school, work, or at camp. Camp offers opportunities for learning, for experimenting under controlled conditions, for helping others, and for helping one self. Challenging camping experiences, such as training as a counselor, a junior counselor, or a senior counselor, appear to improve insight and emotional stability. Other camping experiences, such as mountain climbing, rapelling, or other stressful ventures, help these young people prove to themselves that they are worthwhile and able to manage themselves and their diabetes with supportive counseling from the health team.

DIABETIC EDUCATION

There are many things a parent or child should be taught about the disease. Whatever the initial instruction, continuing education is very important. The approach should be honest and logical and in terms that are easily understood. There should be opportunities for review and return demonstrations. The parents should know, to the best of the physician's or nurse's ability, what diabetes is and what it involves. They should have an understanding of the condition that led to their child's hospitalization and assurance that they can learn how to prevent this from recurring. They should understand that with abnormal blood glucose levels, complications will surely occur and that these complications may be prevented or delayed by attentive care. (See Appendix C for Suggested course outline.)

Supplies and resources

The family and the child should become familiar with the supplies, where to purchase them, and their expected cost. They should be directed to appropriate resources if finances are a problem. They should be told about problems that may occur when applying for insurance and jobs in the future so the preparation and training can begin in the school.

Insulin and glucagon

Insulin is a life-givine medicine, but the family must be able to reconize its untoward effects, such as a rash, insulin resistance, atrophy, or hypertrophy. They must learn to respect insulin by learning as much as they can about how the body reacts to secreted insulin, how it compares with injected insulin, and the importance of giving a correct dose as painlessly as possible. They should learn what glucagon is and how it compares with insulin. They should learn the effective time actions of all insulins in case they are ever in a position where the insulin they are using regularly is unobtainable at the moment.

Parents and children should know how to care for reusable syringes and needles and how to get rid of disposable equipment safely. They will be more careful about rotating injections if the child knows that the doctor or nurse has said they should and if the parents recognize the need for absorption of insulin and prevention of lipodystrophy. If they are mixing or diluting insulin, they must learn how to do so and why they are doing it.

Urine testing

Record keeping and urine testing become meaningless unless their significance is understood. Families of children with diabetes should be able to see and recognize a "pass through" phenomenon as well as what happens to the urine when acetone is not accurately read. They should become familiar with various test methods other than the one they are using, again in case of unavailability. The basic types of specimens and methods of urine testing are described below.

Urine specimens. Basically four kinds of urine specimens' can be chosen for testing: (1) the 24-hour specimen, (2) the fractional specimen (a 24-hour specimen collected in 4 segments), (3) the first-voided specimen (a fractional specimen collected in the bladder [for 6 hours] instead of in a bottle), and (4) the second-voided specimen. The choice of the specimen to test depends on the information that is desired.

The *24-hour specimen* reveals how much carbohydrate is lost in a 24-hour period. This is important information and often useful because it reveals something about overall control. The limitation of this test is that it does not reveal when the glucose spill occurred. Furthermore, if control is good at certain times of the day and very poor at others (as is often the case for individuals on the standard one dose per day insulin schedule) the total spill is diluted out

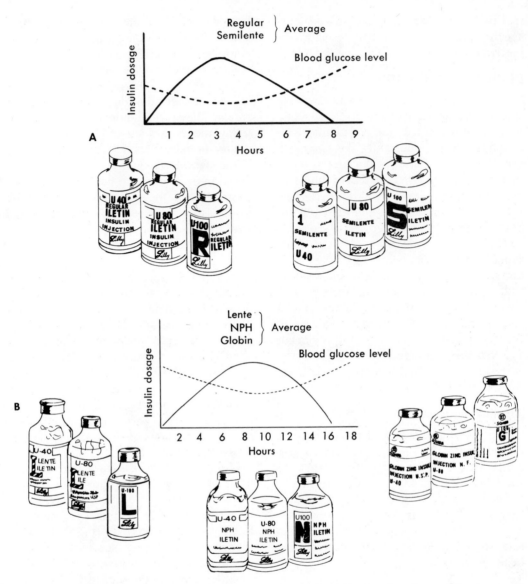

Fig. 4-8. Effective duration of insulin action: **A,** Rapid-acting insulins. **B,** Intermediate-acting insulins.

by the negative urine for a part of the day, and the seriousness of that part of the day when control is poor is lost.

The *fractional urine specimen* corrects the above limitation because the time of the glucose spill can be pinpointed, at least to a 6-hour period, and adjustments in insulin and food to correct the problem for that period can be made. The limitations of the fractional specimen are that it still does not pinpoint precisely the time of the spill and that it is not practical for home use.

The *first-voided specimen* is a reasonable compromise for home use. It represents a fractional urine collected in the bladder. Like the fractional specimen, it does not precisely pinpoint the spill; moreover, it is limited by the fact that not all children can

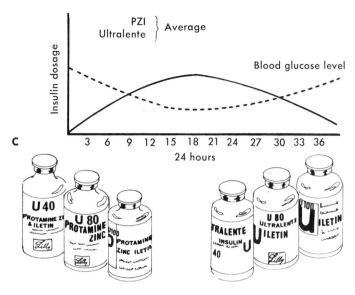

Fig. 4-8, cont'd. C, Long-acting insulins.

hold the urine in the bladder for 6 hours. This is especially true for small children, thus part of the fractional specimen with its attendent information is lost. The first-voided specimen collected before meals and at bedtime, however, is infinitely more useful than the second-voided specimen.

The *second-voided specimen* should, though it does not always, correlate well with the blood glucose level. It gives information about the blood glucose level only for that moment in time and tells nothing of what has gone on for the previous hours since the last specimen. Much information is lost with loss of the first-voided specimen.

We prefer the first-voided specimen as a screen. If it is negative, then we know that the blood glucose level has been below the renal threshold for the time period measured. If there is glucose in a particular specimen persistently, then a second-voided, or spot, specimen, can be collected at different times during the time segment in question, the time of the spill can be pinpointed, and the cause corrected. For example, if the first-voided specimen before lunch is persistently positive for glucose,

spot specimens (second-voided) can be obtained after breakfast, before and after snack, and before lunch to pinpoint the time of the glucose spill. If the spill is found to occur after breakfast, then adjustments in the morning insulin and/or breakfast can be carried out to correct the spill. If the noon urine on a first void is negative, no such worry about this entire time segment is needed. The first void is a screen, the second void the definitive test. It should be remembered that second-voided specimens require time and are difficult for children, especially small children, to collect. They should be avoided if possible in children.

Testing methods. We prefer the 2-drop Clinitest as the most accurate testing method. The 2-drop Clinitest allows testing up to 5% glucose in the urine. The standard 5-drop test allows testing only up to 2%. We find that urine of the diabetic person often contains more than 2% glucose and that a "pass through" phenomenon is therefore a frequent possibility. When urine is tested by the 5-drop method and contains more than 2% (4+) glucose, the "pass through" will occur and lead to a lower estimation of urine glucose than is actually present. This error may result in an underestimation of the required insulin dose. The disadvantage to the 2-drop Clini-test is its insensitivity. It requires more glucose in the urine to produce a positive test result than is true with other tests. We have found it sufficiently sensitive however for everyday hospital and home use.

The paper strip tests have not proved to be useful in our hands. Testape is very sensitive and will pick up minute and insignificant amounts of glucose in the urine, is difficult to read because it shows only shades of color change, measures only up to 2% glucose, and often has variation of color over the length of the strip making interpretation difficult. Diastix and Keto-Diastix have proved even less accurate and less useful than Testape. The positive factor in favor of these methods is convenience. In the presence of acetone, Keto-Diastix will underestimate the amount of glucose in the urine. For all around accuracy, simplicity, and economy, the 2-drop Clinitest is the best test of urine glucose available today.

Parents should be taught the use and the advantages and disadvantages of each of these testing methods. They should also learn how to collect the appropriate and needed specimen and understand the how and why of each specimen.

Hypoglycemia

Hypoglycemia may be the most feared event for the family of the diabetic child. A frank discussion of this problem must be a part of instruction. As parents develop an understanding of the causes of mild, moderate, and severe reactions and the treatments for each, they will develop confidence in their ability to handle these reactions. Careful instructions include why and when the child should be given simple sugar, fruit juice, or milk and when the parents should administer glucagon. Adhering to instructions will pay precious dividends if a reaction should occur. We prefer the following treatment for hypoglycemic reactions:

1. Milk or food from a meal for mild reactions near meal time.
2. Milk for between-meal reactions.
3. Simple sugar or juice for more severe reactions.
4. Sugar or an instant glucose for severe reactions when the swallowing reflex is intact.
5. Glucagon for severe reactions where the swallowing reflex is impaired.

Parents should be assured that a seizure resulting from severely low blood glucose levels is an exception rather than the rule, but they should be prepared with basic first aid knowledge of "seizure care." They should also know how to record all types of reactions and when it is necessary to immediately notify the physician. Most important of all, they should understand how insulin reactions may be prevented by adjustment of food intake with exercise.

Preventing ketoacidosis

Prevention of DKA may prevent future rehospitalization. Again, parents should understand what may cause the imbalance and what to do to prevent the imbalance of diet, exercise, and insulin. They should learn to recognize that during illness, even if food intake is decreased, increased insulin may still be needed if glucose and especially if glucose and acetone are seen in the urine. Information about when the physician or nurse should be notified of the imbalance should be provided so that the child may receive treatment as soon as possible and the imbalance may be prevented from becoming worse. Parents should be instructed to increase insulin dosage, decrease food, and add supplemental insulin in order to keep the urine free of acetone and the urine glucose to 2% (4+) or less in the presence of illness.

Balancing exercise and food intake

Many people recognize the importance of exercise but do not exercise as they should. A child is more often active than inactive, and parents accept this as a natural phenomenon. Parents of a diabetic child must learn to be aware of their child's level of exercise output in order to consciously make appropriate adjustments in food intake. The child follows a general meal pattern on which the insulin dosage is patterned. If exercise is increased or decreased, food intake must vary accordingly. Food may be varied six times a day on a 3 meal–3 snack pattern, and in addition, extra food may be added for extra exercise. Increases in food intake for playing Ping-Pong may not be as large as increases for playing tennis. Playing football and other competitive sports, team or individual, requires more calories during actual competition than in practice. The amount of food to add or take away for more or less exercise is determined by trial and error. The pattern of the urine glucose spill and the presence or absence of hypoglycemic symptoms are used to learn this process of balancing food and exercise. Once this process is learned, a high level of metabolic control without hypoglycemia is possible.

Planning meals

There are many points the families will be able to learn about food. They should be able to use exchanges, calories, or points, depending on food available and amounts of food needed. They will gradually learn to follow a changing meal plan. As their child grows, the parents will find he needs increased calories. If the family knows what to do in certain social situations even before they arise, it will also add positively to the adjustment of the family as a whole.

Keeping records

Daily records should include daily urine checks, insulin dosage, variations from the usual food and activity, and any hypoglycemia. The family may learn to prevent problems by varying the food intake and/or exercise for growth spurts, hypoglycemia, patterned spills, or for changes in health needs and activity. For a child with complete diabetes, illness may be predicted. As the child is becoming ill, more glucose will be seen in the urine. As a girl has a menstrual period, there may be glucose in the urine a few days before or during her period.

Stress from school tests or emotional upsets will cause increased glycosuria. Increased activity without increased food intake may lead to hypoglycemia. Proper adjustments in food intake and/or insulin dosage will prevent these problems from progressing to serious complications.

COURSE IN THE HOSPITAL

The previous discussion has outlined the contents of the instruction to be given to parents during the initial period while the child is hospitalized. During this period of instruction, the child will be steadily improving.

After initial stablization, the child begins to gain weight and replenish lost body stores. Insulin requirements are high (usually about 2 units/kg/day), and the appetite is voracious during this period. The child should be fed to satiety and sufficient insulin given to control glycosuria and provide for proper utilization of the food for repletion. When repletion is complete, food intake will decrease, and insulin requirements will decline 5% to 10% per day as islet cell function temporarily returns.

Depending on the degree of islet cell death before the onset of treatment and the adequacy of the initial treatment, the pancreas may make a remarkable recovery. Occasionally, insulin requirements may decline to very low levels in a few weeks, and there is a temptation to discontinue therapy. Experience has led us to believe that such action is a mistake. A more prolonged remission phase is generally seen if insulin therapy has been continued in adequate doses and in proper distribution. If treatment has been initiated early and has been adequate, the remission, or "honeymoon," phase may be very profound and

MANAGEMENT OF NEWLY DIAGNOSED JUVENILE DIABETES

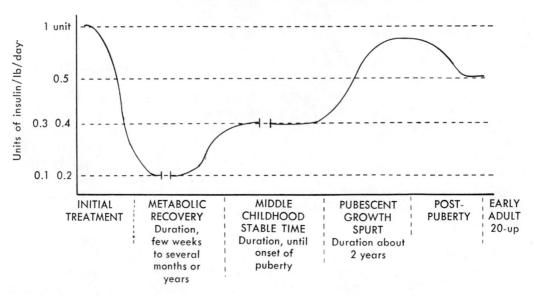

Fig. 4-9. Expected changes in insulin requirements through major periods of childhood.

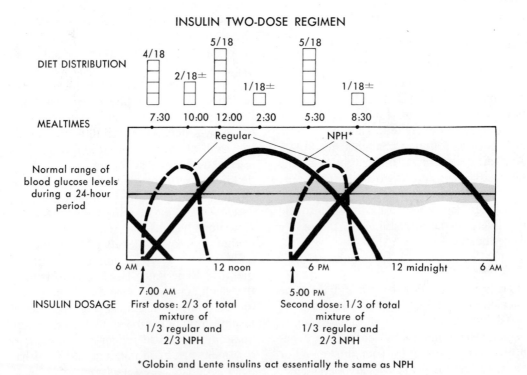

*Globin and Lente insulins act essentially the same as NPH

Fig. 4-10. Basic initial food and insulin pattern.

Table 4-4. Food intake and specific insulin reflected by specific urine test

AM urine reflects	Noon urine reflects	PM urine reflects	Bedtime urine reflects
PM NPH insulin Bedtime snack	AM regular insulin Breakfast AM snack	AM NPH insulin Lunch Afternoon snack	PM regular insulin Supper

Table 4-5. Noon spill, afternoon shock—a common pattern observed in school-age children

AM urine	Noon urine	PM urine	Bedtime urine
N	2%	N—shock	N
N	2%	N—shock	N

Table 4-6. Bedtime spill, AM shock

AM urine	Noon urine	PM urine	Bedtime urine
N—shock	N	N	2%
N—shock	N	N	2%

prolonged, offering a long period of stability during which parents can adjust to the disease and learn from their mistakes without injuring the child. The decreased insulin requirements and stability during the remission phase are apparently a result of the recovery of endogenous insulin production. It is important to preserve this function as long as possible.

As the recovery phase is beginning, we usually initiate a split-dose insulin program. The dietary distribution for this insulin regime is shown in Fig. 4-10. The diet, which was devised first, was based on dietary patters for normal children. The insulin distribution pattern was then planned to provide 24-hour glucose control. The regime, as evolved and recently refined by measuring large numbers of diurnal (round the clock) blood glucose determinations is as follows: $\frac{2}{3}$ of the total daily dose of insulin is given $\frac{1}{2}$ hour before breakfast, and $\frac{1}{3}$ of the insulin $\frac{1}{2}$ hour before supper. A mixture of regular and NPH insulins is given each time. The morning mixture is usually 2 parts NPH and 1 part regular insulin. The evening insulin is the same, a 2:1 mixture or in some cases a 1:1 mixture. If glycosuria is not controlled by these fixed mix-

tures, they can be modified, though we usually prefer to modify the food intake rather than the insulin mixture. Control can be easily accomplished with this regime if a few simple rules are remembered:

1. Food intake should be adjusted with exercise.
2. Food intake should conform to the needs of each individual child and should be modified as those needs change.
3. Insulin dose and distribution can be adjusted and individualized as needed.

Table 4-4 details the relationship between the specific meals and snacks and insulin type to four specific urine tests. If a glucose spill occurs across the board, that is, at all four time periods, the total dose of insulin should be raised. If the urine is negative (N) across the board and reactions are occurring, the insulin should be lowered or the food raised if the child is hungry. If a spill occurs at a particular time in a pattern or if reactions occur at a particular time, then the food and/or the insulin can be modified before that particular time or urine test. Examples of such changes at particular times are shown in Tables 4-5 and 4-6.

In Table 4-5 the spill is at noon and the shock in the afternoon. This is a common pattern seen in school-age children who sit in class all morning and play sports in the afternoon. The solution is to move some food from the morning to the afternoon snack. An alternate solution would be to decrease the morning NPH insulin and raise the morning regular insulin, but this is less satisfactory than changing the food to conform to the individual exercise patterns.

In the example of Table 4-6, the spill is at bedtime and the shock is in the morning. The best solution is a change in the ratio of regular to NPH insulin. Food could be switched from supper to the bedtime snack, but in our experience, this has not always solved the problem. A change from a 2:1 to a 1:1 mixture in the evening has worked very well. We have seen little or no nighttime or early morning hypoglycemia when the 1:1 mixture has been used.

Regular and NPH insulins in these ratios can be premixed in sterile mixing bottles or in old insulin bottles. These mixtures of neutral regular insulin with NPH are stable for long periods of time and reduce the possibility of mixing errors so commonly seen when insulins are mixed in a syringe.

Children with diabetes are commonly treated by a variety of other methods. Most of these regimens use a single injection of an intermediate-acting insulin (NPH, lente, or globin) or a mixture of a short-acting insulin (regular or semilente) and an intermediate-acting insulin. Occasionally, long-acting insulins are used, though this is strongly discouraged because of the prevalence of early morning hypoglycemia with these insulins. Most of these single-dose regimens allow and even encourage frequent and persistent glycosuria; it is well recognized that complete aglycosuria cannot be achieved without hypoglycemia on a single-dose regimen. Data from Metz and Bowers,[10] Jackson and others,[11] and from Horwitzer and others[12] indicate that the presently available intermediate-acting insulins are effective for only 12 to 16 hours so that complete control cannot be attained on a single dose per day.

Because present data indicate that a high degree of metabolic control is necessary to prevent the complications of the disease (short, intermediate, and long term), an alternate regimen is needed. An increasing number of diabetologists in this country and especially in Europe[13] are adopting the split-dose regimen, as previously outlined. A high level of control is desirable and is achievable with this regimen.

Home care

As stability is achieved in the hospital, the child is prepared for discharge and outpatient management begins. The parents then assume the major responsibility for the child's care. Without the supervision they previously had, parents begin to put class instructions into practice.

Through the rest of the child's life, variables will require changes in food intake and insulin dosage, but a basic logical understanding of body responses to insulin will lead to control of the disease. A flexible but regulated control assists in basic good health maintenance. The family's initial knowledge of diet, urine testing, injection giving, and record keeping is expanded to cover daily activities and possible illnesses. Good control is our best method for averting future problems until there are advances in research. It is important for the family to be assisted by the health team to maintain an optimistic outlook as all work together for the improved health of the child with diabetes.

SUMMARY

A high level of diabetic control is needed in the child with diabetes and is attainable with a split-dose insulin regimen and a multiple feeding meal plan, an organized family, a knowledgeable and supportive health care team, and adequate diabetic education. A high level of metabolic control is attainable in most and should be attempted in all children with diabetes mellitus.

REFERENCES

1. Jackson, R. L., and Kelly, H. G.: A study of physical activity in juvenile dibetic patients, J. Pediatr. **33:**155, 1948.
2. Tattersall, R. B., and Pyke, D. A.: Growth of diabetic children: studies in identical twins, Lancet **2:**1105, 1973.
3. Clements, R. S., Jr.: The role of hyperglycemia in the development of diabetic complications. *In* Goodner, C. J., editor: Implications of hyperglycemia, New York, 1972, Pfizer Laboratories, Division of Pfizer Inc., 1972, pp. 6-13.
4. Simond, J. F.: Psychiatric status of diabetic children in good and poor control, paper presented at Third International Beilinson Symposium on the Balance of Diabetes, Tel Aviv, Israel, April 1975.
5. Rasken, P., Fumita, Y., and Unger, R.: Alpha cell dysfunction in human diabetes, Diabetes **24:**410, 1975.
6. Pickens, J. M., Burkeholder, J. N., and Womack, W. N.: Oral glucose tolerance test in normal children, Diabetes **16:**11, 1967.
7. Jackson, R. L., Onafrio, J., Waiches, H., and Guthrie, R. A.: The honeymoon period: partial remission of juvenile diabetes mellitus, Diabetes **20** (Suppl. 1):361, 1971.
8. Simpson, N. E. Multifactional inheritance: a possible hypothesis on diabetes, Diabetes **13:**462, 1964.
9. Fabray, P.: To stay slim, eat little-often Med. World News **15:**25, 1974.
10. Metz, R., and Bowers, M.: Plasma insulin glucose and free fatty acid relationships in insulin treated diabetes, Diabetes **21** (Suppl. 1):325, 1972.
11. Jackson, R. L., and Guthrie, R. A.: The child with diabetes. Current Concepts, Kalamazoo, Mich., 1975, The Upjohn Co., p. 44.
12. Horwitzer, D. L., Kuzuya, H., Stelling, M., and Rosenfield, R. L.: Control of diabetes: variations in response to exogneous insulin, Diabetes **24:**401, 1975.
13. Aegenaes, O.: Insulin once or twice daily. *In* Falkner, F., Kretchmer, N., Rossi, E., and Kayer, S.: Modern problems in pediatrics, vol. 12, Basel, 1975, S. Karger AG, pp. 316-319.

5

The adult

Diana W. and Richard A. Guthrie

Diabetes mellitus in the adult has many variations. There are also many circumstances that may make accurate diagnosis difficult and lead to confusion about what are related and nonrelated problems and complications. Diabetes in the adult may be symptomatic or asymptomatic, insulin dependent or non-insulin dependent. Diabetes often remains undetected because of the asymptomatic nature of the disease in many adults. Younger aged adults tend to be, or soon become, insulin dependent, though the disease is often easier to manage in these individuals than in growing children. Middle-aged adults tend to be non-insulin dependent. In these individuals, there is a marked relationship between the diabetes and obesity.

In the asymptomatic diabetic adult, the diagnosis may be difficult, especially in older individuals because there is a "physiologic" decline in glucose tolerance that may be a part of the normal aging process. Criteria for the diagnosis of diabetes in the adult must therefore be adjusted for age. Whatever standards are used, some modification of the standards must be considered before one makes a firm diagnosis of diabetes in the older individual[1] (Fig. 5-1).

It is known that there is a general decline in body functions with age. Kilo and Williamson[2] noted a gradual increase in the thickening of the capillary basement membrane as nondiabetic men become older and also as women reach the menopause. The decline of bodily function with age affects the secretory mechanisms for insulin as well as the metabolic rates and tissue oxygen consumption and may therefore adversely affect glucose tolerance. Is this decline in glucose tolerance with age simply consistent with the aging process or does it constitute a true diabetic state? The answer is unknown. It is important to find all diabetic individuals and place them under medical care, but it is equally important not to overdiagnose this or any other disease. Glucose intolerance may be noted in a variety of stressful situations, such as stroke, heart attack, or other stresses in the elderly. The glucose intolerance may be manifest in the abnormal results of a glucose tolerance test but may not be distinguishable by notable symptoms.

Many diabetic adults are diagnosed as having diabetes on admission to the hospital for other disorders. Often the ophthalmologist will be the first to note changes in the retina and therefore suspect diabetes. The adult is also in a high-suspect group for diabetes if cuts are slow to heal and if circulation becomes impaired enough to cause pressure sores on the feet or legs. Even though the carbohydrate intolerance may not be as severe as in the youth or young adult, the adult with diabetes may still have complications, especially if the diagnosis is delayed or missed.

CHARACTERISTICS OF ADULT DIABETES

Some young adults will develop insulin-dependent diabetes, which is indistinguishable from juvenile diabetes.

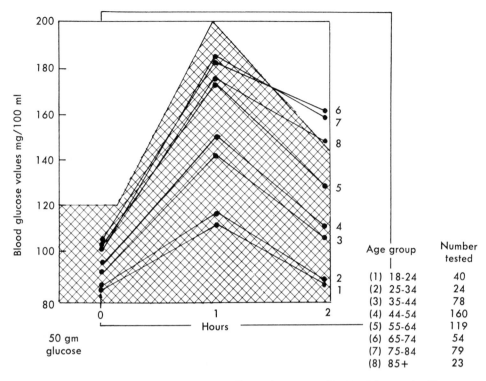

Fig. 5-1. Glucose tolerance by decade. (From Sussman, K. E.: Diagnostic dilemmas. *In* The older diabetic patient, an Upjohn monograph, Jan. 1973., Kalamazoo, Mich., The Upjohn Co., p. 21.)

	FAJANS-CONN CRITERIA* GLUCOSE VALUES (mg/100 ml)		DIAGNOSTIC CRITERIA	**WILKERSON POINT SYSTEM†** GLUCOSE VALUES (mg/100 ml)		POINTS	DIAGNOSTIC CRITERIA
	Whole blood	Plasma or serum		Whole blood	Plasma or serum		
FASTING	—	—		110 or above	130	1	
1 hour	160	185	All levels at or above	170 or above	195	½	Total of 2 points or more
1 ½ hour	140	160		—	—		
2 hour	120	140		120 or above	140	½	
3 hour	—	—		110 or above	125	1	

*Glucose load 1.75 mg/kg ideal body weight as 25% solution
in otherwise healthy and ambulatory individuals under age 50
†Glucose load 100 gm
For all procedures: venous blood, Autoanalyzer (Ferricyanide) or
Somogyi-Nelson method

Fig. 5-2. Interpretations of the oral glucose tolerance test in adults. (From Sussman, K. E.: Diagnostic dilemmas. *In* The older diabetic patient, an Upjohn monograph, Jan. 1973, Kalamazoo, Mich., The Upjohn Co., p. 18.)

Likewise the older diabetic person may develop insulin-dependent diabetes. Symptoms in these individuals are not different from those in the young. Management may vary considerably, however, because older people cannot and should not be as tightly controlled as the younger individuals.

The majority of diabetic adults are over 40 years of age and are somewhat obese. Their disease is mild, relatively stable, and often symptomless. These individuals are usually ketosis resistant. In this form of the disease, the pancreas can produce insulin and in some cases may overproduce. The insulin deficiency is therefore a relative, not an absolute, deficiency. Often if needs can be reduced, the pancreas is capable of meeting the reduced needs, and carbohydrate tolerance improves.

ASSOCIATED PROBLEMS

Hyperosmolar nonketotic coma, in which the person exhibits marked hyperglycemia, may occasionally occur in the diabetic adult. The person may be thought to have DKA and be treated with large doses of insulin, which may be fatal. The patient with hyperosmolar nonketotic coma has a high blood glucose level, increased plasma osmolality, and dehydration. Hyperosmolar nonketotic coma results from a mild deficiency of insulin. Sufficient amounts of insulin are secreted to prevent lipolysis, and thus prevent ketosis, but not enough insulin is present to prevent hyperglycemia. Because most of the symptoms in diabetic coma are produced by the ketosis, acidosis, and electrolyte imbalance, the developing hyperglycemia goes undetected until blood glucose levels are quite high. The very high glucose levels produce a marked osmotic diuresis with a resulting hyperosmolality of the serum. Hyperglycemia and dehydration are marked, but ketones are not present and insulin deficiency is mild. Blood pressure may be low and temperature may be high because of dehydration. Electrolytes may be imbalanced. Other causes for coma, such as a cardiovascular accident (CVA), need to be ruled out, because these causes may be masked when hyperglycemia is marked. Coma could be caused by stroke, kidney failure, or toxic drugs. Treatment of this very serious and potentially fatal illness is massive intravenous fluid therapy, usually with half-normal saline solution and small doses of insulin. Large doses of insulin are not needed and should not be used even in the presence of massive hyperglycemia when ketosis is not present.

If the person is taking biguanides, lactic acidosis becomes a more common occurrence. Lactic acidosis results from hypoxia and may be associated with mild hemorrhage, liver disease, and heart failure as well as with biguanide therapy. Careful diagnostic measures will allow the physician to diagnose and treat this crisis. Electrolyte measurements will reveal the "anion gap" associated with lactic acidosis. It is most important that fluids containing lactate are not administered until lactic acidosis has been ruled out.

A number of problems may become manifest in the older adult and may affect the diagnosis or outcome of the diabetes. Eyesight may have failed or arthritis may have caused joints to stiffen so that even a simple task of giving an injection may become a problem. Hand immobility caused by other conditions may prevent the adult from squeezing a dropper or holding a test strip for urine testing. Memory may fade to the point that the person may not remember taking the injection or oral agents and may repeat the medication just to be sure. Insulin reactions may have more profound physical responses in the older adult than in the younger adult. Aging blood vessels may become weak so that the stress of a severe insulin reaction may cause rupture. Aging or damaged kidneys may cause decreased breakdown and excretion of the oral agents. If the dose of the oral agent is then not decreased, there may be prolonged hypoglycemia.

Urine tests reflect blood glucose levels even lower in the elderly than in the young because the renal threshold is known to rise with age. Therefore urine tests are seldom depended on for major management in the elderly. The action of drugs that potentiate hypoglycemia may be amplified when the patient is receiving oral hypoglycemic agents. Diet therefore becomes an even more important concern and a tool that may be manipulated in a variety of ways.

DIAGNOSIS

The diagnosis of diabetes mellitus in the adult must be made carefully, with consideration given to the many factors listed above. Too often the diagnosis in the adult is determined by glycosuria or moderately elevated fasting blood glucose levels alone. Many factors may cause false positive or false negative urine tests or fasting blood glucose levels, making these tests less precise than desired for proper diagnosis. A 1- or 2-hour postprandial (PPD) or post–glucose load blood glucose level is a more sensitive diagnostic tool, especially in symptomatic individuals.

In the absence of symptoms, the OGTT is the most sensitive diagnostic tool used by many physicians and most diabetes specialists. The OGTT must be properly standardized however, to be a useful tool for the diagnosis of diabetes. Proper standardization and interpretation is mandatory to prevent underdiagnosis or, more importantly, overdiagnosis. The individual to be tested should receive a 300-gm carbohydrate diet for 3 days before the OGTT to stabilize the glycogen reserves and sensitize the pancreas to glucose. A low carbohydrate diet and starvation can produce factitious diabetes. The subject to be tested should be fasting for 8 to 10 hours before the test, and the test should begin in the early morning. A fasting blood glucose level is obtained, and a measured dose of glucose is taken by mouth. The dose of glucose should be 1.75 gm of glucose per kilogram ideal body weight for height up to a maximum dose of 100 gm (see also pp. 12-13).

Drugs, other than life-saving drugs, are banned for a set period of time preceding and during the OGTT, and smoking and coffee or strong tea are prohibited until after the test period has ended. Urine specimens may be collected with each blood specimen or at the time of the 1-hour specimen.

The test results should be compared with properly standardized age-adjusted norms, such as those of Fajans and Conn (see Table 2-1) and evaluated by their criteria or by the Wilkinson point system. These criteria are based on venous plasma or serum. Appropriate adjustments must also be made if arterial or capillary blood is used or if whole blood is used. Capillary and arterial blood have a higher blood glucose content than does venous blood. Blood plasma and blood serum, however, have about a 15% greater glucose content than whole blood because the glucose content of the blood cells is less than that of the fluid plasma portion of the blood.

In the adult, tests that become increasingly more abnormal are more suspicious than a stabilized test pattern seen over the years because declining glucose tolerance indicates declining insulin responsiveness. In the older adult, other causes of hyperglycemia must be ruled out more frequently than in the younger adult. These other causes of hyperglycemia might include diseases of the endocrine glands (such as increased secretion of epinephrine, glucocorticoids, or growth hormone), drugs (such as steroids, diuretics, estrogens, and nicotinic acid), and problems such as starvation. Malnutrition may also cause some mildly abnormal glucose tolerance curves but not as severe as those caused by starvation.

TREATMENT

The treatment of the adult with diabetes varies with the type of diabetes (insulin dependent or non-insulin dependent) and with the age of the patient.

The insulin-dependent adult. These individuals are treated in a similar manner to the child (see Chapter 4).

The insulin-dependent older adult. The older person who develops insulin-dependent diabetes often is not willing to or not able to comply with a rigid schedule of meals, insulin injection, and urine testing. Compromises must, therefore, be developed in these individuals who are relatively set in their ways and have only a few years remaining.

The non-insulin-dependent adult. This group, which constitutes the majority of diabetic adults, can be divided into two groups: (1) those on diet therapy alone and (2) those on oral hypoglycemic agents.

DIET THERAPY GROUP. These individuals are usually over 40 years of age and are usually somewhat obese. They often hypersecrete insulin and can be controlled by lowering the load on the pancreas. Dietary restriction, weight loss, and increased exercise are needed. The dietary management of this problem is discussed in Chapter 13. Achieving compliance with the prescribed regimen is however a very difficult problem. Dietary restriction and weight loss are very difficult to achieve in any individual and are especially difficult in the obese diabetic adult. Careful education is needed to help motivate these people to greater compliance.

ORAL AGENT GROUP. Individuals in this group may have been given oral agents primarily or may have been given them after failure of diet therapy. Oral agents should never be given in place of diet therapy, and their use for any diabetic person is controversial. Most authorities agree that these drugs have at least a limited place in diabetic therapy for those individuals who cannot be controlled by diet alone and either cannot or will not take insulin. The use of the oral agents is discussed in Chapter 10. Diet therapy remains a keystone to management in this group also, and diabetic education must be carried out to achieve compliance.

EDUCATION

Education of the diabetic adult must obviously be individualized because the non-insulin-dependent diabetic person and the insulin-dependent individual need different instructions. Education may also be difficult because the adults are frequently set in their ways, disinterested in education, and often not aware of the seriousness of their problem because their disease may be relatively asymptomatic. Often older adults will not cooperate until they are threatened with loss of a leg or an eye. A diet may become a major threat to existence and be completely ignored. In basic management, the person must be viewed as a whole, and for best cooperation, the present life-style should be disrupted as little as possible.

Initial and continuing education of the diabetic adult should include knowledge of diet, urine testing, action of medications, use of insulin and techniques for administering when appropriate, care of equipment, symptoms of hypoglycemia and uncontrolled hyperglycemia, care of the feet, and complications (historical, prevention measures, and present care). The person should feel secure in being able to contact a team member at any time. Emotional support at the time of initial adjustment as well as ongoing support should be provided by other professionals, such as the community health or visiting nurse. Because emotions cause a stressful situation in the body, adults must recognize that their emotional upsets are as likely to cause problems as any physical illness. Even if they have not been checking their urine frequently when they are well, they should know that when they are ill, urine testing may be used as a tool to incidate when a phone call or visit to the physician is needed to prevent serious trouble.

During clinic visits, reward and punishment for care are not recommended. General discussion and understanding of body responses are more appropriate.

If aging is associated with decreased income, the adult may not be able to afford medication and supplies. Contact with resources for information about services supplied by welfare, Medicare and Medicaid, and those available through the local diabetes association is an important part of the diabetic educational program. Other voluntary health organizations such as the Heart Association and the Association for the Blind may supply assistance with information, books, and volunteers. (See Appendix B.)

In diabetic education, the adequacy of food intake must be stressed. In the obese diabetic adult, a balanced but calorie-restricted meal plan must be stressed. In the older diabetic person, the need not only for a balanced diet but also sufficient calories must be emphasized. The adequacy of food intake, especially in the elderly, may depend on the knowledge of the individual or the resource people associated with the involved person. Eating habits as well as available methods of preparation should be respected. The older adult may be in a controlled environment of a nursing home or eating meals at the local cafe, and these circumstances must be considered in developing both the management and the educational program.

CARE OF THE OLDER DIABETIC

The care of the older diabetic person has special considerations. One of the most stressed points in the education, besides diet and medication, should be preventive techniques. The most important of these is foot care. Foot care, if taught in the hospital, should be part of the person's daily schedule so that habits will hopefully be established before discharge. Lack of feeling in the feet necessitates even closer observation on a daily basis; yet some individuals find it difficult to look at parts of the body if not reminded by discomfort. Obesity in adults may even prevent them from being physically able to view their feet for any type of observation. The community health nurse, neighbor, or family member, who may visit to assist and correct medica-

tion administration, must also be the observers for the specifically handicapped adult.

Podiatrists become valuable members of the team in the management of the older patient. Their careful inspection and routine foot care may prevent complications in older diabetic persons who are not self-disciplined enough to give themselves this care. This intervention also gives the person with diabetes an ongoing contact with education by professionals concerning this particular area of the body. If podiatrists are not available, the nurse, the physician, and the family must be responsible for observation (for bilateral warmth, pulses, color, fluid accumulation, intact skin, and sensitivity of the feet) and for ongoing education of the patient.

Complications in the older adult may lead to other problems. Hospitalization for an amputation or a broken hip may lead to disorientation to time and place. If an active person succumbs to another disease or accident, the diabetes may become much more difficult to manage because of the change in activity patterns. Most often, the patient may shrug off or block out even the observed complication actually related to the disease with thoughts of, "I'll wait a few more days for it to heal," or "They may remove my leg if I report this ulcer on my leg." The older adult, as any diabetic person, should be familiar with laser treatment, or photocoagulation, for retinal hemorrhage in the eye, or vitreophage for removal of the cloudy fluid in the vitreous. They should also be familiar with the possibility of bypass surgery for vascular insufficiency of the legs. They should understand the importance of early management of their problems so that medical intervention will more likely be successful.

If surgery becomes a consideration, the patient's age and physical condition, which may not be an advantage, must be taken into account because even more problems may result from surgery. If possible, surgery should be avoided. For example, one

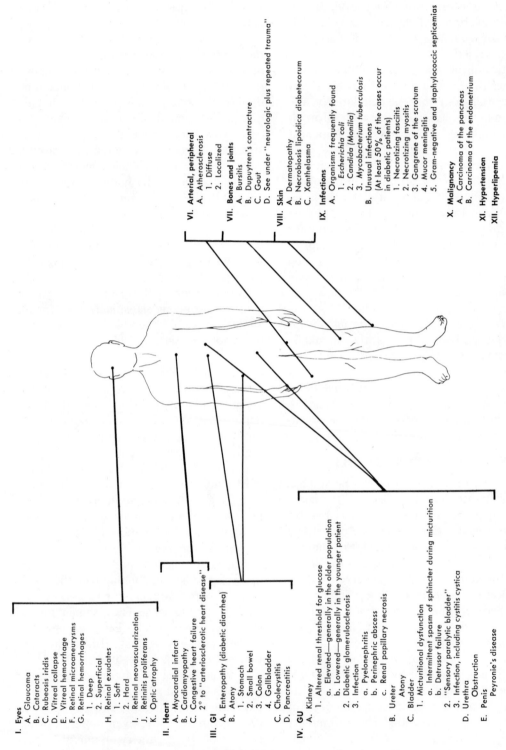

I. **Eyes**
   A. Glaucoma
   B. Cataracts
   C. Rubeosis iridis
   D. Vitreal collapse
   E. Vitreal hemorrhage
   F. Retinal microaneurysms
   G. Retinal hemorrhages
      1. Deep
      2. Superficial
   H. Retinal exudates
      1. Soft
      2. Hard
   I. Retinal neovascularization
   J. Retinitis proliferans
   K. Optic atrophy

II. **Heart**
   A. Myocardial infarct
   B. Cardiomyopathy
   C. Congestive heart failure
   D. 2° to "arteriosclerotic heart disease"

III. **GI**
   A. Enteropathy (diabetic diarrhea)
   B. Atony
      1. Stomach
      2. Small bowel
      3. Colon
      4. Gallbladder
   C. Cholecystitis
   D. Pancreatitis

IV. **GU**
   A. Kidney
      1. Altered renal threshold for glucose
         a. Elevated—generally in the older population
         b. Lowered—generally in the younger patient
      2. Diabetic glomerulosclerosis
      3. Infection
         a. Pyelonephritis
         b. Perinephric abscess
         c. Renal papillary necrosis
   B. Ureter
         Atony
   C. Bladder
      1. Micturitional dysfunction
         a. Intermittent spasm of sphincter during micturition
         b. Detrusor failure
      2. "Sensory paralytic bladder"
      3. Infection, including cystitis cystica
   D. Urethra
         Obstruction
   E. Penis
         Peyronie's disease

VI. **Arterial, peripheral**
   A. Atherosclerosis
      1. Diffuse
      2. Localized

VII. **Bones and joints**
   A. Bursitis
   B. Dupuytren's contracture
   C. Gout
   D. See under "neurologic plus repeated trauma"

VIII. **Skin**
   A. Dermatopathy
   B. Necrobiosis lipoidica diabetecorum
   C. Xanthelasma

IX. **Infections**
   A. Organisms frequently found
      1. *Escherichia coli*
      2. *Candida (Monilia)*
      3. *Mycobacterium tuberculosis*
   B. Unusual infections
      (At least 50% of the cases occur in diabetic patients)
      1. Necrotizing fasciitis
      2. Necrotizing myositis
      3. Gangrene of the scrotum
      4. Mucor meningitis
      5. Gram-negative and staphylococcic septicemias

X. **Malignancy**
   A. Carcinoma of the pancreas
   B. Carcinoma of the endometrium

XI. **Hypertension**

XII. **Hyperlipemia**

Fig. 5-3. Some complications associated with diabetes mellitus. (From Dobson, H. L.: Diagnostic dilemmas. *In* The older diabetic patient, an Upjohn monograph, Jan. 1973. Kalamazoo, Mich., The Upjohn Co., pp. 40-41.)

would allow gangrene of the extremities, especially dry gangrene, to undergo self-amputation or autoamputation rather than expose the elderly person to the rigors of surgery. Wet gangrene, however, is a more serious problem and requires earlier amputation.

COMPLICATIONS OF ADULT DIABETES
Macrovascular disease

The primary concern of adults with the non-insulin-dependent form of diabetes is disease of the large blood vessels, macrovascular disease. The cause of this complication is unknown, but improving control is felt to at least slow the progression of the disease. Macrovascular disease is an accelerating of the aging process, leading to early heart attacks and stroke.

Neuropathy

A second problem often observed in the adult with diabetes is neuropathy. Diabetic neuropathy may have many manifestations. A single nerve or multiple nerves may be affected. Nerves of the autonomic nervous system may also be damaged.

Large nerve disease may cause loss of function of muscle groups with manifestations such as foot drop or ocular muscle paralysis. Neuropathy may also cause hyperesthesia (pain) or hypoesthesia (decreased sensation). The hypoesthesia is especially a problem because decreased sensation leads to decreased perception of injury. Foot ulcers in the diabetic person are more often of neuropathic than of vascular origin. Pressure is not perceived; therefore, the diabetic individual will stand keeping pressure on the ball of the foot longer than usual, leading to pressure ischemia and ulcer formation.

Neuropathy of the autonomic nervous system may lead to various problems including intractable diarrhea, neurogenic bladder, kidney dysfunction, and impotence.

Neurogenic bladder is an especially serious complication. Urinary retention leads not only to overflow incontinence but also to chronic cystitis and pyelonephritis. Glycosuria contributes to pyelonephritis, which may become chronic, leading to renal failure and uremia. Neurogenic bladder can be diagnosed by x-ray studies and by cystometric studies, which are able to measure the urine flow, pressure, and volume as well as residual urine. A suprapubic tap with transabdominal needle insertion into the bladder can also be used to measure pressure, strength of contraction, and sphincter tone of the bladder.

Diabetic individuals with urinary retention from a neurogenic bladder should be taught to void frequently, keep fluid intake to low-normal levels, and to credé the bladder during and after urination. Valsalva's maneuver during urination may also be helpful in emptying the bladder.

Kidney dysfunction may be the final crisis in many elderly diabetic adults. Uremic poisoning caused by renal shutdown may result from thickening of the basement membrane or from chronic pyelonephritis. Another problem to watch for in the older adult with kidney problems is the need for a lowered dosage of insulin or oral agents. Oral agents and, to a lesser extent, insulin are degraded and excreted by the kidney. In the presence of renal failure, the excretion process does not occur and dosage of medication must be appropriately lowered.

Sexual dysfunction is an important problem in the diabetic adult. Sexual impotence in men is the most common manifestation reported. Because sexual frigidity in women is much less often reported than is impotence in men, some experts have doubted an organic cause of male sexual dysfunction. The innervation of the penis and clitoris is the same and should be similarly affected by diabetic autonomic neuropathy. Such is not the case—failure of erection of the penis is a more noticeable problem than clitoral dysfunction. However, it should be pointed out that impotence is common in nondiabetic men of this age group and that diabetic men are subject to all of the organic and psychologic difficulties that may affect nondiabetic men. Thus, the physician must rule out other organic or psychologic causes of impotence or frigidity before assuming that the sexual dysfunction is caused by diabetic neuropathy.

If the sexual dysfunction is related to diabetes, it may be partially reversed in some individuals by improved diabetic control. Silastic penile implants have recently been developed to help this problem. The newest development is a collapsible silastic implant that can be filled from a reservoir when erection is desired and collapsed, reversing the flow through a manual valve, when needed. Counseling has been useful in a number of cases.

Other chronic conditions

The elderly, malnourished diabetic adult may become more susceptible to tuberculosis and, in endemic areas, to histoplasmosis or coccidioidomycosis.

Other chronic conditions may also impose a threat to comfort and management of the disease. The two most common conditions that may occur with diabetes are rheumatoid arthritis and cancer. Rheumatoid arthritis may cause a decrease in physical activity. Cortisone often given for arthritis may cause elevated blood glucose levels, while the large doses of aspirin frequently used may cause nausea, preventing the person with diabetes from eating properly.

Other drugs prescribed for many other diseases may cause unusual responses in urine tests or may result in increased glucose levels in the blood. These drugs should be used with caution, especially by the patient with renal disease.

Cardiovascular disease may curtail activity, and many drugs taken by individuals with cardiac disease may interfere with diabetic treatment. Propranolol, for example, may interfere with epinephrine release, thus preventing the body's normal response to hypoglycemia. Other drugs for cardiac disease may, on the other hand, raise the blood glucose levels. Drugs such as digitalis and quinidine may disturb gastrointestinal tract function, causing anorexia, nausea, and diarrhea and thus interferring with the nutritional control of diabetes.

FOLLOW-UP CARE

The adult with diabetes may be upset simply by being in the physician's office, and this emotional response may be reflected in an elevated blood glucose level, making the single blood value in the office relatively meaningless. Nonetheless, in the diabetic person with a high renal threshold, these blood glucose values may be the only measures of control. Because the person may have many other problems physically associated with diabetes, other follow-up tests (such as x-ray films of the chest, ECG, creatinine clearance, triglycerides, urea, total serum cholesterol, and serum uric acid values) must be obtained and repeated frequently. Determining kidney function and renal threshold, as well as baseline cardiac function and other baseline physical features, will assist in determining diabetes associated and nonassociated problems as they progress.

Diabetic reeducation must be included with each office or clinic visit to fill gaps in the individual's education, to reinforce previous teaching, and to bring the person up to date on new developments. Because changing renal function will alter drug dosages, hypoglycemia must be asked about and searched for at each office or clinic visit.

SUMMARY

Working with the adult patient, especially the elderly, can be difficult but can also be a rewarding experience for those dedicated to the task.

The older diabetic person presents a host of intrusive complications other than those directly related to diabetes, all of which require management that may interfere with the diabetes management. Because diabetes may require a change in life-style, the person with diabetes may withdraw, get angry, block out, or rebel from any outside assistance. The availability of help will certainly be of some support. Any patient with diabetes should never be considered hopeless. As long as that person is alive, the professional should be available, even though the intervention may not be accepted. If adults have lived with the disease for many years, they may either be surprised at how much they do not know and say they had never learned or say that they know all they need to know when diabetic education is attempted. Various approaches to their education may be needed. The use of discussion, audiovisual aids, and other techniques must be individualized so that the client may most comfortably find a way to accept the teaching process and learn in a positive manner. If the learning process ends in a feeling of despair, then the education has lost its main tool, motivation. Knowledge that research is being carried on, even if it means many years of waiting, can still be a positive factor emphasizing that the person with diabetes is not alone. Whatever one attempts in education, communication, or management should be done with dignity, respecting the individual's right to health care and directing the goals toward optimal care in relation to the ability and willingness of the patient to cooperate.

REFERENCES

1. Sussman, K. E.: Diagnostic dilemmas. *In* The older diabetic patient, an Upjohn monograph, Kalamazoo, Mich., The Upjohn Co., Jan. 1973, p. 21.
2. Kilo, C., Vogler, N., and Williamson, J. R.: Muscle capillary basement membrane changes related to aging and diabetes mellitus, Diabetes **21**:881, 1972.

BIBLIOGRAPHY

Bondy, P. K., and Felig, P., editors: Symposium on diabetes mellitus, Med. Clin. North Am. **55**(4), July 1971.

Diagnosis and treatment of maturity-onset diabetes mellitus, Proceedings of the Department of Continuing Education at UCLA, New York, 1976, Pfizer Inc.

Ellenberg, M., and Rifkin, H., editors: New York, 1970, McGraw-Hill Book Co.

Haunz, E. A.: Diabetes mellitus in adults. *In* Conn, H. F., editor: Current therapy, Philadelphia, 1973, W. B. Saunders Co.

James, R. C., and Guthrie, D. W.: A guide to the better understanding of diabetes mellitus for patients and their families, Columbia, 1973, University of Missouri.

The older diabetic patient, an Upjohn monograph, Kalamazoo, Mich., Jan. 1973, The Upjohn Co.

6

Psychosocial implications of diabetes

Betsy S. Desimone

Effective medical management of diabetes, as with control of other chronic diseases, relies heavily on an understanding of how the disease affects the individual psychologically and socially. Although each diabetic person responds to the disease in a unique manner, there appear to be certain universal problems, reactions, and responses. As a result, it is essential for the professional health care worker to recognize these responses and devise comprehensive health care programs that assist the diabetic person and the family in making healthy adjustments and in coping with the stresses of the disease.

The very nature of diabetes and its complications precipitate problems that have varying impact on the individual, depending on his personal development, community resources, and socioeconomic standing. The medical management of diabetes requires restriction and regimentation, without which, the diabetic person is subject to premature death and disability. The diabetic individual often knows this. How he chooses to deal with this reality is often part of the psychologic concomitants of this disease. The social implications of diabetes are also inescapable because the chances are the disease will affect occupational or vocational choices and, as a result, financial security. Diabetes may also strain and stress the interpersonal and social relationships of the diabetic person, depriving him of much needed emotional support.

Whether or not the diabetic individual can cope with these stresses is often dependent on the ability of the health care team to assess individual difficulties and intervene before crisis and needless morbidity develop.

AREAS OF DYSFUNCTIONAL PSYCHOLOGIC RESPONSE

The professional health care worker should be aware that the newly diagnosed diabetic person may have dysfunctional psychologic responses and reactions in at least six areas. The individual may have (1) immediate or delayed response to diagnosis, (2) responses to the impact of regimentation and restriction, (3) unrealistic attitudes or guilty feelings toward the medical regimen, including misinterpretations and fantasies, (4) dependency and reactivation of earlier unresolved emotional conflicts, (5) self-destructive behavior, and (6) difficulties in family interactions. Beyond these, the whole gamut of psychiatric disturbances affecting the nondiabetic population should not be excluded from assessment.

Focusing in on these six specific areas provides some clues regarding their relevance to the diabetic person and their usefulness in the management of the disease.

Diagnosis

The newly diagnosed diabetic person may not immediately feel the impact of the disease and its implications. Initially, he will not really know what having the disease will mean or how it will affect his life and loved ones. This lack of knowledge and uncertainty will almost always produce anxiety. When left with fears and fantasies, the patient may expect the worst and be overcome by severe depression, intense anxiety, and a feeling that he has lost control of his fate. Unfortunately, anxiety and depression are chief problems that accompany diabetes and most other chronic illness.[1] At the same time, these are justifiable emotions, when one considers the life-threatening emergencies, morbidity, and the therapeutic failure rate.

When the medical regimen has been explained to the diabetic individual and he has learned the necessary skills of self-care, his initial anxiety and depression may only increase. Learning to care for the disease may make it a reality that is difficult to deny. Feeling "out of control" and depressed may result from reliance on medication, diet, and exercise.

Diet may become singularly important to the diabetic individual because it is not unusual to associate food with an expression of love and approval and a sense of well-being.[2] In fact, most of us shun this four-letter word, diet, because we link it to restriction and deprivation. The child or adolescent with diabetes may be further hampered by not being able to understand why he cannot eat all of the terrific "junk" that his peers consume.

In addition to diet, if the diabetic person's medical regimen includes dependence on the continuous or intermittent support of insulin, his depression and anxiety may be further intensified. Dependence on the needle and syringe is certain to make him feel "different" or not quite normal. In other chronic illnesses, the individual may receive compensatory attention, consideration, or pity. Very rarely is the diabetic person the recipient of such attentions because the disease is not evident. He feels different, but few people know that his disease may lead to very apparent or serious complications, such as blindness, heart disease, renal disease, or perhaps to the amputation of a limb.

Overwhelmed by anxiety or depression, the diabetic individual may attempt to deny his illness and all of its problems by deliberately neglecting or refusing to take responsibility for self-care. The disease will "not exist" for him or he will consider the diagnosis inaccurate or erroneous.

In spite of all the anxiety, depression, or denial, the professional health care worker must help the diabetic person deal with the reality of the disease and its management. Often, this can be achieved if one supplements teaching with reassurance, patience, and empathy for what the patient is experiencing. Follow-up teaching sessions with the patient *and* his family will give the patient an opportunity to air concerns that were not immediately evident. Such follow-up sessions also give the health care team a chance to assess the patient's prolonged or delayed response to the disease. At this time, it is not uncommon to observe some feelings, possibly resentment and anger, towards the regimentation and restriction that diabetes has imposed and the diabetic now feels.

Regimentation and restriction

Once the diabetic patient has lived with the disease for a while, he becomes aware that he cannot be blasé about when he eats, what he eats, if he exercises, and if and when he should take his medication. The diabetic person must learn to be his own diagnostician, laboratory technician, and registered nurse. He must also know when and where to call for help. All of these requirements may alter his life-style.

For the person with maturity-onset diabetes, whose patterns of behavior may already be deeply ingrained and established, the task of adaptation and change may produce resentment, hostility, and anger. Just the idea of giving up cocktails before dinner may evoke a wide gamut of feelings—not to mention a great deal of backsliding. This should be expected, and the diabetic adult not made to feel guilty. Because restriction and regimentation are essential to good control, enough flexibility must be provided in the management program for individual tastes, lifestyles, and ethnicity. The program should be workable for the diabetic person and expectations realistic. This will usually increase motivations and produce greater adherence to restrictions.

Medical regimen

Beyond the regimentation and restriction imposed by the medical management of diabetes, the regimen itself may cause problems; these may be real or merely imagined. For instance, it is not uncommon for the insulin-dependent diabetic person to fantasize that injections are really a form of self-punishment and self-mutilation. The diabetic individual may think, "What did I do to deserve this?" Or, he may consider the possibility that the "sins of the parents are visited upon the children." In either case, it is tough to reason with such emotional responses. To make matters worse, if the shots are given by someone other than the patient, these subjective feelings may be intensified. The patient may also feel guilty for having these feelings in the first place.

Similarly, the patient taking oral hypoglycemic medication may be confused and frightened about its long-term use. Fearing complications and lacking accurate and consistent information, the diabetic individual may abandon the medication or turn to home remedies or folk medicine.

The whole process of taking medication, testing urine, and restricting diet may be the target of ridicule and misunderstanding from unsympathetic and ignorant peers. The diabetic child or adolescent may be teased and taunted to the point where his self-image and identity are seriously injured and development jeopardized. Reassurance and emotional support, which we all need, are particularly important to the

individual who must live with a chronic illness. A healthy and realistic response and adjustment are best encouraged by open discussion of fears, fantasies, misconceptions, and misinterpretations. Health care workers must disseminate understandable and accurate information, with the realization that it may not completely obviate fantasies and distortions. However, honest discussion, long-term support, and sensitivity by the health care team, family, and friends will go a long way in aiding the diabetic person to view his disease and its management in a realistic manner.

Dependency and reactivation of earlier conflicts

Although the diabetic person is encouraged to be self-reliant in managing his illness, he is often dependent on family members or marital partner when medical emergencies such as acidosis or hypoglycemia arise. The family must recognize and respond to these life-threatening emergencies and provide assistance. Realizing the necessity of such action may provoke fear on the part of the family as well as the diabetic person. Usually, such fear is based on how these individuals respond to the question of dependency. If the question is not appropriately resolved during childhood and the process of maturation, the idea of being dependent or being depended upon can produce or reactivate very negative and dysfunctional behavior.

Family members may accentuate and encourage dependency by being overly solicitous, overly concerned, and overly protective. This type of behavior has many disadvantages. It may have the tragic effect of increasing the diabetic person's sense of being handicapped, abnormal, and particularly vulnerable to premature death. The diabetic individual often interprets such behavior as, "I must be sick and very close to death because everyone treats me too nicely."

The dependency dilemma may be complicated by the diabetic person's wanting to be totally dependent and cared for. He may see it as his "right," considering he must live with this chronic disease, or he may experiment with behavior that is sure to gain attention and security. One way of expressing this desire to be cared for is willful abandonment of the medical regimen. If the diabetic person can get really sick and go to the hospital, there he will find the attention and security he yearns for. Unfortunately, the reality of this behavior is that it is sure to enhance vulnerability to premature death and disability. Working with diabetic persons exhibiting this type of behavior is often very difficult. It is not uncommon for the professional health care worker to feel that the patient is deliberately jeopardizing his health and well-being and thus sabotaging the efforts of the diligent worker to keep the diabetic person out of the hospital and functioning normally. Consequently, the patient may incur the wrath of the health care workers who have not had the opportunity to explore the patient's behavior and its motives. In any case, the patient has partially achieved his goal. He has obtained a response and has been the target of much attention. Often, these patients can be interrupted in their flight toward excessive dependency by early identification of the behavior and the development of a therapeutic milieu under the guidance of a skilled professional. Such guidance will provide the diabetic person with an opportunity to explore the universality of his feelings and subsequent behavior and hopefully discover more constructive methods for handling his dependency needs.

Direct or indirect self-destructive behavior

Another destructive type of behavior is motivated by depression and suicidal ideation rather than excessive dependency. The diabetic individual may abandon the medical regimen in an attempt to escape a troubled home, work situation, or an intolerable life. At the same time, the patient may be ambivalent about taking his own life and will instead be driven by panic to the hospital. This is at least a viable alternative to the distraught individual.

Children will also neglect or mismanage their disease. They may not be suicidal; rather they are intentionally seeking to inflict pain and punishment on family or friends. This behavior is usually quite effective in manipulating individuals in the environment and gaining attention, preferential treatment, or whatever else is desired.

Although direct or indirect self-destructive behavior often works for the patient in attaining what he feels he wants or must do, it is no more constructive than alcoholism or drug addiction. These patients have a problem, and the roots must be found. Therapeutic intervention by a skilled therapist may help the patient cope with these destructive impulses as well as help the health care team to work with these individuals. The diabetic person must be given options in handling his frustrations and impulses if he is to survive.

Family interaction

The way a family interacts will often promote successful management of a chronic disease or magnify existent difficulties between the patient and his family. This is particularly evident in working with the juvenile diabetic. In this case, the parents face the normal everyday problems of raising a child as well as the specific difficulties of raising a diabetic child. Does the diabetic child really comprehend the nature and cause of his illness? Even if the child could comprehend, can the parent or anyone else really explain? Often, all the child really understands is the pain or physical symptoms he feels. Unfortunately, he may interpret these as signs of mistreatment, punishment, or simply as being "bad." It is relatively impossible to deal with these feelings in a rational and objective manner, as might be attempted with an adult.

Compounding the difficulties of raising a diabetic child is the fact that certain behavior evident in some children is difficult to distinguish from some symptoms of diabetes. For example, awkwardness or irritability may be confused with low blood glucose levels, or the reverse might be true. The result of such confusion might be the start of educational problems. Parents may not recognize whether the child is ill or just does not want to go to school. This is a dilemma that is not easily resolved.

In order to help parents and families cope with these problems and promote healthy personality development in the diabetic child, the health care worker must be able to identify some of the signs of dysfunction. The following behaviors are some clues that may indicate the source of difficulties in personal or family interaction:

1. Perfectionistic and aggressive attitudes on the part of parents. Such attitudes may lead to good control of diabetes, but difficult behavior problems may be created.
2. Change in family attitudes toward the diabetic child. The family may become more loving, indulgent, and lax in setting limits and discipline, or may become rejecting and hostile.
3. Fearfulness, inactivity, and lack of outside interests on the part of the diabetic patient.
4. Marked dependency of the diabetic child on a constantly worried and overprotective mother.
5. Overly daring and blatantly antisocial behavior manifest by the diabetic child.

Any or all of the above-mentioned behaviors may result from a family system that is tense, resentful, hostile, guilt ridden, or even overly solicitous. Such a family situation may, in the long run, stifle the child's development, mastery of the skills, and competence necessary for healthy maturation.

Optimally, the child should not be reduced to a state of helpless dependence, but neither should unrealistic expectations or responsibilities be placed on him. The diabetic child should be encouraged to take the primary responsibility for his care, and only necessary and realistic restrictions should be enforced. Regular school attendance and reasonable physical activity should be promoted. Actually these are suggestions for all parents striving for healthy personal and social development of their children.

However, to achieve these results in the diabetic child requires a strong therapeutic alliance between the patient, the family and the health care team. Such a team effort may include helping the parents deal with their feelings about their child, themselves, and the wider constellation of the family. At the same time, it may be the best method for circumventing future problems in the life of the child, his disease, and its impact on family life. Beyond healthy personal development, the diabetic child may also receive the concurrent benefit of being better prepared to face and handle the social implications of his disease.

SOCIAL IMPLICATIONS

Although each diabetic person feels the impact of his disease in various and unique ways, those with fewer community and personal resources usually experience the social implications of diabetes most profoundly. These individuals, often of minority status, may already face limited possibilities economically, vocationally, and educationally. They are further constrained by diabetes and possibly by the lack or inadequacy of local health care services.

In addition the general public is poorly educated regarding diabetes, and this ignorance or lack of information often perpetuates discrimination against the diabetic person. Popular myths, distortions, and fallacies also accentuate the difficulties diabetic individuals encounter in training and education, employment, insurance, health care, and social relationships.

Occupational, educational, and physical complication

Because it is usually imperative to have some source of income in order to survive, the question of employment becomes paramount for most diabetic persons. However, getting a job is likely to be problematic when a physical examination is required. This procedure may be fairly routine and nonthreatening for the nondiabetic individual. However, for the diabetic person, it may be a traumatic event, barring him from employment and exposing him to discrimination. The diabetic individual has no real alternatives when questioned about his health. If he denies that he has the disease, the consequences may be fatal. (In case of an emergency, the employer or fellow workers may not recognize symptoms or initiate life-saving procedures.) However, if the diabetic person admits to the illness, systematic exclusion from the desired position may result. Why hire a diabetic person if the work can be done by a nondiabetic individual?

Nonprofessional workers have a particularly rough time gaining and holding on to employment. Success in finding and keeping a job may be dependent on company regulations and stipulations rather than on the person's ability and motivation. Such is the problem with diabetic truck drivers and heavy machine operators whose livelihoods are strictly controlled by rules and regulations. Further, the nonprofessional worker, while only qualified for a certain occupation, is often rejected because the work requirements are considered to be incompatible with diabetes and its many complications. Often, these kinds of jobs include heavy physical labor or prolonged periods of standing or walking. The diabetic person may also face overt and explicit discrimination when attempting to enlist for military service or enroll in certain technical trade programs. Thus the unskilled, untrained diabetic person is left with very limited employment opportunities—usually the more sedentary occupations. Whether these jobs are actually available and accessible is questionable, particularly during times of economic uncertainty and high unemployment.

On the other hand, the professionally trained and affluent person may not be quite so hampered by diabetes when it comes to getting a job. The prospective employer is more likely to be interested in previous work history and credentials than in medical history.

Regardless of economic status, there are other areas in which a younger diabetic person may be handicapped. The young adult may be unable to perform competitively in an academic environment because of one or more of the diabetic complications. In particular, diabetic retinopathy can be a serious obstacle for the student. As sight diminishes, the student's impaired reading ability reduces his chances of competing with the "sighted" students. This eventuality must be an early consideration. Appropriate counseling must be undertaken to aid these young people in making realistic choices and setting compatible goals that will enable them to earn a living in a meaningful and satisfying manner. Younger children with juvenile diabetes should be given this type of vocational counseling in the early grades so that schooling will be directed toward what is realistic but not inhibiting, oppressive, or demeaning.

Even when the diabetic person has an optimal level of education and employment counseling and the general public is educated, employers and educational and technological institutions hesitate to accept diabetic individuals with the same enthusiasm displayed for those without a chronic disease. This attitude is perhaps understandable. First of all, diabetic patients are admitted to hospitals more often than the nondiabetic persons.[3] It is reported that diabetic persons average 5.4 days in the hospital per year as compared with only 1 day for the nondiabetic individual.[3] In addition, numerous other conditions occur exclusively or with significantly greater frequency in the diabetic individual and often accentuate the severity of the disease.[3]

Financial burdens

As if occupational, educational, and severe physical complications were not enough, the diabetic individual is also often faced with financial strain. Chances are the diabetic person will have many prescriptions to fill at the local pharmacy, the added cost of an adequate and nourishing diet, and possibly the expense of podiatry. How will these expenses be met? If the diabetic person is fortunate enough to qualify for individual or group medical insurance coverage, it will not begin to cover the costs. As an alternative, there is Medicare, Medicaid, and prepaid health plans. However, each program has its own set of eligibility requirements and services, which may or may not be geared to the specific problems of the diabetic person. What often happens is that the diabetic person is faced with the option of no medical insurance coverage, prohibitively high insurance premiums, or very inadequate health care plans. With options like these, the large medical bills from multiple hospital admissions alone will inundate the diabetic individual, possibly resulting in financial disaster.

The expense of proper diet and podiatry will be felt most keenly by those individuals living at a marginal or subsistence level. Although some dietitians would argue that a diabetic diet is not more expensive and that it is really a question of good money management and consumer knowledge, some welfare recipients and individuals on fixed income would heartily disagree. A diabetic person at this level of socioeconomic standing may find it impossible to buy the appropriate foods with his meager income. On the other hand, the more affluent diabetic person may be enticed by dietetic foods available in the local supermarket. They are really an unnecessary expense when compared with the cost and benefit of a sensible, normal diet.

Adequate care of the feet is an additional expense to the diabetic person. As for the individual of lesser means, periodic visits to the podiatrist for removal of corns and nail clipping may be ludicrous luxury rather than good practice. Because of the cost involved, this aspect of diabetic management may go uncared for until it is too late.

Genetic counseling

Genetic counseling may be a service of tremendous importance to the diabetic person. Few diabetic individuals know of the existence of such services and the value counseling can have in answering some questions about passing on the disease, and thus propagating the diabetic population. Helping the diabetic person make reasonable decisions based on facts may also lessen some of the strain and stress on personal and marital relationships, and perhaps prevents crisis or unwanted pregnancy.

CRISIS INTERVENTION

Any service provided by the health care team that helps the diabetic person cope with his disease and its psychologic and social implications may mitigate crisis and keep the diabetic individual out of the hospital and functioning in his community. Perhaps one of the most beneficial services that can be provided by the health care team is recognition of certain events in the life of the diabetic person that are likely to precipitate crisis. Unfortunately, if crises are allowed to develop without appropriate intervention, greater physical and psychologic morbidity may result.

Definition of crisis

First of all, "crisis" must be defined. Gerald Caplan (Rapoport, 1967) has identified disequilibrium, or upset in a person's "steady state," as a crisis.[4] When such crisis occurs, the individual will call upon his coping resources and look for a way to restore his equilibrium. During this period, the individual may become extremely disorganized; at the same time, he may be quite receptive to new or different coping methods that will strengthen or augment existing resources. The level at which the individual is able to reestablish equilibrium is what is important. One of the goals of a successful health care program should be to intervene during the period of disequilibrium and facilitate adjustment.

Events that precipitate crisis

The following list represents events in the life of a diabetic person that are likely to precipitate crisis, or disequilibrium: (1) initial diagnosis, (2) medical regimen, (3) hospitalization and discharge, (4) life-threatening emergencies, and (5) disability. All of these events and their implications require that the diabetic person utilize all of his coping resources to sustain his psychologic and social equilibrium. While an effort may be made by the health care team to prevent these situations from precipitating crises, a certain amount of disequilibrium is inevitable.

Supportive team effort

The health care team should prepare for these situations by developing supportive techniques, which probably require a good deal of teamwork. Such a supportive team effort may engage the services of the family or community and nonprofessional helpers, such as other diabetic persons who have been successful in coping and adjusting. In this instance, the health care team may be required to take on a more passive role, one of coordinating rather than actually providing a direct service.

During the period of disequilibrium, it is essential to identify the precipitating event and discover what it means to the patient. It may be that the diabetic person is concerned about one or all of the above-mentioned events or some of the psychologic or social ramifications of his disease. If this is the case, then offering the patient an opportunity to meet with those caring for him in a casual atmosphere may produce information and solutions that the patient can utilize in coping with the event of concern. The information or solution can sometimes be produced by nontraditional members of the health care team such as attorneys, insurance agents, teachers, school counselors, and clergymen. Above all, it is important to reach out to or engage the services of those individuals most likely to be useful to the particular patient at that particular time.

Because of the chronicity of diabetes, such intervention and support during times of crisis, or impending crisis, must be an on-going effort. Often, the diabetic person will require the continued support and contact with one specific member of the health care team. Usually this can be determined by the quality of the relationship that the patient has with the physician, registered nurse, nurse practitioner, social worker, dietician, or physical therapist. The member who relates best to the diabetic individual can serve as the continuity-of-care liaison. Often this will help in coordinating the patient's care and obtaining maximum participation from the patient in self-care.

SUMMARY

All of the techniques described in this chapter can be used in the physician's office, in the community clinic, and in the large metropolitan medical center. The key word is teamwork—which involves utilizing skills and providing services that are often not included in the provision of acute medical care. The benefits of comprehensive care coordinated by one primary worker, or continuity-of-care liaison, will greatly exceed the output of energy and time. In fact, providing optimal care may keep the patient out of the hospital or reduce the length of a hospital stay when admission is unavoidable. The ramifications for the patient, the health care team, and the hospital will quite possibly be felt in terms of considerable monetary savings.[5] However, these are just fortunate by-products of providing optimal health care services.

Beyond a doubt, the task of providing optimal health care services to the diabetic person is enormous and often frustrating. The potential for medical, social, and psychologic intervention in caring for the diabetic individual is virtually limitless. However, the health care team must remember that assessing the needs and problems of each patient is paramount. Providing appropriate services and resources will help ensure that those individuals least able to carry the burdens of diabetes will be given the necessary supports in resisting and coping with the life-threatening, social and psychologic complications of the disease.

REFERENCES

1. Solomon, P., and Patch, V. D., editors: Handbook of psychiatry, Los Altos, Calif., 1971, Lange Medical Publishers, p. 250.
2. Engelmann, M. W.: The diabetic client. *In* Turner, F. J., editor: Differential diagnosis and treatment in social work, New York, 1968, The Free Press, p. 483.
3. Miller, L. V., and Goldstein, J.: More efficient care of diabetics in a county hospital setting, N. Engl. J. Med. **286:**1388, 1972.
4. Rapoport, L.: The state of crisis: some theoretical considerations. *In* Parad, H. J., editor: Crisis intervention: selected readings, New York, 1967, Family Service Association of America, p. 24.
5. Desimone, B. S.: Study of the utilization and effectiveness of the clinical nurse practitioner in the treatment and management of the diabetic patient, unpublished article, Los Angeles County, 1973, University of Southern California Medical Center.

SECTION THREE

Acute and chronic care

7

Acute care of diabetes

Judy Jordan

One of the most frightening and misunderstood areas in the treatment of the diabetic person involves distinguishing between hypoglycemia (low blood glucose levels) and hyperglycemia (high blood glucose levels) and the treatment of each. The diagram at the bottom of the page demonstrates how the person with diabetes progresses from hypoglycemia and hyperglycemia to coma. Table 7-1 depicts the causes, symptoms, laboratory features, and the treatment for both low and high blood glucose levels.

HYPOGLYCEMIA
Causes

Low blood glucose levels result when there is too much insulin and not enough glucose present. This condition may be caused by too high a dosage of an oral hypoglycemic agent, too much insulin, or by insufficient food intake. Increased exercise without extra food intake may also produce hypoglycemia because the exercise increases glucose utilization, even without insulin, which results in an insulin surplus. If the individual with diabetes misses a meal or snack this too may lead to an insulin surplus and result in low blood glucose levels.

Ingestion of food or drink is important before strenuous exercise in order to prevent hypoglycemia. If the person is overweight or strenuous exercise is prolonged, the health professional may modify the insulin dosage.

Symptoms

The classical symptoms of hypoglycemia include nervousness, shakiness, weakness, sweatiness, headache, blurred vision, and hunger. These are primarily symptoms of falling or moderately low blood glucose levels and of epinephrine release. The importance of these early symptoms is that they should alert the diabetic person to falling blood glucose levels and the need for food intake. If the diabetic person does not eat, the blood glucose levels may continue to fall and true brain symptoms of hypoglycemia may result. Severe headache, blurred vision, disorientation, light-headedness, and finally unconsciousness and convulsions are the result of untreated hypoglycemia. In children, these brain symptoms may appear early. Irritability, anger, belligerence, giddiness, uncontrolled laughing or crying, or a marked or sudden change in mood are often the initial symptoms in children.

It is possible that people with diabetes may not experience any symptoms of low

PROGRESSION INTO COMA

Death—Coma—Shock—Hypoglycemia——Normal——Hyperglycemia—Ketosis—Acidosis—Coma—Death
(Occurs suddenly) ▲ (Occurs gradually)

73

Table 7-1. A comparison of hypoglycemia and hyperglycemia

	Hypoglycemia	Hyperglycemia
Causes	Too much insulin	Too little insulin
	Increased exercise without increased food intake	Eating improperly
	Decreased food intake	Decreased exercise without decreased food intake
	Drugs (oral hypoglycemic agents)	Emotional stress
		Infection
		Drugs
Symptoms	Nervous	Weak
	Shaky	Increased thirst
	Weak	Frequent urination
	Sweaty	Dry mouth and soft eyes
	Headache	Decreased appetite or polyphagia
	Impaired vision	Nausea and vomiting
	Hunger	Abdominal pain
	Irritability	Coma
	Lability of mood	Acetone breath
	Convulsions	
Laboratory findings		
Urine	Glucose—negative	Glucose—positive
	Acetone—negative but may be positive	Acetone—positive
	Diacetic acid—negative	Diacetic acid—positive
Blood	Glucose—60 mg/dl or lower	Glucose—±250 mg/dl
	Acetone—negative	Acetone—usually positive
	CO_2—usually normal	CO_2—<20 vol %
		Leukocytosis—present, may be very high
Treatment	Sugar: ingestion of sweetened fluids, such as soda pop or juice, or 2 tsp sugar	Administration of regular insulin

	Glucagon: ½ to 1 mg given subcutaneously or intramuscularly	Fluid replacement
		    Intravenous
		    Oral

	Glucose: 10 to 20 ml 50% dextrose given intravenously	Frequent monitoring of urine glucose and acetone levels
		Observation for circulatory collapse

blood glucose levels. The body's mechanisms for preventing hypoglycemia (mainly releasing epinephrine from the adrenal glands and/or glucagon from the alpha cells of the pancreas) stimulate the liver to convert glycogen to glucose and to release the glucose into the bloodstream. Occasionally, these conterregulatory mechanisms are faulty, in which case, the fall in blood glucose levels is rapid and unconsciousness sudden, without premonitory symptoms.

Each diabetic person may experience different symptoms. The nurse should determine which symptoms the patient experiences and write these in the chart and Kardex, so that all the staff members are alerted to each patient's particular symptoms.

Laboratory tests

Laboratory tests of urine will usually reveal negative glucose values. However, if the urine has remained in the bladder for a period of a few hours before the drop in blood glucose levels, the urine test may reveal positive glucose values. Usually, the urine test will also indicate negative acetone values.

Laboratory tests of serum will reveal glucose levels of less than 60 mg/dl.

Treatment

Rapid treatment is of utmost importance. The brain is the only tissue of the body that exclusively requires glucose to function. Skeletal and heart muscles derive much of their energy from free fatty acids and ketones. They may not, therefore, be harmed by hypoglycemia. The brain, on the other hand, may sustain permanent damage if hypoglycemia is severe, prolonged, or frequent.

If the patient is conscious and alert, glucose can be given orally in such forms as a sweet drink (containing sugar) or candy. Fluid is absorbed from the gastrointestinal tract much quicker than solids. Therefore, fluids containing sugar are the treatment of choice. The sweetened fluids should not be too concentrated because this will retard absorption. Overtreatment should also be avoided. Ten grams of glucose, which will treat most reactions, is the amount of glucose in 2 teaspoons of sugar, 1 to 2 hard candies, 1/2 glass of orange juice, or 1/4 glass of grape juice.

If the diabetic individual is not alert enough to swallow, forcing fluids by mouth may cause aspiration and lung damage. An injection of 1/2 mg (under 3 years of age) to 1 mg (3 years of age or older) of glucagon can be given at home if the child or adult is not alert enough to drink fluids. Glucagon is a hormone manufactured in the alpha cells of the pancreas. Glucagon triggers the conversion of glycogen (the stored form of glucose in the liver) to glucose. Every diabetic person receiving insulin should have glucagon available in the home, and some family member should be instructed in its use *before* an emergency situation arises.

Knowing how to use this hormone may prevent an ambulance ride to the hospital. If glucagon is not available in the home, or there is poor response to its injection within 25 minutes, immediate transport to an emergency facility where 50% dextrose solution can be administered intravenously is needed. Ten to 20 cc of 50% dextrose solution is usually sufficient to treat most reactions. Overtreatment should be avoided.

Once the patient has responded to treatment, food and drinks should be administered to prevent the blood glucose levels from lowering again. Food or drink with protein, such as milk, cheese, meat, and peanut butter crackers, should be given when the patient is able to eat. Protein is given because it is metabolized at a slower rate than carbohydrate.

HYPERGLYCEMIA
Causes

Hyperglycemia results when there is too much glucose and not enough insulin present. The causes of hyperglycemia are numerous, but the major difficulty is a lack of insulin. This deficiency may be relative or absolute.

A lack of insulin may result when an insulin injection or the oral hypoglycemic agent is forgotten. Hyperglycemia may also develop when the diabetic person deviates from the diet by ingesting large quantities of carbohydrate (such as sweet desserts or starches or increased calories over and above the meal plan), especially when there is not extra compensation by exercise. One of the primary causes of severe hyperglycemia is infection, which almost always causes an elevation in blood glucose levels.

When occupation necessitates heavy labor and the laborer is off work and no longer laboring heavily, increased blood glucose levels may be seen if food intake is not decreased. For example: If the laborer does heavy labor 5 days a week and then is off work for 2 days, his blood glucose level will increase during the 2 days that he does not do heavy labor. Every diabetic person should try to get the same amount of exercise daily or vary diet or insulin on days of changed exercise.

Hyperglycemia resulting from emotional stress is often underestimated. The mechanism causing increased glucose levels during stress is hormonal. When the man, woman, or a child with diabetes is upset, epinephrine from the adrenal medulla is released into the blood, increasing the rate of glycogenolysis and hence the discharge of glucose from the liver. Also, the adrenocorticotropic hormone (ACTH) causes a release of glucocorticoids from the adrenal cortex, promoting gluconeogenesis. Emotional reactions influence adult-onset diabetes to a lesser degree than juvenile diabetes.

Infection and fever also increase blood glucose levels by activating the adrenal medulla and cortex, which produce epinephrine and cortisol respectively. When the diabetic person has an infection, the insulin dosage should be increased until the infection is cleared because increased glucose levels will slow the healing process. Supplemental doses of regular insulin are often given 2 to 4 times per day during severe infections. One must be careful to have the person with diabetes monitor the urine glucose levels carefully so that when the infection is clearing, the supplemental Regular insulin can be discontinued.

Some of the drugs known to increase glucose levels are: (1) thiazides such as Diuril and Hydrodiuril and (2) corticosteroids such as prednisone and cortisone.

Symptoms

Symptoms of hyperglycemia in the earlier stages include polyuria, polydipsia, dry mouth, and increased appetite. Questioning an individual about the number of urinations during the night (nocturia) is often a gross secreening for hyperglycemia.

When a person has an insulin deficiency, fat tissue is broken down, and as a result, ketones appear in the blood and urine.

As hyperglycemia progresses to ketonu-

ria and acidosis, there will be feelings of tiredness, nausea, abdominal cramps, decreased appetite, and Kussmaul's respiration (labored breathing). With the depression of the central nervous sytem, there is headache, drowsiness, stupor, and decreased muscle tone and reflexes. The breath will smell of overripe bananas (acetone breath).

Ideally, the diabetic person should not progress beyond hyperglycemia with mild ketonuria. Instructed properly, the diabetic person can recognize increased urine glucose levels and other signs and symptoms of hyperglycemia, call the physician or nurse, and be treated. The member of the health care team who receives this call should be careful to identify the underlying cause of the hyperglycemia. The most frequent causes are forgotten insulin injection and infection.

Physiology of diabetic ketoacidosis (DKA)

Because we still see patients in ketoacidotic coma, it is important to understand the process of ketoacidosis and acidosis with resulting coma.

Glucose is predominately found in the extracellular fluid when insulin is not present. As hyperglycemia develops, the increased osmolarity causes the water to leave the intracellular space and enter the extracellular compartment. At this point, glucose and water are combined.

Glucose in large amounts enters the renal glomeruli, which normally filter about 100 to 200 mg of glucose per minute. The ability of the nephrons to reabsorb glucose is limited to about the same amount. Glucose in excess of about 200 mg/minute escapes down the renal tubule and impairs the reabsorption of water and electrolytes from the tubular urine. With impairment of water reabsorption, there is increased urine flow, urine concentration falls to about one half of normal, and polyuria develops. Dehydration results from fluid loss. Sodium, potassium, and other electrolytes are lost with diuresis.

As dehydration progresses, hydrogen ions enter the intracellular water compartment and displace potassium to the extracellular fluid; potassium is then lost in diuresis. The intracellular increase in hydrogen ions results in an increased acidity. As the pH falls, the respiratory center is triggered and Kussmaul's respiration ensues in order to remove carbon dioxide and thus reduce carbonic acid and serum acidity. Acidity will not be corrected until the ketones are oxidized or the kidneys are able to excrete the excess hydrogen ions.

Laboratory tests. Tests of urine, which can be performed by the nurse, will reveal postive glucose and acetone values. Blood tests in the laboratory will reveal blood glucose levels usually greater than 250 mg/dl, usually with positive serum acetone levels. A CO_2 content of less than 20 vol% is termed ketosis, and a CO_2 content of less than 15 vol% is termed acidosis.

Leukocytosis is present in nearly all cases of DKA; therefore, white blood cell counts are useless in distinguishing infection from other causes of DKA.

Treatment. Treatment of DKA involves three major steps: (1) restoration of normal carbohydrate, fat, and protein metabolism, (2) restoration of fluid balance, and (3) prompt recognition and treatment of circulatory complications.

In the acute state of DKA, insulin must be administered to restore the body's normal metabolism of carbohydrate, fat, and protein. Regular insulin is the insulin of choice because it has an immediate action and a short duration. The initial dose of regular insulin depends on the patient's blood glucose level, weight, age, and renal status. It may be given one half intravenously and one half subcutaneously. (See Chapter 4 for specifics related to the child.) The entire initial dose is given intravenously if the patient has evidence of circulatory impairment because the insulin uptake depends on circulating blood. Blood glucose values are obtained at varying intervals, after insulin is given, and more insulin may be administered if the blood glucose level is not falling sufficiently. The continuous infusion of low doses of insulin intravenously and the administration of small doses of insulin intramuscularly are new techniques that are being studied and may become the treatment of choice in the future when fully standardized.

Fluid balance is restored by intravenous therapy. Sodium, bicarbonate, potassium, and other electrolytes may be added to the infusion fluids, depending on the patient's electrolyte status. Once the blood glucose level is lowered, an intravenous infusion of 5% dextrose solution should be started to decrease the incidence of hypoglycemia and starvation ketosis. Once the diabetic person is oriented and alert, fluids may be given by mouth as tolerated, and a diabetic diet is gradually resumed.

During the process of giving insulin and replacing fluid, the patient must be carefully observed for circulatory complications. Hypotension, caused by contracted vascular volume from dehydration and decreased blood flow peripherally as well as to the kidneys, is often a problem.

Particular attention should be given to the heart, lungs, and kidneys. Temperature, pulse rate, blood pressure, and respirations, as well as the general level of consciousness, should be charted often. Increased temperature, which may indicate an infection, should be noted so that treatment can be started immediately.

The nurse has a very important role in caring for the individual with DKA. An accurate flow sheet indicating the amount and time of insulin administration, electrolyte and fluid therapy, temperature, respirations, pulse rate, level of consciousness, intake and output, as well as values of urine glucose, urine acetone, and blood glucose should be kept. The success of treatment may very well depend on the nurse's ability to accurately obtain and record these items in the flow sheet (see top of p. 78). The diabetic patient in a severe stage of DKA or coma should be in an intensive care unit

DKA FLOW SHEET

Time	T	PR	R	B/P	Urine test	Insulin dose	Oral intake	IV intake	Blood glucose	Other tests*	Out-put	Conscious level†

*Note by checkmark—for reference to laboratory sheets.
†Conscious level is noted by number: 1—alert, 2—moderately alert, 3—semicomatose, and, 4—comatose.

and carefully monitored. Cardiac monitoring helps in adjusting potassium therapy, and blood glucose levels can be monitored at the bedside with the Dextrostix-Reflectance or Eyetone meter system by the nurse.

OTHER TYPES OF COMA

A person with diabetes is subject to any type of coma that the general population is subject to, but there are two types of coma seen most often in association with diabetes. These are hyperosmolar coma and lactic acidosis.

Hyperosmolar coma

Hyperosmolar coma is most often seen in individuals with maturity-onset diabetes or in those with no previous diagnosis of diabetes. It is most commonly seen in people over 60 years old. The cause of this condition is a relative insulin deficiency sufficient to produce hyperglycemia but not sufficiently severe to allow ketonemia.

The person may have the classical signs of diabetes, that is, polyuria, polydipsia, and weight loss but no ketonemia or ketonuria.

The distinguishing features of this condition are: (1) marked serum hyperosmolarity, (2) very high blood glucose levels (1000 to 2000 mg/dl), (3) frequent hypernatremia, (4) severe dehydration, and (5) coma not associated with ketosis or acidosis.

Treatment consists of restoration of fluid balance and administration of insulin. Less insulin is required with hyperosmolar coma than diabetic acidosis because the patient is not ketotic, but fluid requirements are higher because of the extreme hyperosmolarity.

After recovery, control by diet or diet in combination with an oral agent is often possible.

Lactic acidosis

Lactic acidosis carries with it a high incidence of death. It occurs in the individuals without diabetes as well as those with diabetes. There are increased levels of lactic acid in the blood. However, the major concern is not the increased lactic acid, but the grave underlying problems producing the abnormality.

Lactic acidosis occurs in advanced stages of diabetes especially in individuals who are receiving phenformin treatment (see p. 105) or who have uremia, arteriosclerotic heart disease, pneumonia, acute pancreatitis, chronic alcoholism, and bacterial infection.

Treatment of the diabetic individual with lactic acidosis consists of applying the principles described previously for the treatment of DKA—namely, the administration of insulin, fluids, and sodium bicarbonate. Intravenous administration of solutions containing lactate must be avoided.

BIBLIOGRAPHY

Alberti, K. G. M. M., Hockaday, T. D. R., and Turner, R. C.: Small doses of intramuscular insulin in the treatment of diabetic coma, Lancet **1**:515, 1973.

Crampton, J. H., Reeves, R. L., Steenrod, W. J., and others: Instructions for the diabetic patient, Gainesville, Fla., 1973, The authors, pp. 13-14, 55-58, and 65-68.

Dahl, D.: Diabetic ketosis, Cana. Nurse **55**:1038, 1959.

Eli Lilly Research Laboratories: Diabetes mellitus, ed. 7, Indianapolis, 1955, Eli Lilly and Co., pp. 62-65.

Genuth, S. M.: Constant intravenous insulin infusion in diabetic ketoacidosis, JAMA **223**:1348, 1973.

Martin, M. M.: The unconscious diabetic patient, Am. J. Nurs. **61**:92, 1961.

Martin, M. M.: Insulin reaction, Am. J. Nurs. **67**:328, 1967.

Rosenthal, H., and Rosenthal, J.: Diabetic care in pictures, Philadelphia, 1968, J. B. Lippincott Co., pp. 136-139.

Skillman, T. G., and Thzagournis, M.: Diabetes mellitus, Kalamazoo, Mich., 1973, The Upjohn Co., pp. 24-27.

U.S. Department of Health, Education, and Welfare, Public Health Service: Diabetes, mellitus: a guide for nurses, Washington, D.C., 1962, U.S. Government Printing Office.

Williams, R. H., editor: Diabetes, New York, 1960, Paul B. Hoeber, Inc., pp. 516-548.

Williams, R., editor: Textbook of endocrinology, Philadelphia, 1961, W. B. Saunders Co., pp. 740-753.

8

Chronic complications of diabetes

Judy Jordan

Since the advent of insulin in 1923, the incidence of death resulting from diabetic ketoacidosis has decreased; however, arteriosclerosis still remains a leading cause of death among diabetic persons. Arteriosclerosis occurs in all individuals as age advances, but it occurs with greater rapidity in the diabetic patient. The reason for this is not completely known. Poorly controlled diabetes is believed to acclerate the process of arteriosclerosis, thus resulting in more complications.

Vascular disease in the patient with diabetes affects all vessels of the body, and can be divided into two categories: (1) large vessel disease and (2) small vessel disease.

LARGE VESSEL DISEASE

The chief vessels affected by large vessel disease are those to the heart, the brain, and the periphery—principally to the feet.

Heart

"Coronary disease is the leading cause of death in diabetes, but in juvenile onset diabetes, nephropathy is the most common cause of death."[1]

Angina. The heart is surrounded by a complex of arteries shaped like a crown, hence the name "coronary arteries." These arteries nourish the tissue of the heart with blood. If these vessels are narrowed by arteriosclerosis, an increased load on the heart (such as that from exercise) may cause cramping of the heart tissue because of a decreased blood supply. The cramping is called angina.

Coronary attack. An obstruction of the coronary artery or one of its branches results in a heart attack, or "coronary." With proper treatment that is, with medication, rest, and surgery, the patient may recover from a heart attack and lead a near-normal life.

Brain

Cerebral hemorrhage. The brain is subject to several problems. One problem is the rupture of a cerebral artery with the escape of blood into the brain tissue, which in turn is destroyed. Such a cerebral hemorrhage may come on without warning. Some of the preliminary symptoms may include dizziness, disturbances of speech, anxiety, or numbness of one side of the body. With cerebral hemorrhage, the patient usually loses consciousness and may have convulsions at the onset. Paralysis occurs on the side of the body opposite the hemorrhage. If paralysis is of the right side, then aphasia exists.

Cerebral thrombosis. The second major complication is cerebral thombosis. This condition usually occurs as a result of arteriosclerosis. Symptoms of large vessel occlusion are the same as those for cerebral hemorrhage but may not be as profound. If the occlusion is of a small blood vessel, loss of consciousness does not usually develop. There may be symptoms of mental confusion, headache, and vertigo.

80

Cerebral vascular accident. The nurse must be aware of the impending symptoms of cerebral accident, or stroke, and report these symptoms if they are observed. Of course, if the patient has a stroke, the nurse should be up to date on appropriate treatment. If the patient with diabetes has a stroke, particular caution should be taken to prevent decubitus ulcers, which are caused by pressure on a given area for a period of time. It is especially important to observe the pateint who had a stroke and has no feeling in one side of the body.

Peripheral blood supply

The major complication to peripheral blood supply is partially a result of evolution: walking upright places a tremendous burden on the peripheral blood flow from the feet to the heart. Arteriosclerosis results in decreased circulation so that a cut or traumatized area with decreased blood supply may easily develop infection. Tissue necrosis and gangrene may result. Amputation or bypass surgery may be the only alternative.

Luckily, with the large spectrum of antibiotics available and, more importantly, with education of the diabetic person regarding proper foot care, fewer amputations are seen today than in previous years.

SMALL VESSEL DISEASE
Kidneys

The kidneys are susceptible to two major problems: infection and nephropathy.

Infection. The urinary system is composed of two kidneys, two ureters, one bladder, and one urethra. In the person with uncontrolled diabetes, infection may invade the bladder. This is called cystitis. The symptoms include burning with urination, frequency of urination, and lower back pain. If proper drug therapy is not promptly instituted, the infection may ascend the ureters to the kidney tissue, resulting in pyelonephritis and damaged renal tissue. This can lead to decreased kidney function.

The kidneys are composed of an intricate network of microscopic blood vessels called glomeruli. Their function is to filter waste materials from the blood. The glomeruli are sensitive to changes caused by thickening of the basement membrane of their capillaries. The basement membrane consists of concentric, tightly packed circles of glycoproteins, which are infrequently tagged with galactose and glucose molecules. When insulin levels are inadequate, an enzyme, glucosyltransferase, transfers more glucose and galactose molecules to the basement membranes. These additions permit thickening and separation of the concentric circles of basement membrane material, allowing larger molecular substances to pass through the more porous membrane. This condition may result in edema, hypertension, proteinuria, uremia, and death.

The kidneys normally excrete insulin into the urine. As kidney damage increases, insulin dosage and the dosage of oral hypoglycemic agents must be decreased to prevent hypoglycemia. For example, a diabetic patient who requires 48 units of insulin at age 30 might rquire as little as 6 to 8 units at age 68. Many patients may feel that their diabetes is improving, but it is usually a result of kidney damage.

Nephropathy. There are two types of nephropathy that occur almost entirely in patients with diabetes: glomerulosclerosis and tubular nephrosis. Glomerulosclerosis is most commonly referred to as Kimmelstiel-Wilson syndrome, named after the discoverers of the nodular form of glomerulosclerosis. There is also a diffuse form of glomerulosclerosis believed to cause more functional damage than even the nodule forms.[1] Kidney damage from glomerulosclerosis is probably irreversible, but good blood glucose control is believed to retard or prevent its development. Tubular nephrosis develops in the proximal tubule where glycogen, fat, and mucopolysaccharides are deposited.

With the advent of kidney transplants,

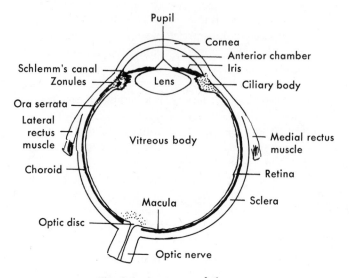

Fig. 8-1. Anatomy of the eye.

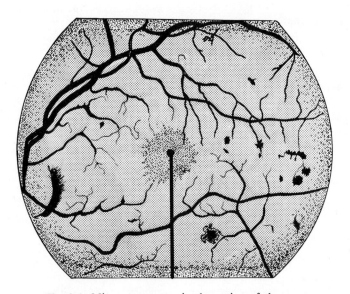

Fig. 8-2. Microaneurysms in the retina of the eye.

the gloomy outlook for kidney disease may become a brighter one in the future.

Eye

The person with diabetes is subject to several changes occurring in the eye. To examine these changes, the physiology of the eye must be reviewed (Fig. 8-1). The macula, the center of the retina, is the area most affected by diabetes.

Retinopathy. "Diabetic retinopathy can be expected to develop in 50% of all cases of diabetes."[2] There are three stages of retinopathy: (1) microaneurysm, (2) exudate and hemorrhage, and (3) retinalis proliferans.

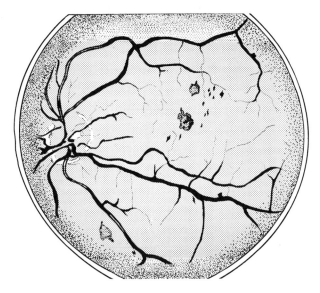

Fig. 8-3. Exudates and hemorrhage in the eye.

MICROANEURYSM. A microaneurysm, a small dilatation of a blood vessel that forms a sac, is caused by pressure exerted by the blood flow on a weakened blood vessel wall. In the macular area of the eye, microaneurysms can be visualized with the ophthalmoscope. They appear as small red dots (Fig. 8-2).

EXUDATES AND HEMORRHAGE. Microaneurysms may hemorrhage into the retina or the vitreous of the eye, causing temporary or permanent blindness. After the microaneurysms are present for several weeks or months, they form waxy deposits called exudates. Through the ophthalmoscope, they appear as waxy areas, yellowish in color (Fig. 8-3).

RETINALIS PROLIFERANS. When there is hemorrhaging into the eye (which occurs in about 25% of the young people with diabetes), a process of neovascularization occurs primarily at the site of the disc. Small blood vessels extend out from the disc in an effort to nourish the tissue with blood. These small blood vessels are subject to hemorrhage. Moreover, these small vessels may compound the problem of neovascularization already present by growing into the vitreous and then contracting, thus causing retinal detachment, the primary cause of blindness in diabetes.

TREATMENT. Earlier treatments for retinopathy included hypophysectomy, or removal of the pituitary gland, which resulted in improvement in the retinopathy. This treatment is now considered to be fairly radical because the removal of the pituitary gland may result in many other chemical imbalances, especially those impairing the individual's ability to combat hypoglycemia. Some of the other earlier treatments for retinopathy included hypophyseal stalk section, radiation of the pituitary, and adrenalectomy.

Newer treatment for retinopathy being performed throughout the country includes photocoagulation and vitrectomy.

Photocoagulation is used in the treatment of diabetic retinopathy to prevent macular edema, fibrovascular ingrowth into the vitreous, vitreous hemorrhage, and retinal detachment. The first instrument developed for photocoagulation was the Ziess Xenon arc photocoagulator. It is used most effectively at the origin of the hemorrhage. If the hemorrhage has resulted in neovascularization into the disc (proliferative diabetic retinopathy), then the argon laser is used to destroy the new vessels and stop neovascularization and retinal detachment.

Vitrectomy is another new form of therapy for diabetic retinopathy resulting from hemorrhage into the vitreous. Vitrectomy is performed when conventional methods have failed or the hemorrhage has not absorbed in 5 to 6 months. In the procedure of vitrectomy, the vitreous of the eye is removed by an instrument called the vitreous-infusion-suction-cutter (VISC). After the vitreous is removed, the vacant cavity is filled with 60% air and 40% sulfur hexafluoride or saline solution. The hemorrhage is removed along with the vitreous fluid.

With all new techniques that are still being documented, complications may result. However, in several years, these new procedures may offer answers to prevent blindness in the diabetic person.

The lens. The lens of the eye is transparent and has no blood supply for nourishment. Its nourishment depends on the aqueous humor; thus the lens reflects changes in the aqueous humor, such as changes in the glucose levels. Glucose levels of the aqueous humor are in turn reflections of the blood glucose levels.

BLURRED VISION. The individual with diabetes may experience sudden changes in refraction and accommodation. Such changes are most often associated with osmotic changes in the lens. The person will complain of blurred vision, which is corrected when the blood glucose level becomes normal and is maintained. Diabetic individuals should not have their eyes examined for glasses until blood glucose levels have been within normal limits for several weeks.

CATARACTS. Cataracts are observed with greater frequency in individuals with diabetes. Cataracts consist of two major types: senile and metabolic.

The senile cataract is a hard opacity of the nucleus of the lens and is usually observed in the aged. Senile cataracts may,

however, occur at an earlier age in persons with diabetes. Therapy consists of surgical removal of the cataract when it significantly reduces vision.

Metabolic cataracts usually occur in young people with diabetes. Through the ophthalmoscope, they appear as small snowflake-shaped areas in the subcapular region of the lens. This form of cataract is preventable with good diabetic control. Metabolic cataracts are caused by hyperglycemia with shunting of the unused glucose into the polyol pathway of metabolism. The resulting accumulation of sorbitol and/or fructose in the lens results in an increase in water content and swelling of the lens. The tissue swelling causes disruption of the lens fibers and cataracts. In their early stages these changes may be reversible if control is improved.

NEUROPATHY

Another degenerative complication that occurs with diabetes is diabetic neuropathy. Diabetic neuropathy is manifested by aching pain and burning of the lower extremities, loss of sensation, loss of autonomic function with bladder paralysis, diarrhea, impotence, and occasionally muscular paralysis. Neuropathy is most often associated with increased blood glucose levels. The pain usually subsides after lower blood glucose levels are established.

Strangely enough, the pain of diabetic neuropathy usually worsens at night while the patient is at rest, and many patients verbalize that they cannot tolerate the slightest stimuli to their feet, not even the bedclothes.

After the individual has had diabetes for 10 to 20 years, painless neuropathy may develop. The ability to feel painful stimuli is decreased, which may result in an injury that the diabetic person does not perceive. Vivid experiences can result. For example, a diabetic person may, in walking barefoot, step on a tack and not find it until taking a bath later that evening. This type of neuropathy, combined with large and small vessel disease, can result in serious damage to the feet and requires constant vigilance in the care of feet (see Chapter 12 on Hygiene).

Diabetic neuropathy can involve one or more large nerves (mononeuropathy or mononeuropathy multiplex), small nerves (ocular neuropathy), and/or the autonomic nervous system. Various mechanisms may be involved, but large and small nerve disease does appear to be related to control. The mechanism of diabetic neuropathy in these nerves appears to be the polyol pathway previously mentioned. Sorbitol and/or fructose accumulation in the Schwann's cells of the nerve tissue results in damage to these cells and decreased myelin production. Without their myelin sheaths, nerves do not function adequately and the clinical manifestations of neuropathy develop.

SUMMARY

The chronic complications of diabetes mellitus may involve the large or small blood vessels, the retina and lens of the eye, and the nervous sytem. Newer data indicate that all of these problems, so devastating to both the quality and quantity of life of the diabetic individual, are preventable by a high degree of metabolic control of the diabetes. Great efforts should be made to accomplish this goal and prevent the destructive complications of the disease.

REFERENCES

1. Williams, R. H., editor: Textbook of endocrinology, Philadelphia, 1961, W. B. Saunders Co., pp. 754, 756.
2. Okun, E., Johnston, G. P., and Boniuk, I.: Management of diabetic retinopathy, St. Louis, 1971, The C. V. Mosby Co. p. 1.

BIBLIOGRAPHY

Dolger, H.: Vascular complications of diabetes mellitus, Bull. Acad. Med. **26:**779, 1950.

Grunnet, M.: Cerebrovascular disease: diabetes and cerebral atherosclerosis, Neurology, **13:**486, 1963.

Herman, M. V., and Gorlin, R.: Premature coronary artery disease and the preclinical diabetic state, Am. J. Med. **38:**481, 1965.

Herman, M. V., and Gorlin, R.: Coronary artery disease and diabetes mellitus *In* Hamwi, G. J., Danowski, T. S., editors: Diabetes mellitus: diagnosis and treatment, vol. 2, New York, 1967, American Diabetes Association, Inc. pp. 185-189.

Kinsell, L. W.: Prevention of vascular disease in the diabetic, Diabetes **4:**298, 1955.

Kronsick, A.: Diabetic neuropathy, Am. J. Nurs. **64:**106, 1964.

Machemer, R.: A new concept for vitreous surgery. Part 2, Surgical technique and complications, Am. J. Ophthalmol. **74**(6):1022, 1973.

Machemer, R.: A new concept for vitreous sergery. Part 7, Two instrument techniques in pars plana vitrectomy, Arch. Ophthalmol. **92:**407, 1974.

Machemer, R., Parel, J. M. and Buettner, H.: A new concept for vitreous surgery. Instrumentation. Am. J. Ophthalmol. **73:**1, 1972.

Mead Johnson and Co. Monograph: Vascular impact of diabetes, Evansville, Ind., 1975, p. 3-17.

Okun, E., Johnson, G. P., and Boniuk, I.: Management of diabetic retinipathy. St. Louis, 1971, The C. V. Mosby Co.

Ostrander, L. D.: The relationship of cardiovascular disease to hyperglycemia, Ann. Intern. Med. **62:**1189, 1965.

Williams, R. H., editor: Diabetes, New York, 1960, Paul B. Hoeber, Inc., pp. 549-623.

Williams, R.: Textbook of endocrinology, Philadelphia, 1961, W. B. Saunders Co. pp. 753-789.

9

Insulin

Elizabeth L. Burke

The administration of insulin has been approached with fear, anxiety, self-pity, and lack of understanding on the part of both the nurse and the patient. Feelings of fear and apprehension are normal for anyone who is doing something for the first time. Some of the lingering anxieties are related to the injection itself and to the nature of insulin. Most nurses have never taken insulin, nor have they given themselves an injection of any kind. Moreover, they have not taught large numbers of persons with diabetes how to give their own injections. Thus nurses feel inadequate in teaching what is obviously so important to the diabetic person. The patient's apprehension is probably related to his attitude about injections or self-injection and the need to take insulin for the rest of his life.

This chapter gives information about various types of manufactured insulin, techniques of injection, and a method for teaching. Also offered is an attitude that will help the nurse approach diabetic patients with confidence and optimism.

GENERAL DESCRIPTION

Insulin is not a drug in the usual sense of the term. It is a hormone, a protein substance, normally secreted by the beta cells of the islets of Langerhans in the pancreas. When there is a deficiency in the production of insulin, for whatever reason, some attempt must be made to make up for the deficiency. When the deficiency is severe, insulin from another source must be given. In this country, the source of manufactured insulin is the pancreas of cattle and hogs. Insulin cannot be taken by mouth because the digestive juices would make its hormonal properties inactive. Therefore, it must be injected. It is this fact that causes considerable apprehension in many patients. Some have been told they will become "hooked" on insulin. Reminding them that they are simply replacing what their body is inadequately producing may help them understand that insulin is not an addicting medication. Presently there is no artificial insulin that can be given to duplicate the action of the body's insulin.[1]

ACTION TIMES

In order to fully understand the effects of insulin, it is necessary to know the action times of the various types of insulin (Table 9-1). Regular, or crystalline, insulin is a short-acting insulin that is clear in appearance. It is most often used in combination with one of the longer-acting insulins but is also used in the treatment of acidosis or other illnesses that make control of diabetes difficult. Semilente has an action similar to regular, but with a slightly longer duration of action. Semilente is usually used in combination with lente or ultralente insulins. The longer-acting insulins have actions that cover a 14- to 24-hour period, or longer. They are all cloudy in appearance, with the exception of globin, which is clear. The intermediate-acting insulins are NPH, lente and globin. Lente is a mixture of 30% semilente and 70% ultralente. Protamine zinc insulin (PZI) has a prolonged action

Table 9-1. Action time and appearance of most commonly used insulins

Type of insulin	Appearance	Action	Previously reported action* (hours)			Revised action† (hours)		
			Onset	Peak	Duration	Onset	Peak	Duration
Regular	Clear	Rapid	$1/2$	2-4	5-7	$1/2$-1	2-4	6-8
Semilente	Cloudy	Rapid	$1/2$	4-8	12-16	$1/2$-1	2-4	8-10
Globin	Clear	Intermediate	1-2	8-10	18-24	1-2	6-8	12-14
NPH	Cloudy	Intermediate	2-4	12-18	24-28	1-2	6-8	12-14
Lente	Cloudy	Intermediate	2-4	12-18	24-28	1-2	6-8	14-16
PZI	Cloudy	Long	4-6	18-26	36-72	4-6	18±	36-72
Ultralente	Cloudy	Long	4-6	18-26	36-72	4-6	8-12	24-36

*These are the standard values for onset, peak action, and duration of action of insulins found in standard medical texts and have been widely accepted for many years. (Data from Eli Lilly Research Laboatories: Diabetes mellitus, ed. 7, Indianapolis, 1973, Eli Lilly and Co., pp. 42-44.)

†These are revised values for insulin action based on careful and accurate diurnal blood glucose measurements in large numbers of diabetic children under carefully controlled conditions of dietary intake and standardized activity patterns. These studies were performed at the University of Missouri and reported in 1975. They represent the latest knowledge in the field. (Data from Jackson, R. L., and Guthrie, R. A.: The child with diabetes, Kalamazoo, Mich., 1973, The Upjohn Co., p. 44.)

but is rarely used today. Ultralente, which also has a prolonged action, is used by some.

It should be kept in mind that the action times of the insulins of Table 9-1 are averages and are not the same in all people with diabetes. It is noted by many diabetes specialists that globin, NPH, and lente insulins do not last 24 hours in many juveniles. The recent studies at the University of Missouri confirm the observation of many scientists that the duration of action of the intermediate-acting insulins is closer to 12 to 14 hours.[2] For this reason many children and young people receive two doses of intermediate-acting insulin each day. The long-acting insulins are too long acting and too variable in their action to be practical in children and young adults and are seldom used.

CONCENTRATION

Insulin is available in U-40, U-80, and U-100 concentrations. For patients needing excessively large amounts of insulin (those who are resistant), U-500 is available by special order. The concentration does not mean that one insulin is stronger than another. One unit of insulin is the same as any other unit of insulin in 1 ml (1 cc) of liquid: U-40 insulin has 40 units of insulin in 1 ml of liquid, U-80 has 80 units of insulin in 1 ml of liquid, and U-100 insulin has 100 units of insulin in 1 ml of liquid. The important point to remember is that whatever concentration of insulin is being used, a syringe of the same concentration is to be used. In other words, when U-40 insulin is being used, a U-40 syringe must be used. When U-100 insulin is used, a U-100 syringe or a Lo Dose syringe which measures up to 50 units) must be used. One should never use a double-calibrated syringe, one with U-40 markings on one side and U-80 on the other. It is too easy to make mistakes with that type of syringe. Hopefully, U-100 will soon be the only insulin available and mistakes in measuring will become a problem of the past.

U-100 insulin has been available since early 1973. It has been manfuctured in an attempt to standardize the concentration in preparation for the metric system, eventually to replace U-40 and U-80 insulin. With only one concentration, much of the confusion about which syringe and which insulin to use will be ended. Currently, the biggest problem in that regard has to do with the accuracy of measurement when taking very small doses of U-100 insulin. It is felt by many that it is impossible to accurately measure less than 10 units of insulin in the U-100 syringe, particularly the disposable syringe. The most accurate syringe for measuring small doses is the glass 0.35-ml (35-unit) syringe, or the new disposable 50-unit Lo Dose syringe. Both syringes measure each unit by 1-unit increments, and it is possible to measure less than 1 unit if necessary. In some programs, U-100 insulin is diluted to U-50, U-25, or U-10, and a tuberculin syringe is used in order to more accurately measure insulin for small children. The new Lo Dose syringe for use with U-100 insulin may obviate the need for these manipulations. This syringe recently marketed by one manufacturer should soon be marketed by others and be widely available within a short time. It has nearly the same overall lenth as a U-100 syringe and the tuberculin syringe but has a smaller internal diameter. Thus it holds only 50 units of U-100 insulin. Because it holds one half as much insulin as a U-100 syringe within a similar overall length, the numbers are spread out, are easier to read, and thus accuracy for small doses of insulin is improved.

STORAGE

The Food and Drug Administration requires that packages of insulin state: "Keep in a cold place. Avoid freezing." This precaution is a warning that insulin can lose its potency under extremes of temperatures (above 90° F or at freezing or lower). Studies have shown that the potency of insulin is very stable at room temperature up to 1 year and even longer for certain types of insulin.[1] Because there is some feeling that cold insulin may be irritating to the tissues (patients do report that the injection of cold insulin is more pain-

ful), it is recommended that the insulin that is currently being used be kept at room temperature and that the extra supply of insulin be kept in the refrigerator. People with diabetes should be instructed to always have on hand at least one extra bottle of each type of insulin they are using. When traveling, patients may use a simple wide-mouth plastic thermos that can hold several bottles of insulin and keep the temperature stable. A container large enough to hold some ice will help if the outside temperature is 90° F or above. When a diabetic person is traveling by public transportation, it is wise to carry insulin and other necessary supplies in hand luggage. The supplies will then be at hand when they are needed and a lot of unnecessary worry will be avoided.

Insulin does carry an expiration date on the label. Although the insulin will not deteriorate overnight, it is a good idea to use it by the date on the bottle. The potency of insulin used after that date can no longer be guaranteed by the manufacturer. There are times when insulin will be found on sale at the pharmacy. This usually occurs when the supply of insulin is reaching the expiration date and the pharmacist wants to sell it out. It is all right to buy this insulin as long as it can be used by the expiration date. If it cannot be used by that date, it should not be purchased. Patients should be instructed to always check the expiration date on the bottle before leaving the drugstore.

EQUIPMENT

There are various kinds of insulin, syringes, and needles available from many different manufacturers; therefore, a decision as to which type to use is often difficult. There is no single syringe to suit all needs. The choice should be made on the basis of the best equipment for the particular situation, after one has had an opportunity to practice with several styles and types of syringes. The features to consider are: cost, convenience, ease of reading the scale, ease of handling the syringe, and accuracy of measurement.

Syringes

There are two main types of syringes: disposable and reusable. The disposable syringe is plastic, individually packaged and sterilized, light weight, and is designed to be used once and thrown away. Most disposable syringes come with a needle attached, usually $1/2$ or $5/8$ inch long. Some do not have a needle, and a disposable needle of desired length may be attached. The reusable syringe is glass, thus it is breakable, needs to be sterilized, (usually by boiling when used in the home), handles somewhat differently, and can be used many times. Needles for glass syringes may be disposable or reusable. Disposable needles that are used once and thrown away are the most frequently used type. They are generally of excellent sharpness and are available in various lengths. (Instructions for determining length are found on pp. 96-97, Length of needle.) Many people still prefer to use reusable needles because they can use them many times, sharpen them, and use them many more times. However, it does take skill to properly sharpen needles, and the modest cost of the disposable

Table 9-2. Disposable vs. reusable syringes

Problem areas	Disposable		Reusable	
	Pros	Cons	Pros	Cons
Cost	←——Approximately \$0.10 to \$0.15 apiece——→		←————— \$4 to \$8 apiece —————→	
	Not very expensive	Too expensive for some; welfare will often not pay for them	Can be used many times to offset cost	Initially expensive
Sterilizing	Presterilized		No need to sterilize daily	Have to be resterilized every week to 10 days
Scale		Lines too close together—difficult for some to read; printing too light or rubs off	Measurement usually darker and spaced more widely	
Measuring	Plunger stays put	Often difficult to remove bubbles causing dead space problems and inaccuracy of measurement, especially when two insulins are mixed in a syringe; small doses difficult to measure except with a Lo Dose syringe	Bubbles easily displaced; small syringe for small doses	Plunger slides too easily at times
Handling	Measured dose not easily displaced; no breakage problem			Measured dose may be displaced; care must be taken not to drop—will break

variety makes their convenience popular.

While the reusable glass syringes are generally preferred and recommended, it is often better for a particular individual to use the disposable variety. In Table 9-2, a list of pros and cons of the reusable and disposable syringes helps identify problem areas.

The pros and cons of the two types of syringes are almost equally divided, thus the decision as to which type to use should be made on an individual basis. When working with patients who are learning insulin injection, the nurse must carefully observe how well they can see the markings, handle the syringe, and accurately measure the insulin dose.

Two controversies

Ecology issue. When disposable equipment of any kind is being discussed, the ecology issue frequently arises. It is true that disposable material does create waste that must be destroyed in some manner. In some areas, plastics are buried; in others, they are incinerated. The ecology question is one that must be resolved by individual conscience.

Dead space. The second controversy regards "dead space." At least two manufacturers now make disposable syringes that they claim eliminates dead space, and one manufacturer has performed some elaborate studies to demonstrate this fact.[3] Dead space refers to the amount of insulin left in the needle and hub when one is measuring insulin and after the injection. When only one kind of insulin is used, the dead space insulin is simply wasted, which does not involve a measurement problem. When one uses two kinds of insulin and measures them in the same syringe, the first insulin left in the needle after measuring is actually included in the measurement of the second insulin. Some observers have felt that the dead space (first) insulin would amount to a significant dosage error. This problem, however, is usually insignificant. If patients always measure insulin in the same way, they will always be getting the same amount of insulin, and they should be taught to do this. If the difference is enough to affect control, then the dosage should be altered to allow for the difference or U-100 insulin should be premixed in volume. The manufacturers have argued that the problem of dead space can be eliminated by the use of a needle that is permanently attached to the disposable syringe is such a way as to eliminate the dead space. Dead space is partially eliminated by reducing the bubbles in the syringe. Bubbles, not dead space, are the biggest problem in insulin measurement, and bubbles are best reduced by use of a glass syringe. Any of the currently available equipment is adequate if care is taken in its use.

Care of equipment

Disposal of syringes. Disposable syringes need no care prior to their use. They are used once and thrown away. Care does need to be taken in the disposal of these syringes. If possible, the syringe should be broken or in some way rendered unusable, and the needle should be broken off from the hub. These actions will help to keep unauthorized persons from using the equipment.

Sterilization of reusable syringes. Reusable glass syringes do need care and the following is a suggested procedure:

1. Take the syringe apart and wash thoroughly with soap and water, being sure to rinse thoroughly. The same is to be done with a reusable needle.

2. Place the syringe parts (and reusable needle) in a strainer that fits into a small pan, and fill with water to cover the equipment. Add 1 tablespoon vinegar or baking soda to the water to prevent the formation of mineral deposits on the syringe.

3. Bring the water to a boil and allow to simmer for 15 minutes. (Instead of being boiled, a syringe may be placed in a double thickness of aluminum foil and baked in a 350° F oven for 15 to 20 minutes.)

4. Remove the pan and pour off the water, returning the strainer to the pan to cool. Meanwhile, a container to hold the syringe should be

prepared in the same manner, or it can be filled with boiling water and allowed to stand for a few minutes.

5. Fill the clean, empty syringe container with 70% isopropyl alcohol. (While some argue that some grades of 70% isopropyl alcohol have impurities that may lead to allergic reactions, such reactions rarely occur.) Glycerine should not be an ingredient in the alcohol. Ninety-one percent alcohol may be more irritating and is not necessarily more bactericidal.[4] For those individuals who do seem sensitive to alcohol, we suggest either boiling the syringe daily or using disposable equipment. Any container tall enough to hold the syringe will do: an olive jar, seltzer bottle, or a test tube with a lid or cork.

6. When the syringe parts have cooled, put them together, loop a string or thread around the top, and immerse parts in the alochol to just below the plunger handle.

The above sterilization procedure needs to be repeated weekly, which makes care of the glass syringe quite simple. Some people choose to use disposable equipment and have no problems with it. However, many people feel they are getting a more accurate measurement with the glass syringe. The above procedure offers a simple method of care, and a choice in the type of equipment that can be used.

When diabetic individuals are ready to give their injections, they should remove the syringe from the container, push the plunger in and out several times to remove any alcohol that might be inside, attach a sterile needle, and measure and give the injection. They then push the plunger in and out several times again to clear any insulin remaining inside the syringe, and put it back into the alcohol container. They should *not* rinse the syringe with tap water before immersing it in the alcohol container. This would render it unsterile. Few individuals have any problems with this procedure, and infections from contaminated equipment are rare.

MEASUREMENT

The accurate measurement of the insulin dose is a critical part of insulin therapy.

The person doing the measuring must be fully instructed and have adequate time to practice before being permitted to do so unsupervised. Whether it is a student nurse, a registered nurse who is not familiar with giving insulin, a diabetic person, or a relative, complete, supervised instruction must take place. The atmosphere of teaching should be unhurried, and accuracy must be stressed. Ideally, the instruction should take place over several short periods. In this way, the patients will not become tired or apprehensive with repeated trials and initial failures. A calm, positive attitude on the part of the instructor is a must.

First, patients should be allowed to become familiar with the equipment. They should handle the syringe, get used to the feel, push the plunger in and out, and be shown the various ways they might hold it. The patients will feel quite self-conscious about the equipment, and the opportunity to explore it before having to perform with it helps them to gain confidence.

When measuring insulin, one should have all equipment at hand: insulin, syringe, needles, cotton balls or alcohol sponges, and alcohol. One must be sure to use a syringe marked for the same concentration as the insulin to be used, that is, if U-100 insulin is used, only a U-100 or a 50-unit Lo Dose syringe may be used. No patient should be taught to convert one concentration of insulin for use in a syringe of another concentration. While that has been done, unnecessary errors have been caused by doing it. There is only one exception to this rule—when one is using U-100 insulin, a tuberculin syringe may be used. The tuberculin syringe is marked the same as a U-100 syringe: each 0.01 ml (0.01 cc) is 1 unit of insulin.

Using one type of insulin

Teach the patient to measure one type of insulin first. The procedure is as follows:

1. Roll the bottle of insulin between the hands. The mixing is necessary to return any particles to suspension. Do not shake

vigorously because this creates many bubbles, which are then difficult to remove.

2. Wipe the top of the bottle with an alcohol sponge.
3. Inject air into the insulin bottle equal to the dosage of insulin to be taken out. The step equalizes the pressure in the bottle to make it easier to withdraw the insulin.
4. Withdraw the insulin into the syringe. Note the air bubbles in the syringe; they will nearly always be there when measuring for the first insulin. Hold the syringe vertically, at eye level, allowing bubbles to rise to the top, or give it a tap. Push the plunger all the way in to inject the bubbles back into the bottle.
5. Withdraw the insulin into the syringe for the second time, adjusting to the required dosage. This time there should be no bubbles. (The problem of having air bubbles in the syringe is that they are taking up space where insulin should be and therefore interfering with an accurate dosage.)

Mixing two types of insulin

When a diabetic person is receiving both modified and unmodified (regular) insulin, the two types can be mixed in the same syringe, thus saving the patient extra injections. (Mixtures of lente insulin with PZI, NPH, or globin insulins result in incompatibility.) When one is measuring two types of insulin, care must be taken not to contaminate one with the other. Follow this procedure:

1. Roll the bottle of modified insulin.
2. Wipe the tops of both bottles.
3. Inject air equal to the insulin dosage into the bottle of modified insulin. Do not withdraw this insulin.
4. Inject air into the bottle of regular insulin equal to the insulin dosage and withdraw this insulin, being certain to remove all air bubbles.
5. Return to the bottle of modified insulin and withdraw the insulin. Take care not to have a bubble in the syringe while measuring this insulin. If an error in measurement is made, redraw the insulin.

Some patients, because of various limitations, cannot be taught to measure two kinds

of insulin accurately. In this situation, it is best to take two injections, have the insulin premixed in the bottle, or have someone else measure the insulin. It is also possible to have a visiting nurse or family member measure the insulin in disposable syringes for a week at a time. There is little or no change in the action properties of the new neutral insulins in periods of a month or more.

Particularly for individuals taking small doses and those on reasonably fixed ratios of unmodified and modified insulins, premixing in a mixing bottle is very advantageous. Premixing a few weeks' supply of insulin dilutes out mixing errors that can be present when small doses are mixed in a syringe and obviates the problem of syringe dead space. It is also convenient for the patient because the insulin can be mixed as seldom as once monthly. Insulin mixing is simple to teach. If for instance a dose of 14 units of NPH insulin and 7 units of regular insulin are to be given, the insulin can be premixed as a 2:1 ratio. 10 ml of NPH and 5 ml of regular can be premixed in a 20-ml presterilized vial. The dose of insulin required, 21 units (14 units NPH + 7 units regular = 21 units) is then simply withdrawn into the syringe and injected. A mixing vial can be reused for about 3 months before it becomes contaminated and the rubber diaphragm wears out. Premixing promotes a remarkable simplicity when insulin ratios can be calculated and when the ratios remain relatively unchanged and is to be highly recommended. Premixing was not possible with the older acid regular insulin but is no problem with the new neutral regular insulin preparations.

MAJOR PROBLEMS FROM INJECTION

There are some major problems resulting from insulin injection: disfigurement caused by hypertrophy or atrophy of subcutaneous fat; localized skin reactions with a hivelike swelling, redness, and itching; and pain caused by the particular site or technique used. Less common problems related to insulin injection are injection directly into a blood vessel and infection at the injection site.

Lipodystrophies

Hypertrophy. It has been found that the greatest problem most insulin-dependent diabetic individuals face is lipodystrophy. The most common lipodystrophy is hypertrophy, or thickening at the site of injection. Lipohypertrophy is probably caused by injecting insulin too frequently into the same area or perhaps injecting too superficially.[1] The result is a raised, thickened area practically devoid of nerve endings (which results in increased use because of its painlessness) and very poor insulin absorption. Insulin builds up in these areas and is released very slowly, thereby causing poor diabetic control.

Atrophy. The second problem is lipoatrophy, or loss of subcutaneous fat, which appears as a depressed hollow or concavity at the site of injection. Rarely do these areas appear in sites other than those being injected. While the cause of this problem is subject to discussion, one program has observed thousands of patients over the years and has come to the conclusion that the injections are either too frequently given in one site or the injection is given too superficially into the fatty tissue. The problem is more common in children and females,[1] and many times a girl seems to outgrow the problem without any treatment.

Watson and Calder[5] recently have shown that lipoatrophy could be treated by injection into the atrophic site by a special injection technique. Wentworth and others[6] believe that the cause of the atrophy is impurities in the insulin. (Highly purified and neutral U-100 insulin became available in 1973.) Believing that the atrophy is caused by impurities and that insulin naturally has a lipohypertrophic effect, Wentworth and associates advocate injecting purified insulin directly into the atrophied sites. The Wentworth technique has worked well,

though the reason it has worked may not be as simple as Wentworth and others believe. Atrophy has for instance occurred (though less frequently) with the purified insulins but has also been cured with the Wentworth technique and the same insulin. This tends to say, though does not prove, that the atrophy is related to injection technique rather than insulin purity, though both may be involved. More research is needed to answer that question. Nonetheless, the injection technique described below is highly curative—to date, approximately 85% of patients with insulin lipoatrophy are showing improvement or cure of atrophied areas when this technique is used.[5,6] For those who have atrophy problems, to either a greater or lesser extent, there is hope beyond waiting months or years for recovery.

INJECTION TECHNIQUE FOR ATROPHY. This technique should be used whenever lipoatrophy is present. Insulin is injected directly into the atrophied area just under the thin layer of skin that covers it. Repeated injections are given around the atrophied area, stripping the skin from the muscle and causing hypertrophy of the underlying fat. Within just a few weeks, mildly atrophied areas are filled in and more severe ones are improved.

Summary. Some observers believe that lipodystrophy problems are simply a part of insulin therapy and there is no prevention. Others believe lipodystrophy is preventable. Countless patients have been seen with one or both lipodystrophic problems, and after using the techniques described above have had no further difficulty.

INJECTION SITES

Throughout the years of insulin therapy, many sites have been used for insulin injection. The most frequently used areas have been the thighs, upper arms, abdomen, and buttocks. The calves and the back of the forearm have also been used. These latter two areas are not recommended because of toughness of the skin, which leads to a more painful injection and a decreased blood supply, which leads to poorer absorption.

There are several reasons for recommending a particular site for insulin injection. In general, the aim is to give a painless injection that will be easily absorbed at a smooth rate and cause no abnormalities in the skin surface. In addition, the site should be readily accessible to either the diabetic person or someone else who will be giving the injections. The best locations for injections to meet the above criteria are the *lateral surface of the thighs, upper abdomen, upper arms,* and *the back.* The midline areas are avoided because of the increased number of nerve endings, leading to increased pain. The buttocks should also be avoided (except in the case of small children) because of the thickness of the fat layer, which decreases absorption. (This is discussed more fully on pp. 96-97.) The four areas described above are relatively painless, easily accessible, have almost equal absorption, and in addition, can be pinched up relatively easily. The areas are large enough to allow the patient a number of injections in each place without using the same site too frequently.

Rotation

Adequate rotation of injection sites is probably the single most important factor in minimizing problems at the site of injection, in spite of the fact that the Eli Lilly Research Laboratories have suggested that rotation may not be as necessary when using the recently purified Lilly insulins.[7] As stated previously, some people have developed lipodystrophies with the purified insulin when using poor rotation or superficial injection techniques.

The suggested rotation pattern to be used should be one that allows use of one area for 1 week at a time, and then nonuse of that area for 4 to 6 weeks. The pattern should be simple enough to be easily followed. The thigh area is scored into two or three rows of seven injection sites each, approximately 1½ inches apart (Fig. 9-1)

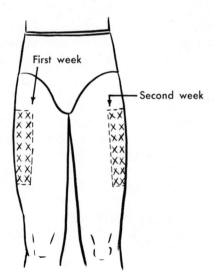

Fig. 9-1. Rotation sites: first and second weeks.

The rows should also be 1½ inches apart. The injection sites may be started just below the groin and continued to about 3 inches above the knee. It is easy to remember where in the pattern the next injection goes when one is using the 1 row–1 week technique: the first injection is given at one end on Sunday, and by Saturday the injection will be at the opposite end of the row. A right-handed individual moves down the right leg and up the left. The opposite is less awkward for a left-handed person.

When the abdomen is being used, injection sites should be on the lower part of the rib cage above the waistline (Fig. 9-2). This area is relatively easy to pinch up and is painless. The skin at the waistline itself is usually tough in adults and makes the injection more painful. The lower area of the abdomen is usually fatter, which makes the technique more difficult. This area is acceptable for use if it is needed when other sites become worn out and is acceptable in children who have thinner skin and fat layers.

Use of the arms and the back needs to be taught to those who are assisting the insulin-dependent person (Fig. 9-2). Some

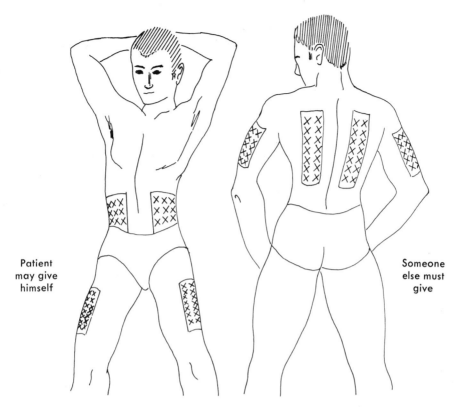

Patient
may give
himself

Someone
else must
give

Fig. 9-2. Rotation sites: suggested plan of rotation allowing a rest of at least 4 weeks before returning to the original site.

persons, especially adolescents, do give their own injections in the arms; however, self-injection into the arms is not as preferable for older less nimble people.

Most people initially feel that the back is taboo. Such is not the case. The back is relatively painless, usually easy to pinch up, and has a wide surface area. Two or three rows of injections can be given on each side of the back. Injection sites are spaced to receive 1 week of insulin in each row. The individual to be injected may either stand, sit, or lie down for the injection. The shoulders need to be in a relaxed position.

The points to remember in the use and rotation of injection sites are:

1. Use as many of the available areas as possible.

2. Do not return to the same site more frequently than every 4 to 6 weeks.
3. Do not use the inside of the thighs or arms or the midline of the abdomen or back.

Inspection

Inspection of injection sites needs to be carried out periodically. The injection sites need to be checked for lumps or hollows or any evidence of infection. The individual should not only look at the areas of injection but should feel them. The best way to do this is by running the flat of the palm down the thighs, across the abdomen, and down the arms. Someone else will have to feel the back. The palm is more sensitive to variations in texture of the underlying tissues than the fingertips alone. If there are lumpy areas, thickening, or hollows felt, the area should be allowed to rest for a time. These areas will soften and return to normal, usually within a few weeks, although it may take 6 months to 1 year or more occasionally. For atrophied areas, the injection technique explained on p. 93 is recommended.

METHODS OF INJECTION

Over the years, several insulin injection techniques have been used. One technique has been injecting at a 45° angle directly into the subcutaneous fat layer. The skin and fat are pinched up, the needle inserted at a 45° angle into the pinched up area, and the insulin injected with a 1/2- to 5/8-inch needle. Another technique is to inject into a deeper subcutaneous layer by injecting at a 90° angle and either stretching the skin taut or pinching it up.[8] The 1/2- to 5/8-inch needle is also recommended with this technique. Both of these techniques use the "dart," or quick, method of penetration. While these techniques may be fine for some people, no one method works for all. The nurse-educator needs to carefully determine individual needs based on the thickness of skin and fat layers and manual dexterity.

A recommended technique

The following technique has been used in a large clinic and hospital for many years.[9] It is not difficult to teach and does accomplish all of the goals of proper injection techniques:

1. It provides a smooth, even absorption rate.
2. It is practically painless.
3. It prevents allergic reactions in most subjects.
4. It prevents lipodystrophies.

Angle and placement of the needle. This method requires pinching up the layer of skin and fat and injecting the insulin into the "space" between the fat and muscle. The injection is given at an angle almost parallel to the skin surface (20° to 45°) at the base of the pinched up area (Fig. 9-3). It is an area rich in capillary blood supply, thus ensuring a smooth absorption rate.

Length of needle. The second part of the method requires a needle that is long enough to reach beneath the fat. Depending on the area used and the person, a 5/8- to 7/8-inch needle is usually recommended. For the thicker fat layer in fatter individuals, a 1- to 11/2-inch needle is used. The only people who should use a 1/2-inch needle are those who have a very thin fat layer (usually men, children, or the elderly).

Many people have given their injections with 1/2-inch needles. Some have used the stretch method with a 90° angle. Many of these people have developed extensive atrophied areas or hard, red, itchy welts at the site of their injections. After accepting

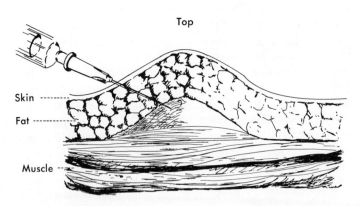

Fig. 9-3. Angle and placement of injection.

the suggestion that they should use a longer needle and inject at a smaller angle to reach the "space" beneath the fat layer, most of them have had no further problems.

How does one determine the length of needle to use? (1) Pinch up the layer of skin and fat. (2) Measure the distance across the base of the fold. This distance is the recommended length of the needle (Fig. 9-4). Disposable needles separate from the syringe so that individuals can use the specific length that is recommended. There are several manufacturers who make needles in various lengths, and it is possible to purchase needles in boxes of 100. With a longer needle, the gauge number should be smaller to permit less bending: 25 gauge is fine for ⁵⁄₈- and ⁷⁄₈-inch needles, 23 gauge for 1-inch, and 22 gauge for 1¹⁄₂-inch needles.

Patients sometimes feel that the larger needle will hurt a lot more, but this is true only to a small degree. The only discomfort felt is right on the surface of the skin, and when the needle point is placed on the skin surface and then pushed through quickly, there is very little pain. In fact, most patients relate that they feel the injection slightly, if at all.

The injection. When giving the injection, take the following steps:

1. Pinch up the skin and fat and wipe the site with an alcohol sponge.*
2. Hold the syringe horizontally, with the thumb on one side and the first three fingers on the other. The little finger holds pressure on the plunger and also injects the insulin.
3. Trace the needle from the top of the "hill" to the bottom, keeping the syringe nearly parallel to the skin surface. This "exercise" prevents guesswork by assuring that the needle is in the right place.
4. With the needle directly on the skin surface, push it quickly through the skin, all the way to the hub. (See Fig. 9-3.)
5. Inject the insulin with the little finger, and release the pinch.
6. Put the cotton ball over the site and pull the needle straight out. (Do not rub the site because rubbing is apt to cause irritation of the tissues.) If the patient has a problem with bruising, hold the cotton ball over the site firmly for 1 full minute. This will usually prevent bleeding just under the skin surface.

Summary. This technique sounds complicated and has been criticized as being too difficult to teach to the person who has

*There has been some question about the practice of special skin cleansing.[10] While this aspect is not overstressed, it is recommended that the person wash hands and use an alcohol wipe at the injection site. Infections are rarely seen when simple cleanliness is observed.

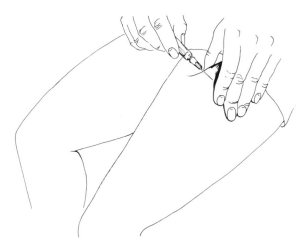

Fig. 9-4. Measurement for choice of needle length.

limited learning ability and may not be capable of always performing the injection in the same way. However, it has been found that people of all educational levels can learn this technique. Recognizing that no one should be taught an injection technique in only one sitting, nurse-educators have noted that with simple repetition and three or four supervised instruction periods, the technique can be mastered.

Special injectors

Automatic injectors. There have been advocates of the use of automatic injectors. The automatic injector works by a push-button spring release of the needle that "automatically" gives the injection with very little participation by the patient. Persons who have used this injector have done so because they "could not learn to give themselves an injection." This is usually because they have some form of denial of diabetes. It has been found in one program that most individuals who use this injector have more lipodystrophy and tougher skin. Most, if not all, people who have fears or other emotional adjustments to diabetes can give their own injections in time, and the use of automatic injectors only perpetuates their fears. It is recommended that the person who has a physical handicap, such as cerebral palsy, use the automatic injector as an alternative aid. However, it is not recommended for others; rather these individuals should be helped to better accept their diabetes rather than depend on crutches.

Jet spray injector. The jet spray injector has been introduced as an alternative to needle injection. It has the advantage of broader distribution of insulin, otherwise the effects at the site of injection are about the same as needle injection.[11,12] Blood glucose curves, chronic inflammatory changes of tissues, and induration at the site of injection are equal in both methods of injection. In the absence of significant benefits and because of the great cost of the jet injector, it is not recommended for general use.

TEACHING OTHERS

Many nurses feel uncomfortable when they have to teach patients or family members how to give insulin. Some nurses do not like to teach at all. However, some simply have not done it often enough to really become accustomed to teaching insulin injection, or they do not know enough about how to teach it. Getting right in and doing it is probably the best way to learn. The following guidelines should be helpful:

Learn as much as possible by reading and talking to nurses and others about insulin injection.

Have self-confidence. Remember, the health professional knows more about insulin injection than the patient, and it will not take very many instruction periods for educators to feel like they have been teaching insulin injection all their life.

Be positive. Assure the individual that they will be able to give the injections. They may tell you that they cannot do it, but be calmly firm and refuse to take "no" for an answer. Do not let them "off the hook." Some people take longer than others to learn, but all will eventually learn. Self-injection is something they have to and will face. Some people are more upset by self-injecting than others. Accept that fact and help them with it. The diabetic person might practice on the nurse first. Most will be saying "I can't do it" while the nurse or doctor is giving directions each step of the way. As they stick the needle, their faces will suddenly change from fear, to surprise, and then to pleasure—pleasure, not from sticking the subject, but from having mastered a task they did not believe they could do. Self-injection is then just one step away.

A bright 4-year-old boy had a mother who was terrified of the injection process. She decided she would have to give herself an injection to realize that it did not hurt, before attempting to give her child an injection. After 1 hour of tears and much self-denial, she was finally able to inject herself. She was so pleased with herself that she asked her son if she could give him a shot even though it was not insulin time and it would have to be a dry run. He pulled up his sleeve and pinched up the skin saying, "Do it right there." He did not even flinch and both of them felt quite pleased with themselves. Rightly so!

Give directions each step of the way. Do not just hand the patients the syringe and expect them to do it. Show how to select the injection site, and help them pinch up the skin and wipe it off. Show them how to hold the syringe and the angle of the needle. Continue detailed instruction until the injection is finished and the needle is out. This will give them assurance that they are not doing something wrong.

Be calm and unhurried. Assure your patients that they will not be released until they are ready.

Use the same basic approach with everyone. Simple language works well with all people. The technique is new to them; thus it does not matter whether they are very intelligent or not. The simple approach can be understood. Medical terms, such as injection, may be used. However, if your students feel more comfortable with "shot," let them use it. Do not use baby talk even with babies; use everyday language.

Always teach patients to inject the thigh first, unless the area is contraindicated. Use of this area seems to be less emotionally charged than the abdomen. They can easily see what they are doing and manipulate the equipment. However, have them use the abdomen once or twice before completing the teaching so that they can get accustomed to the idea.

Begin teaching insulin injection as soon as it is known that the patients will be using insulin. Do not put off injection instruction because it only causes patients the needless anxiety of knowing they will have to learn self-injection but have not begun. In addition, it is helpful to have as much time as possible for practice; if instruction is delayed, the time will be limited.

Do not try to teach the entire injection process at one time. There is too much to

learn, and your patients will become confused or tired. Do it in several short sessions: injection, measurement, review of sites. Begin by teaching the injection procedure first. This may seem backwards, but injection is the cause of the greatest anxiety. If you begin there, the rest will be easier. Occasionally the nurse has slaved over teaching the measurement of insulin and has gotten nowhere because the patient was worrying about self-injection. When the injection was performed, the patient settled down and was able to practice and succeed with measurement. Sometimes the patient can succeed in performing the self-injection but cannot measure because of poor eyesight, shakiness, or related problems. In these instances, teach someone else to measure the insulin and allow the patient to give the injection. This plan certainly helps the patient maintain independence.

Please do not give your students an orange on which to practice injections. It is strongly felt that this allows the denial of the reality of injection. Moreover, it leads them to believe that self-injection is no harder, which is not true. Giving oneself insulin and giving an orange insulin is really not the same. If the patients need a crutch, let them give you an injection first. For young children, the use of a rag doll is suggested. This allows the children to feel they are participating in their care even though they may not be capable of managing self-injection alone. Use of the doll may also serve to encourage the children to act out other feelings they may have about their diabetes.

Allow children to give their own injections as soon as they show interest in doing so. They may not be capable of doing the entire procedure at first. Start them off by letting them hold up the pinch and push in the insulin. Then let them "go for a free ride" by putting their hand on top of yours on the syringe. This helps them get the feel of the action. Next, you "go for the free ride" and let the children do the work. They will think you are helping, when actually they may be doing most of it. Even very young children can do part of the injection with encouragement and praise. Ask them to "help" you. When they trust you, they will usually be cooperative.

Apply these same guidelines when you are teaching family members or others involved in the care of the patient. It is advised to have the family member give themselves an injection before giving their spouse or child one. This practice is the best reassurance for the family member to know they are not hurting their loved one, and it usually frees them from any negative feelings they may have had. In addition, try very hard to involve the whole family in the care of the patient. In this way, one person will not feel that the patient is dependent only on him and that he always has to be available. It should be a shared responsibility.

Use a portion of every hospitalization or outpatient visit as a period of teaching or review. Do not assume that just because patients have had diabetes for awhile they know everything or do what they should. Ask where they inject insulin and show them how to inspect the sites. Review the importance of site rotation. If they have any site problems, make appropriate recommendations—that is, better rotation or different technique. Even though it is a good idea for the nurse to inject an area that patients cannot reach when they are hospitalized, always have them show how they give the insulin at least once during the stay. If there is a question of visual accuracy, ask them to measure their insulin dose for you. Many times these reviews help to identify a problem in control that was not previously recognized.

Develop an attitude of helpfulness, not of criticism. Assure the patients that you want what is best for them and their management of diabetes. Even hostile patients will often come around when they feel you are really concerned and interested in them.

SUMMARY

In summary, insulin injection is an important part of the care and teaching of the person with diabetes. The difference in giving insulin and giving most other medications is the fact that insulin is given every day, therefore maximum maintenance of sites is of prime importance.

The nurse who has a thorough knowledge of diabetes and its management and who has an accepting, positive attitude toward the individuals with diabetes is in a good position to teach them how to accept and give their injections.

There are few times in nursing that give nurses such a feeling of satisfaction as when they have successfully assisted in some area of self-management of a chronic and serious disease. The self-injection of insulin is one of those times. Enjoy it!

REFERENCES
1. Eli Lilly Research Laboratories: Diabetes mellitus, ed. 7, Indianapolis, 1973, Eli Lilly and Co. pp. 38, 48, 88, 90, 106.

2. Jackson, R. L., and Guthrie, R. A.: The child with diabetes, Kalamazoo, Mich., 1973, The Upjohn Co. pp. 44, 45. (Note corrections: on p. 44, peak action in intermediate-acting insulin, 6-8 not 4-6.)

3. College of Pharmaceutical Sciences: A study of dead space and its effect on insulin mixing, New York, 1975, Columbia University Press.

4. AMA Department of Drugs: AMA drug evaluations, ed. 2, Acton, Mass., 1973, Publishing Sciences Group, Inc., pp. 646-647

5. Watson, B. M., and Calder, J. S.: A treatment for insulin-induced fat atrophy, Diabetes, **20:**628, 1971

6. Wentworth, S. M., Galloway, J. A., Haug, E. A., and others: The use of purified insulins in the treatment of patients with insulin lipoatrophy, Diabetes **22** (Suppl. 1):290, 1973.

7. Krall, L. P.: Diabetes forecast, New York, 1974, American Diabetes Association, Inc., vol. 27, p. 11.

8. Coates, F. C., and Fabrykant, M.: An insulin injection technique for preventing skin reactions, Am. J. Nurs. **65:**128, 1965.

9. Burke, E. L.: Insulin injection—the site and the technique, Am. J. Nurs. **72:**2194, 1972.

10. Pitel, M.: The subcutaneous injection, Am. J. Nurs. **71:**78, 1971.

11. Cohn, M. L., Chez, R. A., Hingson, R. A., and others: Use of jet insulin injection in diabetes mellitus therapy, Diabetes **21:**39, 1972.

12. Weller, C., and Linder, M.: Jet injection of insulin vs. the syringe and needle method, JAMA **195:**844, 1966.

10

Oral hypoglycemic agents

Donna Nickerson

The oral hypoglycemic agents have added a new dimension to the treatment of diabetes mellitus since tolbutamide became available in 1956. Recently much controversy has surrounded the action of these drugs and the appropriateness of their use with various types of patients.

Many patients have misconceptions about what oral hypoglycemic medications do and who can take them. Some of these misunderstandings were evidenced in a study of 74 hospitalized patients with diabetes,[1] 66 of whom thought that the pills available for diabetes were, in fact, insulin tablets. Health care personnel often foster such incorrect notions by hurriedly referring to oral hypoglycemic agents as "insulin pills" rather than taking the time to explain the action of these medications.

The oral hypoglycemic medications currently available do not contain insulin, nor are they a substitute for insulin therapy when insulin is indicated. Oral hypoglycemic agents are never a replacement for diet, the cornerstone of all treatment of diabetes.

The oral agents were discovered quite by accident during experiments with sulfa compounds during World War II. It was found that certain sulfa-type drugs could lower blood glucose levels, presumably by stimulating the beta cells of the pancreas to produce insulin. The first sulfonylurea to receive Food and Drug Administration approval was tolbutamide. One year later, in 1957, phenformin, a biguaninde and to-

tally unrelated to the sulfonylureas, became available. The biguanides were believed to have a mainly extrapancreatic effect.

INDICATIONS

The oral hypoglycemic agents are designed for use in controlling diabetes in the patient whose body is still capable of producing some endogenous insulin. The patients most likely to respond to this form of treatment are those with adult-onset, nonketotic diabetes, in whom diet therapy alone has not been successful. These drugs are generally not used for the individual with juvenile-onset, insulin-dependent diabetes. Ketosis is an indication that insulin by injection is required. The oral hypoglycemic agents are also being used in some instances for "prediabetes" and chemical diabetes, as prophylactic agents to improve pancreatic efficiency, but this use remains experimental.

TYPES

The available oral hypoglycemic preparations are of two types—sulfonylureas and biguanides. Several drug companies manufacture hypoglycemic agents; Fig. 10-1 lists them according to generic name, trade name, and strength of tablet or capsule. A description of the properties of each agent listed in Fig. 10-1 follows.

Sulfonylureas

The sulfonylureas act primarily by stimulating the production of insulin by the beta cells, although their mode of action is not completely understood. They may also increase the peripheral uptake of glucose, may inhibit glycogenolysis in the liver, and may have other extrapancreatic effects. However, the extrapancreatic effects of the sulfonylureas will not in themselves lower blood sugar levels in the person who has no pancreatic beta cells. The sulfonylurea-type agents then work in two ways. First, experiments in animals and humans treated with sulfonylureas only briefly disclose an increase in serum insulin levels. However, after several weeks of treatment, serum insulin levels fall. This latter finding suggests that sulfonylureas work by reducing glucose output from the liver or by some other means not related to stimulation of insulin release from the pancreas.

Tolbutamide (Orinase). Tolbutamide is the oldest compound and has the shortest half-life of the sulfonylureas. It is carboxylated in the liver and promptly excreted in the form of an inert metabolite in the urine. Normally, tolbutamide has a half-life of 4 to 5 hours and a duration of action of 6 to 12 hours. Its peak glucose-lowering effect is usually 5 to 8 hours after ingestion. Like the other oral hypoglycemic agents, it is absorbed rapidly from the gastrointestinal tract and has an appreciable effect within 1 hour. At least 75% of the metabolite is excreted within 24 hours.

Orinase is available in 500-mg tablets and

	GENERIC NAME	TRADE NAME AND MANUFACTURER	DESCRIPTION
Sulfonylureas	Tolbutamide	Orinase (Upjohn)	500 mg White tablets
	Chlorpropamide	Diabinese (Pfizer)	100 mg 250 mg Blue tablets
	Acetohexamide	Dymelor (Lilly)	250 mg White tablet 500 mg Yellow tablet
	Tolazamide	Tolinase (Upjohn)	100 mg 250 mg 500 mg White tablets
Biguanide	Phenformin HCl	DBI (Geigy)	25 mg White tablets
		DBI-TD (Geigy)	50 mg 100 mg Blue and white capsule
	Phenformin HCl	Meltrol-25 (USV)	Light blue tablet 25 mg
		Meltrol-50 (USV)	Blue and green capsule 50 mg
		Meltrol-100 (USV)	White capsule 100 mg

Fig. 10-1. Oral hypoglycemic agents in current use.

is usually prescribed in divided doses, generally ranging from 0.5 to 2 gm. The maximum dose is about 3 gm.

Chlorpropamide (Diabinese). Chlorpropamide is the longest-acting oral hypoglycemic agent, having a half-life of 34 to 36 hours and a duration of action of about 60 hours. It is not metabolized but is excreted by the kidney. It takes about 96 hours for 80% to 90% of the drug to be excreted in the urine. Seven to 10 days may be required to achieve a constant serum level of the drug. The prolonged action of chlorpropamide can lead to hypoglycemic reactions, particularly in the older individual who is not eating well. Because of the lengthy action of the drug, the patient should be watched for 3 to 5 days if hypoglycemia occurs.

Chlorpropamide is most often given in single doses, ranging from 100 to 500 mg daily and rarely exceeding 750 mg. Diabenese tablets are available in 100-mg and 250-mg strengths. The usual starting dose is 250 mg, but a lower dose of 100 to 125 mg is often used initially for older clients. Because of the long-acting effect of this drug, the dosage should not be raised more often than every 2 weeks, or overdose may result when full blood levels are achieved.

Acetohexamide (Dymelor). Acetohexamide has an intermediate duration of action of between 12 and 24 hours. The drug is reduced in the liver to *l*-hydroxyhexamide, a metabolite that retains hypoglycemic activity for several hours before being excreted through the urine. The half-life of acetohexamide and its metabolites is about 6 to 8 hours. Renal function should be carefully checked because accumulation of the metabolite may cause hypoglycemia. Acetohexamide also increases the excretion of uric acid and may be useful in patients with diabetes mellitus and gout. This medication is given in single or divided doses, usually ranging from 250 to 1500 mg. Dymelor tablets are made in 250-mg and 500-mg strengths.

Tolazamide (Tolinase). Tolazamide is the newest sulfonylurea to receive Food and Drug Administration approval (1966). It, too, has an intermediate action, with a half-life of about 7 hours and a duration of between 12 and 24 hours. It is metabolized to six major metabolites, half of which retain their hypoglycemic activity. The drug does not accumulate in the blood. An average of 85% of the dose is excreted in the urine. Tolazamide is absorbed more slowly via the gastrointestinal tract than other sulfonylureas, so that peak drug levels occur in 4 to 8 hours after ingestion.

Tolinase is now available in 100-mg, 250-mg and 500-mg tablets. Doses range from 100 mg to 1 gm daily. A total dose of over 500 mg per day is usually given in divided doses.

Precautions. The incidence of toxicity is low when sulfonylureas are given in recommended dosages. Jaundice, hematologic disorders, gastrointestinal disorders, and skin reactions have been known to occur but very infrequently. Occasionally a patient receiving one of the sulfonylureas becomes extremely sensitive to the rays of the sun and will develop a rash, even after a brief exposure, on areas of the skin. As with any other medication, hypersensitivity reactions are possible, and they usually consist of dermatologic symptoms, although a type of serum-sickness may rarely appear. Most allergic reactions take about 3 weeks after the institution of therapy to become apparent.

Intolerance to alcohol, with an Antabuse-like reaction, is seen more commonly than some other side effects. This phenomenon may occur in as many as 30% of the patients taking chlorpropamide and less frequently in patients taking other sulfonylureas. The Antabuse* (disulfiram) reaction is a vasomotor reaction consisting of a sensation of warmth, injection of the conjunctiva, flushing of the face and possibly the trunk, headache, nausea, shortness of

---

*Ayerst, New York, N.Y.

breath, tachycardia, and giddiness. It begins 3 to 10 minutes after ingestion of just a small amount of alcohol, and reaches a peak in about 20 minutes. The symptoms usually disappear within 1 hour but may last longer.

Hypoglycemia can occur with any of the sulfonylureas. These low glucose levels usually can be explained by dietary inadequacies (particularly failure to include snacks in the diet and to distribute food intake properly), by weight loss, increased activity, removal of stress, improper dosage of the oral agent, or impaired renal or hepatic function. Hypoglycemic reactions tend to occur more frequently in the elderly patient. Patients with adrenal or pituitary insufficiency and persons who consume alcohol and decrease their diet are also more prone to hypoglycemia.

Some medications can potentiate the action of the sulfonylureas, thus increasing the risk of hypoglycemia. These drugs include antibacterial sulfonamides, salicylates, dicumarol, phenylbutazone, probenecid, and monoamine oxidase inhibitors (MAOI). Some of the sulfonylureas may prolong the action of barbituatues, and diabetic persons taking both types of medications should be observed closely.

The sulfonylureas are generally not recommended for the following individuals: the person with ketotis-prone, juvenile-onset diabetes; anyone with hepatic, renal, pituitary, or adrenal dysfunction; the pregnant diabetic woman; patients with known allergies to sulfa drugs; or patients undergoing major surgery, severe trauma, infection, or other stress situations. There is, likewise, no real advantage to combining a sulfonylurea with insulin, although one of the sulfonylureas may occasionally be combined with phenformin to achieve a synergistic effect.

Biguanides

The biguanides are completely unrelated to the sulfonylureas. The only biguanide currently available in the U.S.A. is phenformin, its trade names being DBI, DBI-TD (a long-acting form), and Meltrol (Fig. 10-1).

Phenformin. Unlike the sulfonylureas, phenformin has a significant lowering effect on blood glucose levels, even in the absence of the pancreas. Its mode of action is still unclear, but it does apparently increase glucose utilization via muscle and fat in the periphery rather than stimulate insulin production. Phenformin may also decrease intestinal absorption of glucose, may inhibit hepatic glycogenolysis and gluconeogenesis, and may increase anaerobic glycolysis, with a subsequent increase in pyruvate and lactate.

Phenformin has a half-life of 3 hours, with duration of action of 6 to 8 hours, and of 8 to 14 hours with timed-release capsules. Ninety percent of phenformin is excreted through the urine within 24 hours.

DBI and Meltrol tablets come in the 25-mg strength. The timed-release capsules of DBI-TD and Meltrol are available in both 50-mg and 100-mg strengths. The tablets must be given in multiple doses during the day, whereas the capsules can be given in either single or divided doses. The total daily dose usually ranges from 50 to 200 mg.

Phenformin, in light of its extrapancreatic effects, is sometimes used in combination with one of the sulfonylureas to achieve a synergistic effect. Occasionally it is used as an adjunct to insulin therapy to control hyperglycemia, although effectiveness of this combination has rarely proved more successful than insulin alone.

Precautions. There have been reports associating phenformin therapy with some cases of lactic acidosis.[2] A preexisting condition such as impaired renal function can cause the accumulation of phenformin, which decreases the conversion of pyruvate to glucose. The individual who lacks insulin may begin to break down protein, leading to the formation of pyruvate and lactate, and thus augmenting the effects of the phenformin. Lactic acidosis is a serious complication, which requires treatment for restoration of a normal pH and parenteral insulin. There is no evidence that phenformin therapy of itself can cause lactic acidosis.

There have been arguments that phenformin decreases cholesterol[3] although the University Group Diabetes Program study found that this effect leveled off with time (see details below). Phenformin is often used with obese patients with diabetes to assist in weight loss. The drug may inhibit the formation of fat, although this theory has not been fully substantiated. Some patients do experience a bitter or metallic taste when taking phenformin, thus contributing to a loss of appetite. These unpleasant sensations may be a warning of gastrointestinal disturbances, such as nausea and vomiting or diarrhea, in addition to anorexia. No other side effects are generally seen with phenformin. Hypoglycemia is rare when phenformin is given alone. Side effects can best be avoided by taking the medication with meals or by using timed-release capsules.

UGDP CONTROVERSY

The University Group Diabetes Program (UGDP) study is the largest controlled clinical investigation of oral hypoglycemic agents to date. The study was funded by the National Institutes of Health and was conducted at twelve medical centers throughout the United States. Beginning in 1961, newly diagnosed patients with adult-onset diabetes were randomly assigned to tolbutamide, placebo, variable-dose insulin, or standard-dose insulin. In 1962-1963, phenformin was added as one of the treatments. A report by the UGDP[5] revealed that 12.7% of the patients treated with tolbutamide had died of cardiovascular causes as compared with 6.2% or fewer in the groups treated with insulin or diet alone. The UGDP concluded that diet alone would be preferable to diet plus tolbutamide in relation to cardiovascular mortality.[6] As a result, tolbutamide was dropped from use in the UGDP study, and the Food and Drug

Administration recommended that tolbutamide should only be used when diet therapy alone is unsuccessful and when insulin cannot be given. The UGDP subsequently reported findings associating phenformin treatment with increased cardiovascular mortality and other vascular changes.[7] Phenformin was also discontinued from the study.

The UGDP study has been the subject of many headlines, much controversy, and severe criticism. In fact, some critics started legal proceedings to keep the Food and Drug Administration from adversely labeling the oral hypoglycemic agents. Criticisms encompass the selection of patients in regard to life expectancy, the use of a fixed dosage of the oral agents, the use of unfamiliar statistical analyses, and the decision to discontinue the oral agents from the ongoing study.[8]

In view of the criticism that the UGDP had received, the National Institutes of Health charged the Biometric Society with the task of analyzing the scientific quality of the various studies involving oral hypoglycemic drugs. The committee appointed by the Biometric Society concluded that the data available on the oral hypoglycemics thus far had aroused suspicions about toxicity that require further investigation before they can be dismissed.[9] The report did point out that the fixed dosage schedule for the UGDP may not have been comparable to that ordinarily used in private practice.[9] The committee dismissed as noncomparable data that was obtained from nondiabetic individuals showing lower mortality with oral hypoglycemics and data from the Bedford study.[9]

An ongoing study by the Feldman group may shed more light on the effects of tolbutamide and phenformin when used prophylactically in asymptomatic diabetes.[10]

LOOKING TO THE FUTURE

While the controversy regarding currently available antidiabetic agents continues, studies to develop more efficient oral medications are ongoing. Many of these studies involve new forms of the sulfonylureas or the biguanides. For example, glyburide (Micronase*) is a sulfonylurea used in small doses, such as 2.5 to 50 mg. and is reported to have low toxicity and high potency.[11] Burformin is a new biguanide, the action of which is still uncertain.

The goal of many investigations is to perfect new methods for administering insulin. One possibility is the use of highly concentrated oral insulin (such as U-500). The main obstacle is finding a coating for the insulin pill that would prevent breakdown of the insulin by the proteolytic enzymes of the digestive tract. For instance, some studies[12] have employed an ether compound to promote absorption of insulin in the stomach before it reaches the enzymes of the duodenum. Atropine was also administered to decrease gastric secretions. Unfortunately, nausea was reported as a side effect in about 50% of the subjects. Data does indicate that oral insulin, when administered under optimum conditions, causes a significant rise in serum insulin levels and a decrease in glucose levels and is safe. However, use of oral insulin is currently impractical.

The diabetic person taking an oral hypoglycemic agent should be given the opportunity to understand the antidiabetic medication that has been prescribed—how it works and how it differs from insulin per se. A study of hospitalized diabetic individuals revealed that nearly half did not know what therapy they were taking for diabetes.[1] Nurses should become familiar with the oral agents, their appearance (see Fig. 10-1), and their effect so that they can recognize them and their action and relay this information to the patient.

The nurse needs to find out not only what medication has been prescribed but how the patient generally takes the tablets at home and whether this routine goes along with the medical regimen. One should also be aware that hypoglycemic reactions can occasionally occur with these medications. The nurse can often detect symptoms of low blood glucose levels through careful interviewing of the diabetic person and an awareness of the medication and dietary routine.

Diet should not be underemphasized in the patient taking an oral hypoglycemic agent. This medication will usually be effective only when accompanied by diet, to achieve a normal weight and to establish a regular pattern of eating. Encouraging the patient to distribute food evenly in frequent, regular feedings will help to stabilize the glucose curve. Above all, the patient should understand that these agents never replace diet therapy.

An understanding by the diabetic person of the action of the oral hypoglycemic drugs should ease the transition if insulin becomes necessary secondary to a concomitant stress or to pancreatic failure.

REFERENCES

1. Nickerson, D.: Teaching the hospitalized diabetic, Am. J. Nurs. **5:**936, 1972.
2. Dembo, A., Marlis, E., and Halperin, M.: Insulin therapy in phenformin-associated lactic acidosis, Diabetes **24:**28, 1975.
3. Hamwi, G., and Seidensticker, J.: Therapy: oral hypoglycemic agents. *In* Hamwi, G., and Danowski, T. S., editors: Diabetes mellitus: Diagnosis and treatment. vol. 2, New York, 1967, American Diabetes Association, Inc., p. 11.
4. Knatterud, G. L., Klimt, C. R., Osborne, R. K., and others: A study of the effects of hypoglycemic agents on vascular complications in patients with adult-onset diabetes: V. Evaluation of phenformin therapy, The University Group Diabetes Program, Diabetes, **24:**(Suppl. 1):105, 1975.
5. Klimt, C. R., Knatterud, G. L., Meinert, C. L., and Prout, T.: A study of the effects of hypoglycemic agents on vascular complications in patients with adult-onset diabetes: II. Mortality results, The University Group Diabetes Program, Diabetes **19** (Suppl. 2):787, 1970.
6. Schwartz, T. B.: The tolbutamide contro-

*The Upjohn Co., Kalamazoo, Mich.

versy: a personal perspective, Ann. Intern. Med. **75**:303, 1971.

7. Knatterud, G. L., Klimt, C. R., Osborne, R. K., and others: A study of the effects of hypoglycemic agents on vascular complications in patients with adult-onset diabetes: V. Evaluation of phenformin therapy, The University Group Diabetes Program, Diabetes **24** (Suppl. 1):110, 1975.

8. Seltzer, H.: A summary of criticisms of the findings and conclusions of The University Group Diabetes Program, Diabetes, **21**:976-978, 1972.

9. Gilbert, J. T., and others: Report of the committee for the assessment of biometric aspects of controlled trials of hypoglycemic agents, JAMA **231**:592, 599, 1975.

10. Feldman, R.: Progress report on the prophylactic use of oral hypoglycemic drugs in asymptomatic diabetes: neurovascular studies, Adv. metab. Disord. **2** (Suppl. 2):557, 1973.

11. Herrold, J., Tzagournis, M., and Skillman, T.: Acute and chronic studies using a new oral hypoglycemic agent glyburide, Metabolism **20**:414, 1971.

12. Galloway, J., and Root, M.: New forms of insulin, Diabetes **21** (Suppl. 2):643, 1972.

11

Urine testing

Donna Nickerson

Urine testing for glucose and ketones is one tool for estimating diabetes control. Continuous or even frequent blood monitoring has limited practicality; blood glucose levels cannot be monitored over long time periods. Thus urine tests are a reasonable adjunct to blood level determinations.

The usefulness of urine test results depends entirely on the accuracy with which the test is performed. Testing the urine is both a client activity and a nursing procedure. It is generally the nurse who influences the client in selection of method and accuracy of performance of urine testing.

COLLECTING THE SPECIMEN
Semiquantitative urine collections

A semiquantitative test is the most feasible analysis for people with diabetes to perform. The first condition for an accurate test is that the sample be a premeal, second-voided specimen when at all possible in adults.

These terms are frequently used when describing collection of the sample: The *"A" specimen* is the first emptying of the bladder collected 1 hour to 30 minutes before a meal or before bedtime. The *"B" specimen* is the second voiding, collected after the bladder has been emptied, 30 minutes or less before a meal or before bedtime.

There is about a 20-minute lag while urine passes from the gomeruli of the kidney to the ureters. This factor makes the B specimen preferable for testing purposes because the A specimen may represent an overlapping of postmeal and premeal glucose values. However, some physicians do order testing of both A and B specimens. Postmeal samples are mainly useful for detecting intermittent glucosuria rather than monitoring diabetes control. The B sample (second-voided and premeal) is believed by some to be indicative of the continuous state of the blood glucose values. Some authorities even recommend a third-voided specimen for highest correlation with blood glucose values, when the second-voided sample is positive. See Chapter 4, The child, p. 44 for an expanded discussion of the meaning and usefulness of first- and second-voided urines in children.

The following steps should be followed in collecting the B specimen:

1. The patient empties the bladder 30 minutes to 1 hour before the test is to be performed. This urine is the A specimen and should be discarded, unless testing of both A and B samples has been ordered.
2. Patient may drink a glass of water if he has difficulty in obtaining a second specimen.
3. The patient empties the bladder again. This urine is the B specimen.
4. The B specimen is tested.

Quantitative urine collections

Often an assessment is made of the total quantity of glucose spillage in the urine for a time period of between 4 and 24 hours. This value correlates higher with venous blood glucose values than a semiquantitative analysis does. All of the urine that the patient excretes during the specified time is collected in a container. The collection begins with a second-voided urine and ends with a first-voided urine.

Twenty-four hour urines. If the urine collection is to be from 8 AM on Monday to 8 AM on Tuesday, this procedure would be followed:

1. At 8 AM on Monday the bladder is completely emptied. This urine is discarded, because it does not represent excretion during the specified time period.
2. All urine excreted thereafter until 8 AM Tuesday is saved in a clean container, including samples used for semiquantitative tests.
3. The bladder is completely emptied at 8 AM on Tuesday, and this urine also goes into the container. Now the collection is complete.
4. Urine volume is measured in milliliters.
5. Tests for ketone and glucose levels are performed. If the nurse is to do these tests, she can follow the same procedure as with any smaller sample. The 2-drop Clinitest method best approximates the quantitative measurement of glucose.
6. The result of the test for glucosuria, stated in a percentage, is multiplied by the total volume of the 24-hour urine to obtain the amount of glucose spillage in grams for the time period. For example, if the result is a 3% glucose concentration with moderate acetone levels for a 1000-ml sample, 30 gm of glucose have been lost during the 24-hour period ($1000 \times 0.03 = 30$).

If the results of a 24-hour urine are to be accurate and used as the basis for one's judgments regarding diabetes treatment, particular care should be made by the nurse to ensure that, especially in the case of children, all urine voided is placed in the container.

Fractional urine collections

Block urines. Sometimes there is a need to test urine for shorter time intervals within the 24-hour period, particularly for purposes of adjusting insulin therapy. These fractional collections are sometimes referred to as "block" urines when a collection time in terms of hours is blocked off.

The following steps are taken to measure glucose lost from 1 PM to 5 PM and from 5 PM to 9 PM:

1. The patient empties the bladder at 1 PM and discards the urine.
2. The patient saves all urine voided from then until 5 PM.
3. At 5 PM the patient empties the bladder and places that urine in the container.
4. The urine is tested for glucose concentration, the results multiplied by the total volume of urine in the container, and the urine discarded.
5. A second collection is made of all urine excreted from after the first collection is finished until 9 PM.
6. The patient empties the bladder at 9 PM and places that urine in the container.
7. Testing is done again, and the results are multipled times the volume of the second collection.

Aliquots. Another situation that may be encountered is the fractionalization of a 24-hour period into four aliquots. The bladder is completely emptied before breakfast, and then urines are collected and tested at the following times:

Collected	Tested
From after breakfast to lunch	Before lunch, after B (or A) specimen has been tested and added to container
From after lunch to supper	Before supper, after B (or A) specimen has been tested and added to container
From after supper to bedtime	Before bedtime, after B (or A) specimen has been tested and added to container
From bedtime to breakfast	Before breakfast, after B (or A) specimen has been tested and added to container

The urine is discarded (unless a 24-hour collection is in effect) and the container rinsed after each aliquot is done. The volume of each aliquot is measured, testing is performed, and results are multiplied times volume. For example, if a 300-ml sample from breakfast to lunch tests at 1% glucose concentration, that aliquot shows a spillage of 3 gm of glucose (300 × 0.01 = 3). Aliquot testing is also referred to by some authors as fractional testing.

TESTING FOR GLUCOSE LEVELS

The excretion of glucose depends on the concentration of glucose in the afferent arteriole of the glomerulus. When blood glucose levels are sufficiently increased, the glucose filtration rate of the glomeruli exceeds the reabsorption rate of the renal tubules, the renal threshold is attained, and glucose is excreted through the urine. There are conditions that alter the renal threshold, but the mean renal threshold in the normal population is a blood glucose level of 180 mg/dl, and it is unlikely that glucosuria will appear at levels below 130 mg/dl. The fasting blood glucose level is 60 to 110 mg/dl, with the random range never exceeding 170 mg/100 ml in normal persons, even shortly after ingestion of a glucose load. Therefore, under normal circumstances and given a normal renal threshold, glucose should never appear in the urine, even postprandially.

From as early as the 5th century until the 18th century, the only diagnostic test available for diabetes was the tasting of urine for sweetness. In the late 18th century the material in the urine of diabetic persons was identified as sugar and later as grape sugar. In the 1840's cupric oxide tests for glucose were developed. These tests formed the basis for the present Benedict's and Clinitest methods.

Reduction methods

Benedict's test. Benedict's test is based on the reduction of cupric sulfate to cuprous oxide in an alkaline solution. Eight drops of urine are added to a test tube containing 5 ml of Benedict's quantitative solution and boiled for 3 minutes. If the color changes, the solution is boiled an additional 2 minutes. The color ranges from green (1+) to red (4+) as the blue cupric ions are reduced to brick-red cuprous ions when heated in the presence of an aldehyde group, such as the one in glucose or any other reducing substance. The excessive time and bulky equipment required for this procedure make it unnecessary in this day of newer easier methods.

Clinitest. There are many different tests for glucosuria, but we will review only those that the nurse is most likely to encounter. The Clinitest method is a modification of the older Benedict's test. The Clinitest tablet contains anhydrous copper sulfate. It generates heat when combined with urine and water in a test tube, causing the liquid to boil. The 5-drop Clinitest procedure is the traditional method, utilizing the chart packaged with the Clinitest kit. The 2-drop and 1-drop Clinitest procedures require the same equipment as the 5-drop test, plus a special 2-drop chart or packaged insert.

FIVE-DROP CLINITEST. The following critical elements must all be included by the tester when the Clinitest 5-drop method (Fig. 11-1) is used:

1. Place 10 drops of water (tap water is satisfactory) in a clean, dry test tube.
2. Place 5 drops of urine in the test tube.
3. Put the water into the test tube first or rinse the dropper after putting the urine in.
4. Hold the dropper vertically, so that drops fall into the bottom of the tube rather than sliding down the sides.
5. Next, drop 1 Clinitest reagent tablet into the tube, without touching the tablet, so that the hands are not burned and there is no contamination of the tablet.
6. Hold the tube still while boiling occurs. (Carbon dioxide entrapped in bubbles prevents added oxygen in the atmosphere from entering into and changing the chemical reaction occurring in the test tube.)
7. Wait exactly 15 seconds after boiling stops to read the results, but observe color changes that occur during the reaction.
8. Read results correctly according to the 5-drop chart.
9. Record results.

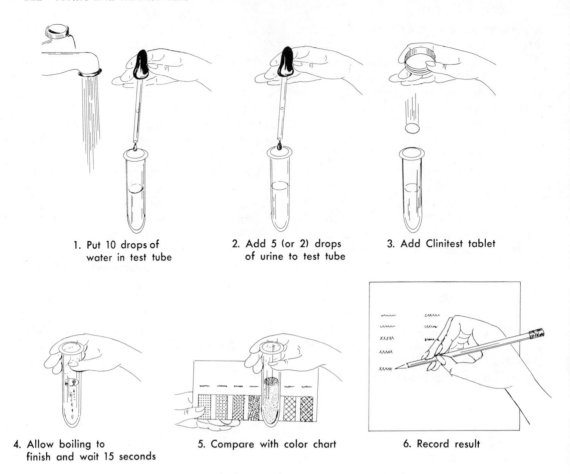

1. Put 10 drops of water in test tube   2. Add 5 (or 2) drops of urine to test tube   3. Add Clinitest tablet

4. Allow boiling to finish and wait 15 seconds   5. Compare with color chart   6. Record result

Fig. 11-1. Clinitest—5-drop (or 2-drop) method.

The 5-drop Clinitest method quantitates only up to a 2% (4+) glucose concentration in the urine. A pass-through, or burn-through, phenomenon occurs whenever the glucose concentration exceeds 2%. This phenomenon necessitates careful observation of the reaction's color, which passes from bright orange to dark greenish brown within the 15-second timing period. This factor may cause errors in the reading of the reaction if not carefully observed or if interpreted incorrectly as a lower value. This reaction should be read as greater than 2% (5+).

ONE- AND TWO-DROP CLINITESTS. The 2-drop Clinitest has one major advantage that none of the other glucosuria determinations

can offer—it quantitates glucose concentrations up to 5% (not to be confused with 5+) and up to 10% if the 1-drop method is used with the 2-drop chart.

The 2-drop test is exactly the same as the 5-drop test except that only 2 drops of urine are used, and the results must be read on a special 2-drop package insert or card. The tester uses the same Clinitest equipment packaged with the 5-drop chart, discarding the 5-drop chart, or obtains a specially marked 2-drop Clinitest kit with a 2-drop chart. The nurse and client must be cautioned to use the proper chart for the technique performed. The 2-drop chart has color blocks and directions that are larger and easier to see than those on the packaged 5-drop chart, although enlarged 5-drop charts can also be obtained for patients who would benefit by them.

The 2-drop Clinitest should include the following behaviors:

1. Place 10 drops of water in the test tube.
2. Next place 2 drops of urine in the test tube.
3. Hold dropper vertically so that the urine falls directly into the water.
4. Next drop 1 Clinitest reagent tablet into the tube, without touching the tablet.
5. Allow the solution to boil until it stops, but do not shake the tube.
6. Wait exactly 15 seconds; shake.
7. Compare the color with the 2-drop color chart.
8. Record results.

The 1-drop test is used whenever a 5% reading is obtained by the 2-drop test (a burn-through greater than 5%) or when the solution passes from orange and then drops back to greenish brown within the 15 seconds. The 1-drop test employs the same method, materials, and total volume as the 2-drop test but merely dilutes the urine more to see how much greater than 5%, if at all, the glucose concentration is.

The 1-drop Clinitest is performed as follows:

1. Place 11 drops of water in the test tube.
2. Add 1 drop of urine (carefully so that it mixes with the water).
3. Add 1 Clinitest reagent tablet to the solution.
4. Allow the boiling to finish; do not shake tube.
5. Wait 15 seconds after the boiling stops.
6. Compare the reaction to the 2-drop color scale.
7. Multiply the results on the 2-drop scale by 2 because of the dilution.
8. Record the results, using the highest value (occasionally the 1-drop test shows 4% when the 2-drop indicates 5%). EXAMPLE: Suppose the 2-drop test indicates a 5% glucose concentration, and a 1-drop test is performed. If results from the 1-drop method show a 3% glucose concentration, multiply 3% by two (3% × 2 = 6%). Six percent is greater than 5%; thus, a glucose

value of 6% is recorded. If results from the 1-drop method indicate a 2% glucose concentration, multiply 2% by two (2% × 2 = 4%). Four percent is less than 5%; therefore, a glucose value of 5% is recorded on the diabetes record.

A COMPARISON OF METHODS. The major advantage of the 2-drop and 1-drop Clinitest methods is the capacity to quantitate glucose levels as high as 10%. Therefore, results from these tests are a more complete guide to regulation of diabetes control when there is glucosuria. Attempting to reduce glucosuria on the basis of other tests, which are more sensitive to glucose or which have 2% (4+) as the upper limit of glucose, may actually be harmful for some patients. For example, 2% glucosuria is considered an acceptable level in children with diabetes by some pediatric diabetologists,[1] though not by others.[2] The lowered renal threshold in pregnant women also changes the interpretation of glucosuria findings. On the other hand, renal threshold generally increases with age; thus in the older patients, more sensitive tests might be preferable.

Glucosuria represents a loss of calories through the urine, resulting in weight loss and polyphagia. The greater the testing range, the greater the perspective of how many calories are actually being lost. For example, if one takes into account that 1 gm of carbohydrate is equivalent to 4 calories, a 24-hour urine showing glucose levels of 2% (the maximum value on most tests), with a volume of 1000 ml, would mean a loss of 20 gm of carbohydrates, or 80 calories (1000 × 0.02 = 20 × 4 = 80). However, the same urine collection showing glucose levels of 10% by the 1-drop test indicates a loss of 100 gm, or 400 calories (1000 × 0.1 = 100 × 4 = 400), a loss significantly higher than 80 calories.

PRECAUTIONS. Several precautions must be taken when Clinitest reagent tablets are used. The tablets are very hydroscopic, so the bottle should be tightly capped after each use to avoid a loss of potency when the tablets are exposed to moisture. Dark blue or black tablets should not be used. The tablets should also be kept away from direct sunlight and direct heat. Individually foil-wrapped tablets cut down on the potency loss, provided that the seals are not accidentally broken. Particular care should be taken that Clinitest tablets are kept out of the reach of children, because ingestion can cause esophageal strictures. The tablets are similar to other pills that are taken as medication and have been mistaken for aspirin by older children.

Clinitest, like the Benedict's test, is sensitive to reducing agents in general. False-positive tests can be produced by other reducing agents such as galactose, fructose, pentose, or lactose. Large amounts of ascorbic acid per day can reduce the Clinitest. Tuberculin and penicillin therapy can both affect Benedict's test, but Clinitest is affected only by nalidixic acid, cephalosporins (Keflin), and probenecid.

Diastix method. The newest reduction test for measuring glucose levels in the urine is the Diastix method. This procedure consists of a dipstick with a block of reactive paper. The color scale is similar to that of Clinitest, with positive glucose values ranging through green to brownish orange at its maximum of 2% (4+).

The following steps must be included in the Diastix procedure:

1. Hold stick at the bottom, not touching the reactive paper.
2. Dip the stick into the urine.
3. Remove the stick immediately from the urine and wait exactly 30 seconds to read the results.
4. Continue to hold the stick; do not set it down before reading it.
5. Read results correctly according to the proper chart.

A variation of Diastix is Keto-Diastix, which includes a Ketostix paper for ketones. Particular caution must be taken in timing this combination test because the Ketostix portion is timed for only 15 seconds, while the Diastix part is timed for 30 seconds.

PRECAUTIONS. The Diastix reactive strips are subject to spoilage like other types of testing materials. The bottle should be kept in a cool, dry place, the desiccant packet must be kept in the bottle to absorb moisture and the cap must be replaced promptly and tightly. Note carefully that the Diastix reading will be depressed if ketones are present in the urine. The Diastix and Keto-Diastix methods of urine testing are not recommended for testing urine in children.

Glucose oxidase methods

The newer glucose oxidase tests provide simpler but more sensitive techniques for detecting glucosuria. The enzyme glucose oxidase converts glucose to gluconic acid, making these tests specific for glucose.

Testape and Clinistix. Testape consists of a dispenser roll of paper impregnated with reactive material; when a strip is dipped into urine that contains glucose, it changes from yellow to dark green, depending on the glucose concentration.

The following critical elements should be included when one uses Testape:

1. Tear a 1½-inch strip of tape off the dispenser.
2. Touch only the end of the tape not dipped into the urine.
3. Dip the tape into the urine.
4. Remove the tape from the urine and wait exactly 60 seconds to read the results.
5. Hold the tape; do not set it down until the reading is made.

Testape values range from 0.1% to 2% glucose concentration. Since positive readings range among various shades of green, it is important that the individual performing the test be able to distinguish small differences on the color scale. Testape, like Clinitest, must be protected from moisture, heat, and direct light. Moreover, Testape may not change color when it is spoiled, so that the user has no way to check its potency unless it is dipped into some known glucose-containing substance. However, an expiration date is printed on the Testape package, and instructions indicate that Testape should be discarded after being open for 4 months or longer.

The Clinistix test utilizes a plastic stick, the tip of which is covered with a square of paper impregnated with reactive material. This method is probably the easiest to perform. The following steps must be included in the Clinistix procedure:

1. Hold the stick at the bottom, not touching the reactive paper.
2. Dip the stick into the urine.
3. Remove the stick immediately from the urine and wait exactly 10 seconds to read the results.
4. Continue to hold the stick; do not set it down before reading.
5. Read results correctly according to the proper chart.

The paper strip turns from pink to purple to dark blue in the presence of glucose. The chart estimates the amount of glucose in terms of "light," "medium," and "dark" color, rather than numerical quantities. The maximum level represents a glucose concentration of 2% or higher, and the sensitivity detects as little as 0.1% glucosuria.

As with other methods, the Clinistix user should avoid exposing the test strips to light, moisture, or touch. The Clinistix paper has also been incorporated into multiple-test strips, such as in Uristix, Labstix, and Bili-Labstix.

PRECAUTIONS. Although the glucose oxidase methods are specific for glucose, they can produce false-positive and false-negative results and are subject to interference from various substances such as ascorbic acid. It has also been found that any potent reducing agent, such as large doses of levodopa or salicylates in the amount prescribed for arthritic patients, can produce false-negative results in the glucose oxidase tests.[3] It is also possible that patients with carcinoid may produce metabolites that could interfere with these procedures. The nurse should be aware of the possible effect that the client's condition and therapeutic regimen could have on urine testing. These tests are highly sensitive to small amounts of glucose and are too sensitive for use in children.

TESTING FOR KETONES

What are ketones? In any fasting state, including states of uncontrolled diabetes, the body is, in effect, starving; as a result, lipolysis occurs. When glucose is not available (either because of inadequate intake or lack of insulin) for the body to oxidize for energy, fat breaks down. Fatty acids are converted to ketones. Ketones, produced in the liver, are acetoacetic acid, beta-hydroxybutyric acid, and acetone. Therefore the presence of ketones would indicate fat breakdown, decreased carbohydrate intake, even self-induced dieting, or lack of insulin to metabolize carbohydrates.

When is it necessary to check for ketones? Generally speaking, it is important for diabetic individuals to check for ketones in the urine when glucose concentration is 2% or higher or when another disease process is apparent and may increase the need for insulin. Acidosis and unnecessary hospitalization can often be avoided if the urine is routinely checked for ketones. Checking for ketones is also used as an adjunct to dieting in some people without diabetes.

There are two tests generally used in measuring ketonuria. In both cases, a purple color indicates a positive ketone test and quantitation is in terms of small, moderate, and large.

Ketostix. Ketostix are plastic strips with squares of paper impregnated with reactive material. The following steps should be included in the Ketostix procedure (Fig. 11-2):

1. Hold stick at proper end, not touching reactive paper.
2. Dip stick into the urine.
3. Remove the stick immediately and wait exactly 15 seconds to read the results.
4. Continue to hold the stick; do not set it down before reading it.

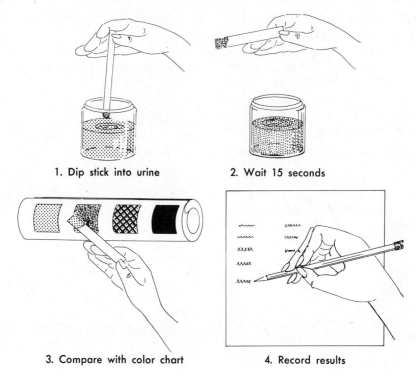

1. Dip stick into urine   2. Wait 15 seconds

3. Compare with color chart   4. Record results

Fig. 11-2. Ketostix procedure.

5. Read the results correctly according to the chart on the bottle label.
6. Record results.

PRECAUTIONS. The reactive paper is a manila color before testing. If a strip has turned dark brown, it is no longer good and should not be used. Because Ketostix are subject to spoilage, the bottle cap should be replaced tightly and the bottle kept away from moisture, heat, or direct sunlight. A Ketostix test is also included in Keto-Diastix, Labstix, and Bili-Labstix.

Acetest. The Acetest procedure utilizes a small white tablet. The following critical elements should be included in the Acetest method:

1. Set tablet on clean surface (such as on a paper towel or tissue) without touching the tablet.
2. Drop 1 drop of urine on the tablet.
3. Wait exactly 30 seconds to read the results.
4. Read the results correctly according to the proper chart.
5. Record the results.

PRECAUTIONS. Particular care should be taken to time this test accurately. Because the hands are free, nurses and clients often tend to set the tablet down, place the drop of urine on the tablet, and leave it while performing the test for glucosuria. Both tests for ketonuria will show a darker purple as time progresses. Because the degree of ketonuria is often used to determine emergency therapy, an accurate test is a necessity. (False-positive results are produced with levodopa,* phenylketones,* bromsulphalein,* and salicylates.)

Because the presence of moderate to large concentrations of ketones with glucosuria in a B specimen usually indicates a serious situation, it is not enough for the person with diabetes to know when and how to check for ketones but what to do with the information. If ketone and glucose values are positive in a B specimen, another B specimen of urine should be

*False-positive results when Ketostix are used.

checked 4 hours later. If the ketone concentrations are moderate to large, a physician should be contacted because more insulin is probably needed. Some patients can be taught to give themselves supplements of regular insulin, but all diabetic individuals should at least know that ketonuria indicates the need to seek medical advice. If ketonuria persists and the personal physician is not available, emergency facility treatment should be sought.

EVALUATION OF TECHNIQUES

One of the first things that people with diabetes tend to be careless about is urine testing. A study of 74 hospitalized patients with diabetes revealed that only 5 people were able to test urine correctly with the method of their choice. The demonstrations showed that these patients usually failed at least several critical points, making particularly gross errors in timing.[3] Leifson's studies[5] with patients using either Testape or the 5-drop Clinitest at home showed that 26% failed to use a color chart when testing, and 87% stored testing equipment improperly.

Nurses often tend to become careless when urine testing is routine. The more effectively the nurse carries out a testing procedure, the more likely the patient will be impressed with the importance of testing correctly.

There is no substitute for actual demonstration when evaluating or teaching a procedure. As indicated by the studies mentioned previously,[4,5] having performed urine tests for years is no guarantee of accuracy of performance. Asking clients to describe in words how they perform the test is not sufficient either. A demonstration, ideally with the person using his own equipment, is necessary. When teaching urine testing, the nurse should demonstrate step by step and then ask for a return demonstration. Samples can be prepared with glucose and acetone added, so that the patient who has never tested can see what

a positive reaction, particularly a burn-through, looks like.

When evaluating techniques, it is handy to use a checklist of the critical elements of the procedure, such as those listed in the previous sections for each method. If the performance fails on any point, the results could be inaccurate and the demonstration should be considered incorrect. It helps to give the person a written checklist to follow at home. The written instructions will reinforce the demonstration and practice.

Persons with diabetes should be encouraged to perform the urine tests themselves from the start, even during hospitalization. This experience provides not only practice and accurate evaluation but also the opportunity for the individual to relate changes in therapy to test results.

KEEPING AND INTERPRETING URINE RECORDS

It is most important to remember that urine testing is not in itself a goal but a guide to treatment. Keeping an accurate record of tests is almost as important as performing the procedures.

When urine records are used as a guide to regulating chronic care and treatment of diabetes, the *pattern* of test results is far more valuable than single, isolated tests. During the initiation of treatment, testing should be done 4 times daily—before breakfast, lunch, supper, and bedtime—on B (second-voided) specimens or as directed.* If B specimen cannot be obtained, the tests should be noted for A (first-voided) specimens. Testing 4 times a day is especially important for patients receiving insulin, so that a pattern of absorption and peak effect can be determined for each individual.

Testing 4 times a day is often impractical and, once diabetes control has been estab-

---

*See Chapter 4 for a differing opinion on the use of first- and second-voided specimens in children.

Table 11-1. Urine records

Date	Insulin	Time	Before breakfast		Before lunch		Before supper		Before bedtime		Reactions	Comments
			G*	K†	G	K	G	K	G	K		
A	30 U lente	7 AM	0	—	0	—	3%	N	1%	—		
	10 U lente	6 PM	0	—	0	—	5%	N	3%	N		Ate piece
			0	—	0	—	2%	—	0	—		of cake
												at 4 PM
B	20 U lente	8 AM	0	—	2%	—	0	—	0	—		
			0	—	3%	N	0	—	0	—		
			0	—	2%	—	0	—	0	—		
C	20 U NPH	7 AM	5%	N	3%	N	0	—	0	—		
	5 U NPH	6 PM	3%	N	1%	—	—	—	0	—		
			2%	—	0	—	0	—	0	—		
D	50 U lente	8AM	0	—	0	—	0	—	0	—	5 PM	
			0	—	0	—	0	—	5%	N		
			0	—	0	—	0	—	5%	Small		Missed
			0	—	0	—	0	—	0	—		supper

*Glucose values.
†Ketone values.

lished, is not as necessary in the adult as in the child (see Chapter 4). At this point, testing 4 times a day, 2 or 3 days a week, becomes more acceptable to most people and still provides the physician or nurse with the needed information. When test results are elevated or infection or other bodily stress is present, testing 4 times a day should be resumed to direct management of acute diabetes problems.

The urine record (Table 11-1) should include space for noting insulin reactions and for comments, such as irregularity in eating patterns, the presence of infection, menstrual periods, changes in activity, or emotional flare-ups. For example, a family argument may cause a temporary elevation in urine glucose levels. This reading may not be indicative of the usual state of control and, therefore, the circumstances should be noted.

Looking at recurring patterns in urine records can give clues to factors that are affecting diabetes control. For instance, a student may be aglycosuric all of the time except before lunch, at which time he consistently spills 3% glucose, despite changes in insulin. Upon inquiry, one learns that he has a math class in which he is doing poorly at 11 AM. The underlying problems must be determined and resolved in some cases before glycosuria can be eliminated.

Urine test patterns, as those in Table 11-1, are useful in modifying insulin therapy to reduce glycosuria. In example A, the morning dose of insulin may be increased to bring down the presupper glycosuria, or perhaps the afternoon snack may be changed. In pattern B, short-acting regular insulin may be added, or breakfast may be modified. In example C, the evening dose of insulin may be increased.

Urine records can also be used to determine patterns and causes of hypoglycemic reactions. Writing down on the record the times when reactions occur may help to pinpoint such things as deficiencies in snacks, inadequate food intake for high activity periods, or too much insulin.

Analyzing the pattern of glycosuria can even help to detect hypoglycemia when the patient is not aware of actually having reactions, though glycosuria is present. This phenomenon is called the Somogyi, or re-

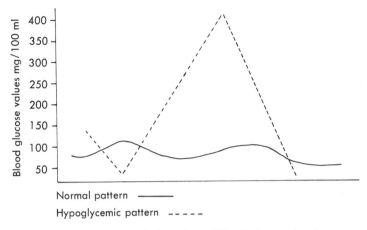

Fig. 11-3. Rebound elevation of blood glucose levels.

bound, effect. The urine record would probably look something like pattern D in Table 11-1. Reactions might or might not be recorded. The series of negative results followed by an elevated glucose level could indicate that a hypoglycemic reaction has occurred and that the body's own defenses, such as epinephrine and glucagon, have increased glycogenolysis. Sometimes this mechanism overshoots the body's need for glucose and leads to a rebound elevation of blood glucose levels (Fig. 11-3) and glycosuria, or even rebound ketonuria.[6] If testing reveals only the intermittent glycosuria, dangerous overtreatment could result. Thus, the complete urine record helps to evaluate the true situation.

Persistent glycosuria is far more easily differentiated from intermittent glycosuria when urine records are kept regularly at 4 readings a day. Positive glucose values, even without ketones, at every test for 2 to 3 days' duration would probably warrant an increase in the daily insulin dose. Two or more reactions, unexplained by unusual circumstances, require a decrease in insulin dosage. Many patients can learn to modify their insulin dosage, with the aid of accurate records.

Interpretation of urine tests is also significant in acute situations. Keeping records of ketone levels can often prevent hospi-

talization if moderate to large readings on one to two tests are reported to the provider of health care. In this case, single tests are very important until ketosis has been broken with increased insulin and carbohydrate intake.

Interpretation of urine tests should always include consideration of the type of individual being tested and the circumstances surrounding the test. For instance, the higher renal threshold in elderly patients means that glucosuria probably represents a very elevated blood glucose level. The same change in threshold may occur in patients with renal disease. On the other hand, glucosuria may be acceptable in pregnant women with diabetes who have lower thresholds. The general health of the patient and the emotional climate, as well as the patient's attitude toward testing, should be carefully noted. Some people become so emotionally upset by performing urine tests that they actually trigger an epinephrine response, leading to elevated blood glucose levels and glucosuria. It is advisable to have such compulsive individuals test their urine less frequently. There are also some individuals who feel that the results of testing must please the physician or nurse; thus they do not report their true findings. The nurse can help by focusing in on the faulty attitudes.

SUMMARY

For most individuals, the 2-drop Clinitest and the Acetest are the recommended testing methods because they represent a reasonable compromise between simplicity and accuracy. For some individuals, other testing methods may be better. When the most suitable testing procedure for the individual is used and performed accurately and when proper emphasis is placed on the results, urine testing can serve as a valuable guide for the therapeutic control of diabetes mellitus.

REFERENCES

1. Rosenbloom, A.: Stability and control of diabetes mellitus in children, South. Med. J. **64:**728, 1971.
2. Jackson, R. L., and Guthrie, R. A.: The child with diabetes. Current concepts, Kalamazoo, Mich., 1975, The Upjohn Co.
3. Feldman, J., Kelley, W., and Lebovitz, H.: Inhibition of glucose oxidase paper tests by reducing metabolites. Diabetes **19:**337, 1970.
4. Nickerson, D., Teaching the hospitalized diabetic, Am. J. Nurs. **72:**936, 1972.
5. Leifson, J.: Glycosuria tests performed by diabetics at home, Public Health Reports **84:**31, 1969.
6. Service, F., Molnar, G., and Taylor, W. F.: Urine glucose analyses during continuous blood glucose monitoring, JAMA **222:**298, 1972.

BIBLIOGRAPHY

Beland, I. L.: Clinical nursing: pathophysiological and psychological approaches, New York, 1970, The Macmillan Co.

Belmont, M. V., Sarkozy, E. S., and Harpur, E. R.: Urine sugar determination by the two-drop clinitest method, Diabetes **16:**577, 1967.

Crampton, J.: Diagnosis: urine testing and postprandial blood glucose. *In* Danowski. T. S., editor: Diabetes mellitus: diagnosis and treatment, vol. 1, New York, 1964, American Diabetes Association, Inc.

Derr, S.: Testing for glycosuria, Am. J. Nurs. **70:**1513, 1970.

Dobson, H. L., Saffer, K., and Burns, P.: Accuracy of urine testing for sugar and acetone by hospital ward personnel, Diabetes **17:**281, 1968.

Fajans, S., Levine, R., and Moss, J.: The diagnosis of diabetes: the fasting blood glucose test and the oral glucose tolerance test, Gen. Practition. **34:**133, 1969.

Fajans, S., Levine, R., and Moss, J.: The diagnosis of diabetes: identifying the diabetes suspect, Gen. Practition. **34:**133, 1969.

Fajans, S., Levine, R., and Moss, J.: The diagnosis of diabetes: an introduction to the pathophysiology of diabetes, Gen. Practition. **34:**133, 1969.

Fajans, S., Levine, R., and Moss, J.: The diagnosis of diabetes: standardization of oral glucose tolerance test procedure; prognostic significance of mild abnormalities in the oral glucose tolerance test; the two-hour postprandial blood glucose test; urinalysis for glucose, Gen. Practition. **34:**141, 1969.

Gates, E.: Therapy: teaching of the patient. *In* Donowski, T. S., editor: Diabetes Mellitus: diagnosis and treatment, vol. 1, New York, 1964, American Diabetes Association, Inc.

Genierser, N., and Becker, M.: Clinitest strictures of the esophagus, Clin. Pediatr. **8**(Suppl. 17A):7, 1969.

Haunz, E. A.: The role of urine testing in diabetes detection, Am. J. Nurs. **64:**102, 1964.

Leifson, J.: Glycosuria tests performed by diabetics at home, Public Health Reports **84:**28, 1969.

Logan, J. E., and Haight, D. E.: An evaluation of some commercial test papers and tablets for the determination of glucose in the urine, Can. Med. Assoc. J.**91:**11, 1964.

MacNeil, A.: Urine testing when the diagnosis is diabetes, Am. J. Nurs. **61:**67, 1961.

McFarlane, J., and Nickerson, D.: Two-drop and one-drop test for glycosuria, Am. J. Nurs. **12:**939, 1972.

Nickerson, D.: Teaching the hospitalized diabetic, Am. J. Nurs. **72:**935, 1972.

Rosenbloom, A.: Stability and control of diabetes mellitus in children, South. Med. J. **64:**728, 1971.

Service, J. F., Molnar, G., and Taylor, W. F.: Urine glucose analyses during continuous blood glucose monitoring, JAMA **222:**298, 1972.

Schmitt, G. F.: Diabetes for diabetics, Miami, 1965, The Diabetic Press of America, Inc.

Williams, R. H.: Diabetes, New York, 1965, Paul B. Hoeber, Inc.

Williams, R., editor: Textbook of endocrinology, Philadelphia, 1968, W. B. Saunders Co.

12

Hygiene in diabetic care

Judy Jordan and Donna Nickerson

The individual with diabetes is more prone to infection than the general population. This susceptibility is due to decreased circulation, increased glucose concentrations, abnormalities in immunolgic responses, poor white blood cell activity in the presence of high glucose concentrations, and perhaps other as yet unidentified factors.

Consequently, the diabetic person should be instructed in the general area of hygiene and infection prevention, paying particular attention to foot care. We, as health professionals, can decrease the complications resulting from infection if we alert ourselves and the diabetic person to the prevention of these complications.

CARE OF THE TEETH

Individuals with diabetes are subject to many problems of the oral cavity. According to Comroe and others, these oral manifestations include:

1. Dryness of the mouth and thirst.
2. A deep red color of the mucous membrane.
3. Swollen, highly inflamed, dark red gums, frequently detached from the teeth; chronic gingivitis almost always present.
4. Pus readily expressed from periodontal pockets and gum papillae; pyorrhea almost universal among poorly controlled diabetics.
5. Teeth frequently become loose; this may seem to occur almost overnight.
6. Increased sensitiveness about the necks of the teeth.
7. Ready bleeding from the gums on slight trauma.

8. Frequent formation of salivary calculus.
9. At times, an enlarged, thick, fissured, raw ham-colored tongue.
10. Frequent occurrence of dry sockets.
11. Presence of acetone on the breath when the diabetes is not under control (this is not pathognomonic of diabetes mellitus).*

Recent studies have shown that diabetic individuals have fewer caries than nondiabetics.[1] One part of the diabetes management that could account for this finding is emphasis on a well-balanced, nutritious diet with restriction of concentrated sweets.

The following list from Comroe and others is a summarization of recommended dental care:

1. The diabetic patient should be examined by a dentist at least every three or four months [every two months in children].†
2. Local conditions within the mouth cannot be successfully treated without careful control of the diabetic status by a clinician.
3. Rigid oral hygiene must be carried out with the frequent removal of accumulated calcareous deposits.
4. Loose teeth may become tightened after control of the diabetes has been established.
5. Complete mouth roentgen-ray should be performed yearly.

---

*From Comroe, A. B., Collins, L. H., Jr., and Crane, M. P.: Internal Medicine in dental practice, Philadelphia, 1946, Lea & Febiger, p. 263.
†Editors' note: It has been the experience of the editors that if the diabetes is well controlled only routine dental examination as per the nondiabetic individual is needed.

121

6. All tissues should be handled very gently with a minimum of trauma.
7. Any extensive work should be divided into several stages.
8. Sudden looseness of a tooth may result from an apical abscess.
9. No dental work should be undertaken without the full consent of the medical consultant.
10. Teeth with periapical infection should be removed, and root canal treatment should be attempted.
11. Extensive infiltration with local anesthesia should be avoided if possible.
12. Great care must be taken in the construction of artificial dentures in order to avoid trauma; some patients may have difficulty in wearing dentures because of pressure pain.
13. Surgical asepsis must be employed in extractions as the diabetic patient is very susceptible to infection. Epithelial ulceration and bony necrosis are not infrequent.
14. If an anesthetic is required, local anesthesia with procaine is first choice. If nitrous oxide is used, the greatest of care must be exercised. Epinephrine should not be used in large amounts, as this substance tends to raise blood glucose. In diabetic patients, ether should be avoided because it may reduce the liver glycogen.
15. An abscessed tooth is a distinct liability, the removal of which may improve not only the general health but also carbohydrate tolerance.*

If oral surgery is required, it is generally performed in the early morning, preferably 2 to 3 hours after breakfast. If the diabetic person is receiving insulin therapy, the physician may give the entire dose, one half of the dose, or withhold the insulin, depending on the person's ability to eat before and after the surgery. (See Chapter 16, Surgery and diabetes.)

In the postoperative period, it is important that the urine be tested frequently, 3 to 4 times daily, and that the physician be consulted should increased glucosuria develop.

After oral surgery, coke, juice, or other sugar-containing fluids may be given. Solids are not tolerated. This is especially important when insulin is taken because lack of food may result in hypoglycemia.

Antibiotic therapy is often begun after tooth extraction to help prevent the possibility of infection. It is often started 2 to 3 days before oral surgery.

No dental surgery should be performed until the physician states that blood glucose levels are under adequate control. The reasons for restricting surgery are: (1) The increased infection is observed with poorly controlled diabetes. (2) The healing process is slower with increased glucose levels. (3) Diabetic acidosis is possible if infection does develop or healing is slow.

CARE OF THE SKIN

Persons with diabetes are more prone to attack by staphylococci, beta-hemolytic streptococci, and fungi. Furuncles and carbuncles are very common and usually increase the requirement of insulin. The infecting organism should always be cultured and antibiotic therapy instituted. Infections that are associated with fever and leukocytosis result in hypermetabolism, thereby necessitating an increase in insulin requirement.

Several lesions of the skin are often observed in people with diabetes. One of the most common skin lesions, diabetic dermopathy, occurs in diabetic individuals after age 30 (Fig. 12-1). It commonly occurs as a result of localized trauma and is most prominent on the shin. Diabetic dermopathy may appear as hyperpigmented areas, usually tan in color. They are not painful but are cosmetically unattractive. There is no treatment for this type of lesion.

Another lesion observed on the lower extremity is necrobiosis lipoidica diabeticorum (Fig. 12-2). It is not a common disorder, and may occur in subjects who do not have diabetes, but is considered symp-

*From Comroe, A. B., Collins, L. H., Jr., and Crane, M. P.: Internal medicine in dental practice, Philadelphia, 1946, Lea & Febiger, p. 264.

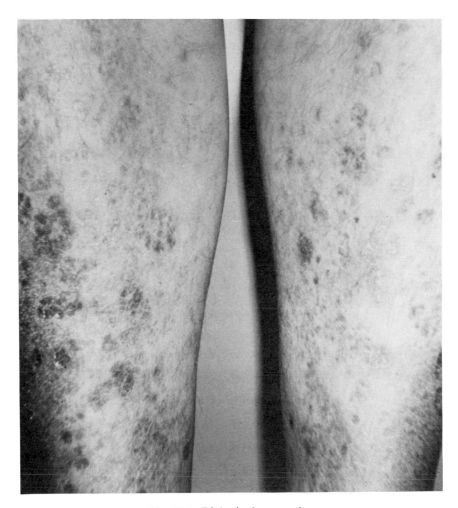

Fig. 12-1. Diabetic dermopathy.

tomatic of diabetes. The lesion occurs most commonly among women before age 40. It starts much like an area of dermopathy, enlarges to form a plaque, and may cover the entire lower leg. It is often a result of trauma, and ulcerations may be located within the area. Treatment may include injection of hydrocortisone; however, this treatment is painful, and remission tends to be temporary.

Another lesion of the skin occasionally observed is xanthoma diabeticorum. With this condition, the pateint has marked hyperlipemia when blood glucose levels remain elevated for a long period of time. The

lesion appears as firm nodules in scattered papules, which are pinkish yellow in color. The papules are predominantly located on the buttocks, extensor surfaces, palms and soles and are not painful. Treatment of xanthoma diabeticorum consists of lowering blood glucose levels, which in turn reduces the serum lipid levels.

Gangrene of the feet is more prevalent in diabetic persons, and prevention of gangrene and amputation is a special challenge to medical personnel. (See discussion of foot care on subsequent pages.)

One of the most common infections observed in women with diabetes is candi-

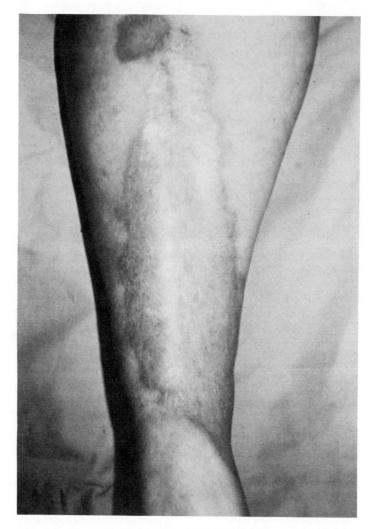

Fig. 12-2. Necrobiosis lipoidica diabeticorum.

diasis (moniliasis). The presence of vaginal candidiasis should prompt investigation for diabetes. *Candida (Monilia)* organisms are normally present in the vaginal mucosa, and with the increased concentrations of glucose in the urine, the *Candida* multiply rapidly, causing vulvovaginitis in combination with severe pruritis. The labia may become swollen and red, and a cheesy-white discharge is often present. Candidiasis may also appear in the oral mucous membranes, axillary areas, and under the breasts if they are pendulous. Treatment of candidiasis includes the use of topical powders, vaginal suppositiries, or oral medication. The best treatment is the control of blood glucose levels. A *Candida* infection, which prompts an individual to see the physician for diagnosis and treatment, is often an index to the physician or nurse that blood glucose levels are elevated.

CARE OF THE FEET

The most important aspect of foot care for the person with diabetes is the prevention of serious problems. The feet of the diabetic person are prone to vascular insufficiency (particularly small vessel disease), neuropathy, and infection secondary to trauma. The "diabetic foot," as Max Ellenberg refers to it, is not much different from the foot of any other person with advanced vascular disease, except for one outstanding feature—diabetic neuropathy[2]—which interferes with the perception of trauma or pressure. Preventive foot care is based on knowledge of these possible complications of diabetes and has two aspects: (1) hygiene and other means of active prevention and (2) avoidance of trauma.

Hygiene

People with diabetes should wash and soak their feet daily. Lukewarm water should be used for this purpose. Since the temperature receptors in the lower extremities of the diabetic person may be impaired, the water should always be tested with the wrist or elbow, or by another family member. Mild hand soaps are best, but those with an antibacterial agent added give extra protection against infection. Particular care should be taken to gently but thoroughly pat the feet dry and to dry well between the toes. A bland foot powder can then be applied if the feet tend to perspire. If dryness is noted, lanolin, baby oil, or even corn oil can be rubbed gently into the skin. Applying lotion routinely also provides an opportunity for inspection of the feet. Immediately after soaking is the best time to cut toenails or to care for corns or callouses, because the warm water has softened them. One should cut toenails straight across and square, without digging into the corners and without cutting below the end of the toe, unless there are thickened folds of skin on either side of the nail. (Ideally at this point, the podiatrist should be involved because the manner of toenail cutting is quite different for diabetic individuals.) Nail scissors or, ideally, clippers should be used in preference to a knife or other sharp object, which may slip and injure the foot. If the patient cannot see well or if the nails are extremely hard, a podiatrist should perform the job. Callouses or

corns should be soaked and then rubbed gently with a soft towel or pumice stone. These areas should never be treated with corn remedies, which are usually harsh, or cut with a knife, scissors, or razor blade. A podiatrist can usually provide the best treatment for these problems and should be informed about the diabetes.

Daily inspection of the feet. The person with diabetes should carefully insepct the feet daily. Daily hygiene provides a regular time for this examination, which should include the tops and the soles of the feet, the heels, and the area between the toes. If the patient cannot see well enough to do this himself, another person in the family can make the inspection. Even a minor injury to or a change in the feet, such as a small reddened area, should be checked by the physician or the nurse clinician. Many serious complications can be avoided if slowly healing wounds or other problem areas are reported early, before they develop into ulcerations. Ulcerations can evolve rapidly; therefore, no foot problem should be taken lightly. The person with diabetes cannot rely on pain or discomfort as a clue to injury, because neuropathy impairs sensation. In fact, neurogenic ulcers are painless. Thus, daily examination is imperative.

Proper shoes and socks. Clean socks or stockings and properly fitting shoes should be worn every day and changed frequently. Inspection of the feet can reveal areas that may be irritated by the shoes being worn. New shoes should be broken in carefully and slowly, and old shoes and slippers should be checked periodically to ensure that they are intact and still fit well. Shoes should not be worn without hose or socks, and the socks should be free of holes or darns. Even a curled thread in a sock can cause an irritation if unnoticed. If indicated, bunions, hammer toes, and pressure points should be protected by insoles to avoid pressure sores. Lambs wool can be used between toes that rub or overlap.

Improving circulation

Active prevention of foot and leg problems should include measures to improve the circulation in the lower extremities. Buerger's exercises offer one method of stimulating circulation to the legs. These exercises consist of (1) maximal lowering of the feet below heart level and leaving them until the veins fill, followed by (2) elevation of the feet at the least height and for the shortest time that will empty the foot. For example, the patients may sit down dangling their feet over the side of the bed for 1 minute, extend both legs and hold them parallel to the floor while lying on their backs for 1 minute, and then rest in a supine position for 1 minute, repeating the entire process as indicated. If the patients are unable to exercise themselves, an oscillating bed can provide the effect of active Buerger's exercises. Buerger's exercises also include elevation, rotation, flexion, and extention of the foot at the ankle.

Walking slowly can be a form of Buerger's exercise if the vein valves work properly. Muscle contraction forces blood up the deep veins, venous pressure decreases as the muscles relax, and the high arterial pressure produced by gravity fills the veins. Walking slowly should be strongly encouraged, especially in patients with occlusive arterial disease. If the patient has intermittent claudication, periods of rest can be alternated with walks. The person with venous insufficiency may require bed rest several times a day.

In addition to walking, abstinence from the use of tobacco helps the circulation in the vasoconstricting extremities that may already have vascular impairment in the person with diabetes.

Avoiding trauma

Trauma to the foot can lead to infection, and infection requires an increased blood supply and increased insulin, both of which the diabetic person may be lacking. The easiest way to avoid setting up this vicious circle is to prevent trauma.

The possible impairment to sensation because of neuropathy should be kept in mind. Temperature sense, vibration sense, and proprioception may all be impaired in diabetic individuals. They should avoid heat from hot water, heating pads, hot water bottles, or other devices and also keep their feet away from open fires or stoves. Dry heat is dangerous because the diabetic person may lack sensation and be afflicted with vasculopathy. Since blood acts as the body's cooling agent, decreased blood flow due to vasculopathy may lead to overheating and a severe burn. The patient should be encouraged to use warm socks and extra covers if he has difficulty keeping warm. Frostbite may occur if the patient's circulation is poor or humidity is high and temperature is 40° F or less. The body tends to conserve warmth by decreasing circulation to the extremities when the trunk is cold. The nurse should question her client carefully about heating methods employed at home, because hot water bottles or even hot bricks are not uncommon devices. Medical personnel also need to be educated about foot care. Nurses working in hospitals are often guilty of leaving ice packs or hot soaks on patients with diabetes and forgetting to check them, thus allowing burns to occur.

The feet should be protected at all times from cuts, bruises, introduction of foreign objects, and fractures. Such protection can usually be accomplished if the diabetic person wears shoes (or well-fitted slippers) that are sturdy and closed in at all times. Many amputations have resulted from the entry of an object, such as a staple into the foot, without the diabetic patient noticing it. It is not uncommon for minor fractures to go unheeded by the individual with neuropathy. Instead of protecting the injured foot, the person with decreased sensation will continue to use it for weight bearing, which leads to further deterioration, multiple fractures, and even Charcot's joint. The person with diabetes should never go barefoot, even around the house.

If an accident involves the foot, the medical team should check for possible injury regardless of lack of pain.

Socks or stockings should be worn in such a way that adequate circulation is maintained. Tight-fitting socks or stockings may lead to minute trauma or mechanically cause a process of pathology. Tight elastic bands, circular garters, or twisted hose should never be used. Crossing the legs at the knees for long periods of time will also decrease circulation to the lower extremities.

Minor cuts should be kept clean and dry. Alcohol may be applied, but all harsh antiseptics and chemicals should be avoided. For instance, iodine, Merthiolate, Mercurochrome, or liniment should not be used on the feet. Corn pads and corn plasters can lead to ulcerations and should be considered taboo. Likewise, home remedies for cuts—known to range from spider webs, to motor oil, to bleach—can be extremely dangerous. If in doubt, the patient should consult the medical team before any first-aid measures are instituted.

The integrity of the skin on the feet should never be broken purposely in caring for toenails, corns, or callouses, even by an expert, without recommendation of the physician treating the person with diabetes. Ingrown toenails should be promptly treated by a podiatrist, as should fungal infections of the nails. Fungus on the skin also requires medical attention. Athlete's foot should not be taken lightly, because if left untreated, it can lead to ulceration.

Avoidance of trauma should be of special consideration when a localized amputation, as of a single toe, has already been performed. In this case, the remainder of the extremity may be off balance and more subject to stress in certain areas. Shoes and padding must be carefully selected.

TREATMENT OF TRAUMA AND LESIONS. Conservative treatment of trauma to the foot of the person with diabetes has met with increasing success, particularly when problems are detected early and when vasculopathy is not advanced. However, the patient and the nurse must be compulsive in carrying out the therapy indicated. Frequent, cleansing foot soaks are usually ordered. Bed rest and high doses of antibiotics are generally prescribed for foot lesions, as are dry, sterile dressings. Resting the affected part is probably the most important element of treatment and must be strictly enforced. Bed rest may be necessary for as long as 3 to 9 months. Careful monitoring and control of the diabetes is particularly important in overcoming infection, because poor diabetes control will prolong the infectious process. Buerger's exercise may be helpful in healing the foot (see p. 126). Tobacco should be avoided. Vasodilators may be prescribed occasionally, although they have the potential of actually shifting blood flow away from the ischemic part. Debridement of a lesion with a bland solution may be carried out, even on an outpatient basis, if treatment is begun early and circulation is fairly good.

Amputation is usually indicated when gangrene has set in, infection is uncontrollable, pain is unrelenting, tissue has been destroyed, or an ulcer will not heal. Amputations can range from a single toe to an entire limb. With proper rehabilitation therapy, amputation can often restore the patient to a more productive life.

Nursing measures

Despite the serious consequences that can result from improper foot care, this area of therapy is frequently overlooked by nursing personnel during history-taking, examination, and teaching. Nurses seem to shy away from the first, quickest and easiest step—inspection of the patient's feet. Teaching preventive foot care is often delayed, because it is not perceived to be as immediate a need as insulin technique. This delay is particularly observed in the treatment of young patients. A survey of patients treated for neuropathic lesions by the Joslin Clinic group showed that 38% were less than 50 years old.[3] The lack of emphasis on foot care was reflected in the results of a study of patients hospitalized at the University of Florida teaching hospital, in which 82% were using improper first-aid treatment of feet at home.[4]

Nursing care should begin with an assessment of what the patient is currently doing in terms of foot care.

A. *Inspection of the feet should be frequent* and include the following considerations:
   1. What is the condition of the shoes?
   2. How well do the shoes fit?
   3. Is the patient wearing socks or stockings? Are they clean? In good repair? Fit well?
   4. Is the patient using circular garters? Twisting hose? Wearing tight elastic bands?
   5. Are the feet clean?
   6. Are the feet warm to the touch?
   7. Do the feet have good color?
   8. Is there hair growing on the feet?
   9. Is there any edema?
   10. What is the condition of the toenails? How are they cut?
   11. Are there any corns, callouses, or bunions? (In examining for fissures, one gently separates the toes as there is a possibility of creating fissures in the examination process.)
   12. Are there any cuts? Fissures? Bruises? Ulcerations? If so, does the tissue appear ischemic or gangrenous?
   13. What is the general condition of the skin? Is it dry? Any rashes? What about the area between the toes? The heels? The soles?
   14. Are there any apparent pressure points?
   15. Do the toes overlap?
   16. Can the peripheral pulses be palpated? Are they strong? (See Fig. 12-3.)
   17. Does the patient have sensation to pain? Vibration? (One can test with a pin or tuning fork.)
   18. Are the leg muscles atrophied?
   19. Is there any abnormality in gait?

B. *Observation of the foot-care routine with the client's own equipment* is the ideal way to assess the usual procedure for hygiene. The nurse can gain the most information by going into the patient's residence, where she can assess the home facilities for bathing, such as the water supply. Watching the patient actually carry out the foot-care regimen is far more revealing than simply having patients state what they do.

   If the nurse is unable to go into the client's homes, she can ask them to bring the foot-care equipment to the health care facility. The nurse should have the opportunity to see:
   1. Soap or other material used for washing or soaking feet.
   2. Lotion or powder.
   3. Articles used for trimming toenails.
   4. First-aid remedies for cuts, bruises, or infection.

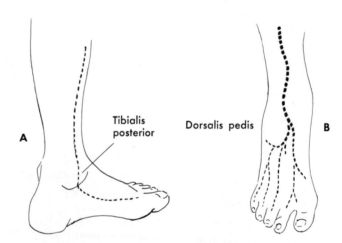

Fig. 12-3. Sites of palpable arteries. **A,** Tibialis posterior. **B,** Dorsalis pedis.

5. Preparations, if any, used for corns or callouses.
6. Anything else applied to the feet or used in foot care.
7. Bedroom slippers and shoes worn most often.
8. Equipment used for keeping the feet warm.

C. *Interviewing regarding foot-care practices* can begin with general questions: What has the patient already been told about proper foot care? Why is foot care important for the person with diabetes? Whether or not the nurse is able to observe the foot-care regimen, she should inquire:

1. How often are the feet washed or soaked? What is used? What temperature is the water? How is it checked? Is anything applied to the feet after washing? How are the feet dried?
2. How are the toenails trimmed and how often is this done?
3. How are cuts and bruises treated?
4. What is done about corns and callouses?
5. Is anything else applied to the feet?
6. How are the feet kept warm?
7. What is worn on the feet around the house? Does the patient ever go barefoot?
8. How often are the feet inspected?
9. Is a member of the health care team ever consulted for treatment of the feet?

D. *Eliciting information about symptoms* can pinpoint potential foot care problems. For instance, the nurse might consider the following questions:

1. Is there any numbness or tingling in the lower extremities? A burning sensation?
2. Is there calf pain (intermittent claudication) when walking?
3. Is there rest pain in the lower extremities?
4. Is there decreased sensitivity to temperature?
5. Is there lack of pain with injury?
6. Is there nocturnal pain in the lower extremities?
7. Is healing slow?

Teaching

A thorough assessment of the foot-care regimen helps the nurse to focus on the areas for which teaching should be done.

The first step in instruction must be the *rationale* for good foot care. The "do's" and "don'ts" of foot care make sense to patients once they understand how complications of diabetes can affect the feet. Health care personnel often forget to emphasize the "why" when instructions are given. A study of 74 hospitalized diabetic persons revealed that 42 patients, including several with foot lesions, had no idea why foot care is important.[4]

Demonstration is the best method for teaching routine foot hygiene and treatment of problem areas. The nurse can have the patients soak their own feet with her supervision. This procedure gives the diabetic individual the opportunity to learn such things as how to accurately check the temperature of the water. The nurse can inspect the feet, explaining each step to the patients, and can show them how to wash and pat dry the feet. If the toenails need trimming or if corns or callouses are present, the procedures for care of these problems can be demonstrated, as can dressing changes or other therapy prescribed for more serious problems. Having the patient's own equipment on hand makes it easy to select the best items to use and to suggest changes.

If demonstration and practice with the individual is not feasible, many films and slides are available and provide a visualization of proper foot care. Pictures of various foot problems also aid the patients in examination of their own feet and detection of potential trouble.

Written "do's" and "don'ts" of foot care give the patient a handy list to refer to when a question is encountered at home. A list of positive steps to take in daily hygiene and in treating injuries, as well as a list of situations to avoid, should be included in such a guide:

Do	Don't
Examine feet *daily*— tops, soles, heels, and between toes.	

Do	Don't
Wash feet *every day* with mild hand soap and *warm* water—check temperature with wrist or elbow.	Do *not* use hot water to wash feet or bathe in.
Pat feet thoroughly dry, especially between the toes.	Do *not* leave feet wet, or dry them roughly.
Apply bland powder if feet perspire.	
Apply lanolin, oil, or bland lotion to dry feet.	
Cut toenails after soaking—straight across with clippers or scissors—file corners smooth with an emory board.	Do *not* cut toenails short or dig into the corners. Do *not* use a knife to cut nails.
Rub corns or callouses gently with a soft towel after soaking; consult podiatrist if they persist.	Do *not* use corn pads or corn plasters. Do *not* cut corns or callouses.
Wear clean socks or hose every day.	Do *not* wear socks or stockings with holes or loose threads.
Wear pantyhose or use garter belt or girdle.	Do *not* wear round garters or twist hose to hold them up.
Wear good, sturdy shoes that are comfortable.	
Wear shoes *all* the time, inside and outside the house.	Do *not* walk barefoot.
Treat minor cuts or bruises with gentle cleansing and alcohol.	Do *not* use iodine, Merthiolate, Mercurochrome, liniment, or antiseptics on cuts or bruises.
Use warm socks and extra covers to keep feet warm.	Do *not* use hot water bottles, heating pads, hot bricks, other heating devices, or ice packs on the feet.

Summary

Diabetic patients should be told to consult their medical team if they notice a cut that does not heal, a sore, a reddened area, a rash, or an ingrown nail. If in doubt, they should always call the doctor or nurse clinician.

The most important idea to leave with the diabetic person is that any foot problem can become a serious situation and that a physician should be contacted immediately.

The nurse's responsibility may not stop at checking the patient's feet and imparting information about good foot care. She often has the opportunity to assess the materials and facilities available to the patients for adequate foot care and should guide them in utilizing or altering these items withing their means.

Preventive nursing care is essential if the person with diabetes mellitus is to avoid serious foot problems.

REFERENCES

1. Comroe, A. B., Collins, L. H., Jr., and Crane, M. P.: Internal medicine in dental practice, Philadelphia, 1946, Lea & Febiger, pp. 263, 364.
2. Ellenberg, M.: Diabetic foot, N.Y. State J. Med. **73:**2778, 1973.
3. Krall, L., Goldstein, H. H., Graham, C., and Rosobotharn, J.: Foot lesions in diabetics, Hosp. Med. **9:**66, 1973.
4. Nickerson, D.: Teaching the hospitalized diabetic, **72:**936, 1972.

BIBLIOGRAPHY

Adams, R. D., Braunwald, E., Isselbacher, K. J., and others, editors: Harrison's principles of internal medicine, ed. 7, New York, 1974, McGraw-Hill Book Co.
Binkley, G. W.: Dermopathy in the diabetic syndrome, Arch. Dermatol. **92:**625, 1965.
Bortz, E. L., and Burroughs, D. L.: The control of infections in diabetic patients, Am. J. Nurs. **54:**1348, 1954.
Burket, L. W.: The interrelationship of oral and systemic disease, Dent. Clin. North Am., July 1958, pp. 465-469.
Comroe, A. B., Collins, L. H., Jr., and Crane, M. P.: Internal Medicine in Dental Practice, Philadelphia, 1946, Lea & Febiger, pp. 262-264.
Diabetes mellitus: a reference for nurses, Durham, N.C., 1969, The Diabetes Consultation and Education Service of the Association for the North Carolina Regional Medical Program, pp. 43-54.
Ellenberg, M.: Diabetic neuropathy. *In* Ellenberg, M., and Rifkin, H., editors: Diabetes

mellitus; theory and practice, New York, 1970, McGraw-Hill Book Co.

Ellenberg, M.: Diabetic foot, N.Y. State J. Med., **73**:2778, 1973.

Fitzpatrick, T. B.: Dermatologic lesions and diseases associated with diabetes. *In* Williams, R. H., editor: Diabetes, New York, 1960, Paul B. Hoeber, Inc. Chapter 42.

Haimovici, H.: Peripheral arterial disease. *In* Ellenberg, M., and Rifkin, H., editors: Diabetes mellitus: theory and practice, New York, 1970, McGraw-Hill Book Co., Inc., p. 890.

Joslin, E. P., Root, H. F., White, P., and Marble, A.: The treatment of diabetes mellitus, ed. 9 Philadelphia, 1952, Lea & Febiger, pp. 30, 186, 446, 447.

Krall, P., Goldstein, H. H., Graham, C., and Rosobotharn, J.: Foot lesions in diabetics, Hosp. Med. **9**:66, 1973.

Locke, R. K.: Foot care for diabetics Am. J. Nurs. **63**:107, 1963.

Oakley, W., Catterall, R. C. F., and Martin, M. M.: Aetiology and management of lesions of the feet in diabetes, Br. Med. J. **2**:953, 1956.

Pohl, M.: Teaching function of the nursing practitioner, Dubuque, Iowa, 1968, William C. Brown Co., Publishers.

Rosenthal, H., and Rosenthal, J.: Diabetic care in pictures, Philadelphia, 1968, J. B. Lippincott Co., pp. 165-183.

Sindoni, A., Jr.: The role of the dentist in diabetes mellitus, J. Dent. Med. **9**:205, 1954.

Skillman, T. G.: Peripheral vascular disease. *In* Hamwi, G. J. and Danowski, T. S., editors: Diabetes mellitus: diagnosis and treatment, vol. 2, New York, 1967, American Diabetes Association, Inc.

Sussman, K.: Peripheral vascular disease, *In* Sussman, K. editor: Juvenile-type diabetes and its complications, Springfield, Ill., 1971, Charles C Thomas, Publisher.

Whitehouse, F. W., and Block, M. A.: The problem of the diabetic foot, J. Am. Geriatr. Soc. **12**:1045, 1964.

Williams, R. H., editor: Diabetes, New York, 1960, Paul B. Hoeber Inc., pp. 623-641.

Williams, R. H., editor: Textbook of endocrinology, Philadelphia, 1968, W. B. Saunders Co., pp. 779-782.

13

The meal plan

Virginia Stucky

Nutrition is important in the overall management of the patient with diabetes. Nutritional care for the patient can be fraught with frustration for the patient and the health professionals. The health professionals are presented with varied information that quickly becomes obsolete. At the present time the most universally used tool for dietary control is "Exchange Lists for Meal Planning." (See Table 13-13 and also refer to Appendix F for details of the revised ADA exchange list.) The American Dietetic Association and the American Diabetes Association plan for continued revision of "Exchange Lists for Meal Planning" or for a program that utilizes a completely different procedure. Plans for revision have been a project of the two organizations for many years.

Another frustration is the promise of good health as a result of good diet control, which does not always materialize. The individual's ability to interpret "cause and effect" is often less than scientific. Too often patients who are given a diet may not actually follow that diet yet fail to recognize poor diet control as the cause of health problems.

Following are several other dilemmas in nutritional care:

1. The 1964-1965 National Health Survey indicated that 25% of the diabetic patients surveyed did not follow a diet. Fifty-three percent of the patients said that they followed a diet, *but* only one-third of these patients could recall the number of food exchanges permitted.[1]

2. Physicians in many areas are ignoring the exchange list, offering free diets and allowing jelly and sugar. Others advocate free diets but advise patients to avoid concentrated sweets such as jams and sugar.

3. The exchange list is rigid and does *not* always consider the patients' life-styles and their economic situations.

4. The exchange list was written for the person with diabetes, yet we have universally accepted it for obese individuals also.

5. Dietitians know *how* to make variations in the diet and may add carbohydrate, protein, and fat in foods such as pizza, but they do not always adequately explain how this can be done to the patient.

6. The person with diabetes may require control of saturated and unsaturated fats.

7. The carbohydrate allowance may not need to be as restricted as was once believed.

Diet is probably a major part of diabetic treatment, but the best diet has not been conclusively determined. Gaps in our knowledge are many. We have an inadequate number of controlled studies that would give us the answers for ideal dietary control. Among authorities in the field, there is much discussion about the necessity for "changing" from the exchange list to something more appropriate. Some authorities suggest dietary consideration for conditions in addition to diabetes, such as endogenous hyperglyceridemia or hypercholesterolemia. The new exchange list

Those who offered valuable suggestions for this chapter were Catherine McCarty. Shelia Cochron. Sharon Mallory, and Francis Rogers.

does take these other conditions into account.

In their special report, the Committee on Food and Nutrition of the American Diabetes Association describes the principle of nutrition and dietary recommendations for the patient with diabetes.[2] By using their report and information that has become available since the report, one can draw a few conclusions: It is generally agreed that "nutritional care" implies that the patient should have a diet that supplies all the necessary calories and nutrients for normal growth, development, and activity. Beyond this point, it becomes difficult to decide how to minimize fluctuations in blood glucose levels or how important this goal is for everyone. Perhaps there is more than one way to meet everyone's nutritional needs. There definitely is not one diet for all persons any more than there is one insulin for all persons.

Perhaps all the objectives for dietary treatment have not been determined. Dietary treatment depends on many factors, especially the individual, the individual's consistent exercise pattern, and insulin therapy. The majority of health professionals wish to return the patient's blood glucose to normal levels. Others attempt to improve levels of blood lipids, fluid retention, and hypertension and to use diets that may slow the development of complications. The following are essential objectives for the health professional:

1. Identify the nutritional needs of the patient (Sections I, II, III, and IV).*
2. Use tools and methods that assist in meeting the nutritional needs of the patient (Sections V, VI, VII).
3. Evaluate problems that interfere with meeting the nutritional needs of the patient (Section VIII).

For health professionals to adequately meet these objectives, it is essential that they consider the patient. Etzwiler has said

*Roman numerals refer to subsequent referenced sections.

that "the health professional does not do most of the care, . . . it is the patient." We cannot forget that the patient is part of the team.[3]

Often we use the term "individualization" very inadequately because we are not sufficiently individualizing the dietary treatment. When we consider the individuals and attempt to meet their demands, they may adhere more closely to their diet. When the health professional respects the patient's life-style, values, and beliefs, the professional will give primary consideration to the patient in the nutritional planning and make only the dietary changes that are absolutely necessary. Throughout this discussion the emphasis will be on the patient as an individual. As our concern for the individual becomes more evident in prescribing diets (meal patterns) and interpreting dietary prescriptions, we will see greater responsibility taken by the patient.

• • •

As we emphasize individuality, the patient develops responsibility.

SECTION I: ADEQUATE NUTRIENTS

All persons of normal weight who have diabetes require the same amount of nutrients as their normal weight counterparts who do not have diabetes. The Food and Nutrition Board of the National Research Council (NRC) recommends daily dietary allowances of many essential nutrients for various individuals (Table 13-1 and boxed material on p. 136).

Nutritionists often recommend a Basic-4 meal pattern as found in Table 13-2. The recommended protein for adults is 0.8 gm for each kilogram of ideal body weight. The "average man" of 70 kg who needs 56 gm of protein can receive this amount with the food and servings shown in Table 13-2. Too often we overemphasize and increase the consumption of protein. An increased consumption of protein often results in a greater consumption of fat when the protein eaten is principally meat and cheese.

Table 13-1. Food and Nutrition Board, National Academy of Sciences, National Research Council, nutrition of practically all healthy people in the U.S.A.*

	Age (years)	Weight kg	Weight lb	Height cm	Height in	Energy (kcal)[b]	Protein (gm)	Fat-soluble vitamins — Vitamin A activity RE[c]	Vitamin A activity IU	Vitamin D (IU)	Vitamin E activity[e] (IU)
Infants	0.0-0.5	6	14	60	24	kg × 117	kg × 2.2	420[d]	1400	400	4
	0.5-1.0	9	20	71	28	kg × 108	kg × 2.0	400	2000	400	5
Children	1-3	13	28	86	34	1300	23	400	2000	400	7
	4-6	20	44	110	44	1800	30	500	2500	400	9
	7-10	30	66	135	54	2400	36	700	3300	400	10
Males	11-14	44	97	158	63	2800	44	1000	5000	400	12
	15-18	61	134	172	69	3000	54	1000	5000	400	15
	19-22	67	147	172	69	3000	54	1000	5000	400	15
	23-50	70	154	172	69	2700	56	1000	5000		15
	51+	70	154	172	69	2400	56	1000	5000		15
Females	11-14	44	97	155	52	2400	44	800	4000	400	12
	15-18	54	119	162	65	2100	48	800	4000	400	12
	19-22	58	128	162	65	2100	46	800	4000	400	12
	23-50	58	128	162	65	2000	46	800	4000		12
	51+	58	128	162	65	1800	46	800	4000		12
Pregnant						+300	+30	1000	5000	400	15
Lactating						+500	+20	1200	6000	400	15

[a]The allowances are intended to provide for individual variations among most normal persons as they live in the United nutrients for which human requirements have been less well defined.

[b]Kilojoules (kJ) = 4.2 × kcal.

[c]Retinol equivalents.

[d]Assumed to be all as retinol in milk during the first six months of life. All subsequent intakes are assumed to be half as and one fourth as β-carotene.

[e]Total vitamin E activity, estimated to be 80% as α-tocopherol and 20% other tocopherols.

[f]The folacin allowances refer to dietary sources as determined by *Lactobacillus casei* assay. Pure forms of folacin may be

[g]Although allowances are expressed as niacin, it is recognized that on the average 1 mg of niacin is derived from each 60

[h]This increased requirement cannot be met by ordinary diets; therefore, the use of supplemental iron is recommended.

Recommended daily dietary allowances,[a] revised 1974. Designed for the maintenance of good

Water-soluble vitamins							Minerals					
Ascorbic acid (mg)	Folacin[f] (μg)	Niacin[g] (mg)	Riboflavin (mg)	Thiamin (mg)	Vitamin B₆ (mg)	Vitamin B₁₂ (μg)	Calcium (mg)	Phosphorus (mg)	Iodine (μg)	Iron (mg)	Magnesium (mg)	Zinc (mg)
35	50	5	0.4	0.3	0.3	0.3	360	240	35	10	60	3
35	50	8	0.6	0.5	0.4	0.3	540	400	45	15	70	5
40	100	9	0.8	0.7	0.6	1.0	800	800	60	15	150	10
40	200	12	1.1	0.9	0.9	1.5	800	800	80	10	200	10
40	300	16	1.2	1.2	1.2	2.0	800	800	110	10	250	10
45	400	18	1.5	1.4	1.6	3.0	1200	1200	130	18	350	15
45	400	20	1.8	1.5	2.0	3.0	1200	1200	150	18	400	15
45	400	20	1.8	1.5	2.0	3.0	800	800	140	10	350	15
45	400	18	1.6	1.4	2.0	3.0	800	800	130	10	350	15
45	400	16	1.5	1.2	2.0	3.0	800	800	110	10	350	15
45	400	16	1.3	1.2	1.6	3.0	1200	1200	115	18	300	15
45	400	14	1.4	1.1	2.0	3.0	1200	1200	115	18	300	15
45	400	14	1.4	1.1	2.0	3.0	800	800	100	18	300	15
45	400	13	1.2	1.0	2.0	3.0	800	800	100	18	300	15
45	400	12	1.1	1.0	2.0	3.0	800	800	80	10	300	15
60	800	+2	+0.3	+0.3	2.5	4.0	1200	1200	125	18+[h]	450	20
80	600	+4	+0.5	+0.3	2.5	4.0	1200	1200	150	18	450	25

States under usual environmental stresses. Diets should be based on a variety of common foods in order to provide other

retinol and half as β-carotene when calculated from international units. As retinol equivalents, three fourths are as retinol

effective in doses less than one fourth of the recommended dietary allowance.
mg of dietary tryptophan.

NUTRIENT POINTS*
For good health, eat each day

Persons	Protein points ♡ Reds	Carbohydrate points ◇ Whites	Fat points ▭ Blues	Calcium points ◯	Iron points ◼	Vitamin A points △	Thiamin points Grey	Riboflavin points White	Niacin* points Black	Vitamin C points C
Man†	7	29	40	4	4	4	9½	4	4½	3
Woman†	6	20	28	4	7	3	7	3	3	3
Boy (10-18)	6	29	39	6	7	4	9½	4	4½	3
Girl (10-18)	6	22	30	6	7	3	7½	3½	4	3
Preschool	3	15	21	4	5	2	5	2	2½	2½
School age	4½	24	32	4	4	3	8	3	4	2½
Baby 2-6 mo	1½			2	4	1¼	2	1	1	2
Baby 6-12 mo	2			2½	6	1½	3	1½	2	2
Mother-to-be	+4	+1	+4	6	7+	4	+3	+1	+½	4
Nursing mother	+2½	+4	+6½	6	7	5	+2	+1	+1	4
USRDA				5	7	4	10	4	5	4
Under 4 yr				4	4	2	4½	2	2	3
Pregnancy, lactation				6	7	5	10	5	5	4

*Based upon part of niacin coming from protein (tryptophan).
†After age 51—man = ◇ = 23; ▭ = 32. Can reduce vitamin B's ½ to 1 point.
  After age 51—woman = ◇ = 17; ▭ = 24; ◼ = 4. Can reduce vitamin B's ½ to 1 point.

Also use iodized salt, sea foods, or foods from iodine-rich soil.

A plus (+) *before* a number means these points should be *added* to the normal requirements shown for a specific age of a woman who is not pregnant or nursing a baby.

A plus (+) *after* a number means that these points *or more* should be eaten.

Most averages in the chart above are taken from recommended dietary allowances reported by the Food and Nutrition Board, National Research Council (NRC). The precise figures are found in their publication from National Academy of Sciences, Washington, D.C. Our niacin amounts are lower because some niacin comes from tryptophan (protein). Carbohydrate and fat are our suggestions and may vary considerably to meet individual calorie needs.

A point is a simplified unit of weight that allows one to use smaller numbers than usually found in nutritive value charts. When computing the nutritive value of a food, recipe or daily diet we have used the simpler "points." The weight (grams or milligrams) is different for each nutrient. See "Point equivalents" below.

Point equivalents

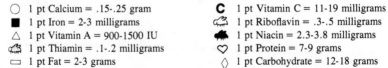

◯ 1 pt Calcium = .15-.25 gram

◼ 1 pt Iron = 2-3 milligrams

△ 1 pt Vitamin A = 900-1500 IU

🦗 1 pt Thiamin = .1-.2 milligrams

▭ 1 pt Fat = 2-3 grams

C 1 pt Vitamin C = 11-19 milligrams

🐛 1 pt Riboflavin = .3-.5 milligrams

🐜 1 pt Niacin = 2.3-3.8 milligrams

♡ 1 pt Protein = 7-9 grams

◇ 1 pt Carbohydrate = 12-18 grams

*From Stucky, V.: Nutrition for the nation, Wichita, Kan., 1976, Diet Teaching Programs, Inc.

Table 13-2. Basic-4 meal pattern*

Basic-4 requirements (servings or units)	Group	Servings or units	♡	◇	▭	○	■	△	🐭	🐇	🐗	C
2	Milk	3	4	2	12	5		1	1	3		
		2	2	1	8	3		1	1	2		
		1	1	1	4	2				1		
6	Meat, beans, nuts, etc.	6	5	2	11	1	2	1	2	1	4	
		4	4	2	8		2		2	1	2	
		2	2	1	4		1		1		1	
		1	1		2						1	
4	Fruits and vegetables	6	1	5	1	1	2	2	4	1	2	6
		4	1	3			1	1	2		1	4
		2		2			1	1	1		1	2
		1		1					1			1
4	Bread and cereal	8	2		8	2	1	2	5	1	2	
		4	1		4	1	1		2	1		
		2	1		2	1	1		1			
		1		1					1			
Total nutrients in Basic-4 requirements			9	10	20	4	4	3	7	3	6	4

The equivalents for one serving or unit are:

Milk: 1 serving = 1 cup milk, two 1-inch cubes cheddar-type cheese, 1½ cup cottage cheese, 1½ cup ice cream or ice milk.

Meat, beans, nuts, etc.: 1 unit = 1 oz meat or fish, ½ cup legumes, 1 egg, 2 Tb peanut butter.

Fruits and vegetables: 1 serving = ½ cup of vegetable or fruit or a portion as ordinarily served, such as, 1 medium apple, banana, orange, or potato, half a medium grapefruit or cantaloupe, or the juice of 1 lemon.

Bread and cereal: 1 serving = 1 slice of bread, 1 oz ready-to-eat cereal, ½ to ¾ cup cooked cereal, cornmeal, grits, macaroni, noodles, rice, or spaghetti.

Specifically, this group includes: Breads, cooked cereals, ready-to-eat cereals, cornmeal, crackers, flour, grits, macaroni and spaghetti, noodles, rice, rolled oats, and quick breads and other baked goods if made with wholegrain or enriched flour. Parboiled rice and wheat also may be included in this group.

*From Stucky, V.: Don't read this . . . unless, Wichita, Kan., 1976, Diet Teaching Programs, Inc.

POINT EQUIVALENTS*
Vitamins and minerals

One point of calcium equals

1 ounce
American or cheddar cheese

1½ ounce
Sardines

3 ounces
Salmon with bones

½ cup
Almonds
Pudding
Soybean seeds

¾ cup
Collards
Custard
Dandelion greens
Macaroni and cheese
Milk
Rhubarb
Turnip greens
Yogurt
Half and half

1 cup
Baked beans (no pork)
Cottage cheese
Ice cream
Mustard greens
Oysters
Spinach

Portions
Blackstrap molasses, 1½ Tbs
Bread, whole wheat, 7 slices
Bread, white, 8 slices
Cheese pizza (⅛ of 14-inch d),
  1½ pieces
Corn muffins, 2
Pancakes (4-inch d), 3
Parmesan cheese, 3 oz
Processed cheese food, 2 Tbs
Tortilla (not refined corn), 2½
Waffle (7-inch d), 1

One point of niacin equals

1 ounce
Chicken
Salmon
Tuna

*Whole grain or enriched.

2 ounces
Beef
Lamb
Salami
Sardines
Veal

3 ounces
Fish

½ cup
Almonds
Catsup
Chili (no beans)
Mushrooms
Oysters

¾ cup
Beef-vegetable stew
Bulgur*
Dates

Portions
Avocado, ¾
Bagel,* 2
Beef pot pie, ½
Braunschweiger (2-inch d),
  3 slices
Bread,* 4 slices
Buns,* 3
Frankfurter (8/lb), 2
Liver, ½ oz
Blackstrap molasses, 6 Tbs
Muffins,* 4
Peanuts, 2 Tbs
Peanut butter, 1 Tbs
Pizza* (⅛ of 14-inch d),
  4 pieces
Potatoes, 1½
Potato chips, 25
Potatoes, french fried (2 ×
  ½ × ½ inch), 15
Sunflower seeds, 2 oz
Tomatoes, 2
Tortilla,* 8
Waffles,* 4
Shredded wheat biscuits,* 2

One point of thiamin equals

½ ounce
Pork

1 ounce
Salami

2 ounces
Heart
Liver

3 ounces
Lamb

4 ounces
Veal

6 ounces
Chicken
Beef
Fish

¼ cup
Soy beans, cooked

⅓ cup
Cowpeas
Peanuts

½ cup
Beans, dry cooked
Beans, baby limas
Catsup
Collards
Dandelion greens
Green peas
Macaroni*
Noodles*
Nuts (almonds, walnuts)
Orange juice
Rice*
Spaghetti,* cheese and tomato
  sauce

¾ cup
Baked beans (no pork)
Dates
Macaroni and cheese*
Oatmeal*
Spaghetti,* meat balls and
  tomato sauce

1 cup
Asparagus
Beet greens
Bran flakes*
Broccoli
Cauliflower

*From Stucky, V.: Don't read this . . . unless, Wichita, Kan., 1976, Diet Teaching Programs, Inc.

POINT EQUIVALENTS—cont'd
Vitamins and minerals—cont'd

One point of thiamin equals—cont'd

Cocoa
Cornflakes*
Farina*
Grits*
Hominy*
Mustard greens
Pineapple
Potato, mashed
Squash
Tomato
Turnip greens

Portions

Avocado, ½
Bagel, 1
Biscuits,* 2
Bread,* 2 slices
Bun,* hamburger or frank-
    furter, 1
Cantaloupe, 1
Eggs, 2
Frankfurters, 2
Grapefruit, 1
Green peppers, 2
Orange, 1
Muffins,* 2
Pancakes,* 3
Pizza* (⅛ of 14-inch d),
    3 pieces
Pork link, 1
Potato, 1
Potato chips, 30
Potatoes, french fried, 15
Shredded wheat biscuits,* 2
Sunflower seeds, ¼ oz
Sweet potato, 1
Tangerines, 2
Tomato, 1
Tortilla,* 3
Waffle* (7-inch d), 1
Watermelon (4 × 8 inches),
    1 wedge
Wheat germ, ⅓ oz
Yeast, brewer's, ¼ tsp

One point of vitamin C equals
(See also Table 13-3)

⅓ cup
Catsup
Cranberry juice
Tomato

*Whole grain or enriched.

½ cup
Asparagus
Beans, baby limas
Beet and dandelion greens
Berries, not strawberries
Green peas
Pineapple juice
Sauerkraut
Squash, winter
Turnip

Portions

Banana, 1
Cucumber, ½
Liver, 2 oz
Okra, 8
Potato, medium (3/lb), ¾
Potatoes, french fried (2 ×
    ½ × ½ inch), 10
Radish, 6
Watermelon (4 × 8 inches),
    ½ wedge

One point of riboflavin equals

1 ounce
Braunschweiger
Heart

1½ ounce
Parmesan cheese

2 ounces
Blue or Roquefort
Cheese spread

3 ounces
American cheese

4 ounces
Swiss cheese

¼ cup
Almonds

½ cup
Mushrooms

¾ cup
Cottage cheese

1 cup
Broccoli
Chili (no beans)
Cocoa
Collard greens

Custard
Macaroni and cheese*
Milk
Pudding
Turnip greens
Yogurt
Half and half

Portions

Avocado, 1
Bagel,* 3
Braunschweiger (2-inch d),
    3 slices
Bread, white, 6 slices
Buns,* hamburger or frank-
    furter, 5
Cheese food, processed,
    4 Tbs
Eggs, 2
Frankfurters (8/lb), 3
Liver, ⅓ oz
Muffins,* 4
Rolls,* hard, 3
Waffles (7-inch d), 2

One point of iron equals

¼ cup
Prune juice

⅓ cup
Almonds, walnuts

½ cup
Asparagus, canned
Dry beans, cooked
Chili (with beans)
Dates
Peas, split, cooked
Soybeans, cooked
Spinach
Raisins

¾ cup
Chili (no beans)
Cowpeas
Blackeye peas, cooked
Dandelion greens
Spaghetti,* meat balls and
    tomato sauce

1 cup
Bean and pork soup
Beef-vegetable stew

Continued.

POINT EQUIVALENTS—cont'd
Vitamins and minerals—cont'd

One point of iron equals—cont'd

Beet greens
Catsup
Green beans, canned
Green peas
Mustard greens
Spaghetti,* cheese and tomato
   sauce
Tomato juice, canned

Portions
Bagel,* 2
Banana, medium, 3
Beef, 3 oz
Blackstrap molasses, ¾ Tbs
Braunschweiger (2-inch d × ½
   inch), 4 slices
Bread,* white, 4 slices
Bread,* whole wheat, 3 slices
Buns,* frankfurter or ham-
   burger (1½ oz), 3
Chicken, 5 oz
Dill pickles, 3
Eggs, large, 2

Figs, 3
Frankfurters (8/lb), 3
Grapefruit, 2
Heart, 1½ oz
Lamb, 5 oz
Liver, 1 oz
Molasses, 2½ Tbs
Muffins* (3-inch), 4
Oranges, 4
Peaches (dried, halves), 6
Peanut butter, 7 Tbs
Pears, 4
Pizza, cheese (⅛ of 14-inch
   d), 3 pieces
Pork, 3 oz
Potato, 3
Shredded wheat biscuits, 3
Sorghum, 1 Tbs
Soybean seeds, 2 Tbs
Sunflower seeds, 1 oz
Sweet potato, 2
Tomatoes, 3
Tortilla,* 2½

Veal, 3 oz
Waffles* (7-inch d), 2
Watermelon (4 × 8 inches,
   ¹/₁₆ of 2 lb), 1 wedge

One point of vitamin A equals
(See Table 13-4)

Portions
Apricot, 1
Braunschweiger (2-inch d ×
   ¼ inch), 2 slices
Butter or margarine, 3 Tbs
Cheese (made of whole milk),
   3 oz
Eggs, 2
Milk, whole, 3 cups
Parsley, 3 Tbs
Peach (yellow flesh), 1
Peppers, green, 3
Tomato, ¾

*Whole grain or enriched.

Because of the higher intake of saturated fatty acids that usually occurs with increased meat consumption, it may be prudent to decrease meat. Some scientists are advocating an increase in breads and vegetables. Because the foods recommended in Table 13-2 represent only one way to eat, the health professional should attempt to offer other foods with the *same* nutrients to replace those foods that are not accepted by the patient. The boxed material on pp. 138-140 and Tables 13-3 and 13-4 can be used with such a goal in mind. The patient can choose from a variety of foods that will provide the required nutrients. The amount consumed determines how much nutrient is received from the food. All of the foods listed in a given nutrient section are equal to a predetermined simplified unit of measure called a *point.*

Use of the nutrient point lists, boxed material on pp. 138-140, and Tables 13-3 to 13-4 allows for more individualization and gives the patients the opportunity to take responsibility for their own health care.

• • •

Good control requires adequate nutrition.

SECTION II: CALORIE CONTROL

"Kilocalorie" is the correct term for calorie. However, for easier reading, this discussion uses the more common term, "calorie."

Obese patients

Calories do count and may be the most important consideration for patients with diabetes. Obese or overweight patients with diabetes often improve their condition by reducing their weight. The procedure is the same as that for overweight patients who do not have diabetes—that is, to consume 500 calories less than will be utilized

Table 13-3. Number of points in foods high in vitamin C*

Food	Amount†	Number of vitamin C points
Broccoli	1 cup	9
Brussels sprouts	1 cup	9
Cabbage, cooked	1 cup	3
Cauliflower	1 cup	4
Collards	1 cup	6
Kale	1 cup	4½
Mustard greens	1 cup	4½
Pepper, sweet green	1 pod	5
Pepper, mature red	1 ounce	7
Spinach	1 cup	3
Tomato, raw	1 (3-inch d, 2½ inches high)	3
Tomato, canned	1 cup	3
Tomato juice	1 cup	2½
Turnip greens	1 cup	4½
Cantaloupe	½ (5-inch d)	4
Grapefruit	½ (3¾-inch d)	3
Grapefruit juice	1 cup	6
Orange	1 (2⅝-inch d)	4
Orange juice	1 cup	8
Papaya	1 cup	7
Strawberries	1 cup	6
Tangerine	1 (2⅜-inch d)	2
Tangerine juice	1 cup	4

*From Stucky, V.: Don't read this . . . unless, Wichita, Kan., 1976, Diet Teaching Programs, Inc.
†Usually the serving listed will give all the vitamin C that is needed for the day.

Table 13-4. Number of points in foods high in vitamin A*

Food	Amount†	Number of vitamin A points
Apricot, dried	1 cup	7
Beet greens	1 cup	6
Broccoli	1 cup	3
Cabbage, spoon, pakchoy	1 cup	4
Carrots	1 cup	10
Collards	1 cup	8½
Dandelion greens	1 cup	17½
Kale	1 cup	7
Liver	1 ounce	12½
Mustard greens	1 cup	7
Pepper, mature red	1 ounce	4
Pumpkin	1 cup	12
Spinach	1 cup	12
Squash, winter	1 cup	7
Sweet potato	1 cup	14
Turnip greens	1 cup	7
Cantaloupe	½ (5-inch d)	5
Grapefruit juice, red only	1 cup	1
Papaya	1 cup	2½
Peaches, dried	1 cup	3

*From Stucky, V.: Don't read this . . . unless, Wichita, Kan., 1976, Diet Teaching Programs, Inc.
†Usually the serving listed will give all the vitamin A that is needed for the day.

each day. This should result in an average weight loss of about 1 pound each week. Greater weight loss is achieved with increased exercise. If the overweight patients are *not* requiring injected insulin, their carbohydrate, protein, and fat consumption is not as crucial as is the total calorie consumption. For example, the calories could come from margarine or fruit, providing they consumed the recommended total calories for the day and ate a diet that provides necessary protein, vitamins, and minerals. However, if they are using insulin and the physician believes that the insulin should be balanced with an exact amount of consumed carbohydrate or carbohydrate, protein and fat, the exchange of 1 teaspoon of margarine for one serving of fruit is not appropriate, even though both foods contain equivalent calories. Changing margarine for fruit considerably changes the available glucose, carbohydrate, and/or fat in the diet. Correctly changing calories while ignoring the carbohydrate in food prevents consistent intakes of glucose. Inconsistent blood glucose levels affect the dosage of insulin.

Older obese patients who do not require insulin and do not follow the diet, which controls carbohydrate, protein and fat, appear to follow a diet better when counting only calories.

Nonobese patients

Nonobese patients require adequate calories to maintain ideal weight. It is essential that they *never* receive inadequate calories. Too often the person who is not obese receives a prescription of reduced calories because the health professional is accustomed to restricting calories for the obese patient. In the hospital, inactive patients may say they are getting adequate amounts of food. Because of their inactivity and the greater bulk in low calorie foods they may think their diet is adequate. Later they will find it necessary to cheat because their calorie intake is less than their body requires. They have inadequate adipose tissue to compensate for the deficiency in calorie consumption. They soon discover that they feel better when cheating. How can they be convinced to remain on a diet to prevent *later* complications when they were never

Table 13-5. Suggested weights for heights and basal metabolic rates (BMR) of adults*

| Height | | Men | | | Women | | |
| | | Median weight | | BMR (kcal/day) | Median weight | | BMR (kcal/day) |
in	cm	lb	kg		lb	kg	
60	152				109 ± 9	50 ± 4	1399
62	158				115 ± 9	52 ± 4	1429
64	163	133 ± 11	60 ± 5	1630	122 ± 10	56 ± 5	1487
66	168	142 ± 12	64 ± 5	1690	129 ± 10	59 ± 5	1530
68	173	151 ± 14	69 ± 6	1775	136 ± 10	62 ± 5	1572
70	178	159 ± 14	72 ± 6	1815	144 ± 11	66 ± 5	1626
72	183	167 ± 15	76 ± 7	1870	152 ± 12	69 ± 5	1666
74	188	175 ± 15	80 ± 7	1933			
76	193	182 ± 16	83 ± 7	1983			

*Data from Food and Nutrition Board, National Academy of Sciences, National Research Council: Recommended dietary allowances, ed. 8, Washington, D.C., 1974, U.S. Government Printing Office, p. 29. Weights were based on those of college men and women. Measurements were made without shoes or other clothing. The ± refers to the weight range between the 25th and 75th percentile of each height category.

Table 13-6. Adjustment of calorie (kcal) allowance for adult individuals for various body weights and ages, assuming light physical activity*

| Median body weight of men | | Daily calorie allowances according to age | | | Median body weight of women | | Daily calorie allowances according to age | | |
lb	kg	22	45	65	lb	kg	22	45	65
110	50	2200	2000	1850	88	40	1550	1450	1300
121	55	2350	2150	1950	99	45	1700	1550	1450
132	60	2500	2300	2100	110	50	1800	1650	1500
143	65	2650	2400	2200	121	55	1950	1800	1650
154	70	2800	2600	2400	128	58	2000	1850	1700
165	75	2950	2700	2500	132	60	2050	1900	1700
176	80	3050	2800	2600	143	65	2200	2000	1850
187	85	3200	2950	2700	154	70	2300	2100	1950
198	90	3350	3100	2800					
209	95	3500	3200	2900					
220	100	3700	3400	3100					

*Data from Food and Nutrition Board, National Academy of Sciences, National Research Council: Recommended dietary allowances, ed. 8, Washington, D.C., 1974, U.S. Government Printing Office, p. 29.

given adequate calories to meet *present* needs?

Inadequate calories result in damage to the body that is similar to conditions found in people in underdeveloped countries. A nonoverweight person receiving an adequate protein or high-protein diet with inadequate calories will not benefit from the protein intake because the protein will be used to supply calories. The protein-sparing action of calorie foods prevents the body from using exogenous or endogenous protein as a source of calories. Protein cannot be used for essential body functions (other than for energy) if a nonobese person receives deficient calories. No one can tolerate conditions of calorie deficiencies unless they are overweight. Nonobese pa-

tients have a protein deficiency if they have a calorie deficiency.

Kilocalorie requirements

Tables 13-5 and 13-7 from NRC[4] can be used to determine kilocalorie requirements for adults. Calorie allowances based on light physical activity are adjusted for weight, height, age, and sex. The amount of exercise is a very important factor in determining kilocalorie needs. The more recent publication of the NRC[5] advocates use of these tables. To determine calorie needs of an individual, one first uses Table 13-5 to find the median weight that corresponds to the patient's height. One then uses that body weight (in pounds or kilograms) in Table 13-6 to find the number of calories

Table 13-7. Examples of daily energy expenditures of mature women and men in light occupations*

Activity category	Time (hr)	Men, 70 kg		Women, 58 kg	
		Rate (kcal/min)	Total kcal (kJ)	Rate (kcal/min)	Total kcal (kJ)
Sleeping, reclining	8	1.0-1.2	540 (2270)	0.9-1.1	440 (1850)
Very light	12	Up to 2.5	1300 (5460)	Up to 2.0	900 (3750)
Sitting and standing activities, painting trades, auto and truck driving, playing musical instruments, sewing, ironing					
Light	3	2.5-4.9	600 (7520)	2.0-3.9	450 (1890)
Walking on level 2.5 to 3 mph, tailoring, pressing, garage work, electrical trades, carpentry, restaurant trades, working in cannery, washing clothes, shopping with light load, golfing, sailing, playing table tennis or volleyball					
Moderate	1	5.0-7.4	300 (1260)	4.0-5.9	240 (1010)
Walking 3.5 to 4 mph, plastering, weeding and hoeing, loading and stacking bales, scrubbing floors, shopping with heavy load, cycling, skiing, playing tennis, dancing					
Heavy	0	7.5-12.0		6.0-10.0	
Walking with load uphill, tree felling, working with pick and shovel, playing basketball or football, swimming, climbing					
TOTAL	24		2740 (11,500)		2030 (8530)

*Data from Durnin, J.V.G.A., and Passmore, R.: Energy, work and leisure, London, 1967, Heinemann Educational Books Ltd.

allowed in the age column that most nearly approximates the patient's age.

To determine the daily energy need of an individual, one allows for hours of sleep at 90% of the BMR in Table 13-5 and for time periods engaged in various activities as indicated below. Data are expressed as kilocalories per kilogram per hour.

Activity	Men	Women
Very light	1.5	1.3
Light	2.9	2.6
Moderate	4.3	4.1
Heavy	8.4	8.0

For example, a 50-kg woman who is employed as an agricultural worker and maintains a home might have the following needs:

Activity	Time	Energy need
Sleep	8 hours	420 (1399 × 0.9 × ⅓)
Very light	6	390 (1.3 × 6 × 50)*
Moderate	10	2050 (4.1 × 10 × 50)*
Total	24 hours	2860 kcal

Some professionals determine the caloric requirements for ideal weight by using the following: 25 calories per kilogram of ideal weight for a bed patient; 30 calories per kilogram for light work; 35 calories per kilogram for moderate work; 40 calories per kilogram for heavy work.

Others have suggested basal energy needs as being 1 calorie per kilogram of ideal weight per hour (+20% of basal energy needs for very sedentary activity, +40% for moderate activity, and +50% for very vigorous activity).

The caloric requirements for children with diabetes are no different from the calorie requirements of nondiabetic children and vary with age, growth rate, body size, and activity pattern. Commonly the child is given 1000 calories plus 100 calories per year of age. This method of calorie calculation presupposes that all children of the same age are the same size and have the same activity patterns. Such an assumption is, of course, not true because body size

*Kcal × hours × kg.

Table 13-8. Approximate calorie (kcal) needs for children

Age	Calorie needs (kcal/lb ideal weight)
Birth	55
Infant to 1 year	45-50
Children to 10 years	35-40
Adolescent males	22-30
Adolescent females	16-25

at any given age varies tremendously in children as does activity patterns. Table 13-8 gives the average caloric requirements for children of different ages and body weights.

The preferred method for calculating calorie requirements is based on ideal body weight. As a beginning point, 30 calories/pound (about 60 calories/kilogram) is an average requirement. Variations are then made to compensate for differing activity patterns: the active child may need more than 30 calories/pound and the relatively inactive child only 20 to 25 calories/pound. The postpubescent girl who is no longer growing in height usually needs a marked reduction in calories, often 10 to 15 calories/pound (20 to 25 calories/kilogram) to prevent adolescent obesity. The most important aspect of diet control in the child is that the intake should be flexible to allow for the marked changes in activity patterns that occur from day to day and within a given day in the child.[6] Table 13-1 gives recommendations for various ages as suggested by the NRC. NRC also recommends a "level of 120 kilocalories per kilogram at birth to 100 kilocalories per kilogram by the end of the first year. The energy allowances for children of both sexes declines gradually to about 80 kilocalories per kilogram through ten years of age. After age 10, energy allowances gradually decline further to 45 kilocalories per kilogram for adolescent males and 38 kilocalories per kilogram for adolescent females."[4]

Special considerations

The single most important goal in diet therapy for the obese diabetic patient is a control of calories. West[7,8] has reviewed many studies that indicate that a decrease in glucose tolerance occurs with an increase in obesity.

The NRC recommends an increase of calories, proteins, and some other nutrients for the pregnant patient (see Table 13-1). NRC requires an extra allowance of 300 kilocalories each day during pregnancy for most women and an increase of 500 kilocalories for the mother nursing her baby. The diabetic pregnant woman or the diabetic child who is not obese require the same calories that are necessary for those who are not diabetic.

• • •

Good control means normal weight for height. Make dietary changes in kilocalories that will result in ideal weight.

SECTION III: CARBOHYDRATE, PROTEIN, AND FAT CONTROL

After determining the caloric requirements for the patient with diabetes, it may be necessary to determine the amount of carbohydrate, protein, and fat that is necessary within the specified caloric requirements.

The NRC recommends that adults receive 0.8 grams of protein per kilogram of ideal weight. Table 13-1 shows children, infants and prenatal women to have higher requirements. Physical activity does not significantly increase the protein requirement.

Research does not adequately substantiate the need for the extremely large amounts of protein that have been used in diets for the patient with diabetes. Economic situations may demand that less of the costly proteins be used. The protein consumed is often in the form of meat, which might also contain high amounts of saturated fats. If most of the protein requirement consumed is from vegetable ori-gin, it may be necessary to increase the 0.8 gram of protein per kilogram of body weight because it is more difficult to receive complete proteins that offer all the essential amino acids from vegetable sources. Usually the protein intake will account for 10% to 20% of the total calories. As stated earlier a protein deficiency occurs with an extreme deficiency in caloric intake.

Each gram of protein yields 4 calories when metabolized as does each gram of carbohydrate. A gram of fat yields 9 calories when metabolized.

Generally, a daily amount of fat that yields 30% to 35% of the total caloric intake is most often recommended. The trend is to recommend that 30% of the total calories be fat calories. The trend to decrease saturated fatty acids is discussed in Section VIII, p. 173.

Much controversy is related to the amount of carbohydrate required in a diet for the patient with diabetes. Recent research demonstrates improved glucose tolerance with high carbohydrate diets, provided the caloric requirement is met and obesity does not occur. Recent writings appear to recommend that 40% to 60% of total daily calories should be carbohydrate calories. The average proportion of carbohydrate calories consumed by people in the United States is 45%. The increase of carbohydrate intake does not appear to increase insulin requirements of diabetic individuals if the intake of calories or simple refined sugars is not increased. The increasing of total carbohydrate intake is a trend toward increasing starch, not glucose.[8] Desirable results are not always reported when the increase of carbohydrate is achieved with refined sugar. The more rapidly absorbed disaccharides and monosaccharides (such as sucrose, lactose, glucose, and fructose) are not the favored carbohydrates. The favorable results that have been reported generally involve starches as the principle carbohydrate.

Careful experimentation with children over the years at the University of Iowa and the University of Missouri[6] has shown that the most important factors in dietary management are the total calories and the distribution of the calories according to the absorption pattern of the insulin and the activity pattern of the child. It has been found that the composition of the diet is less important than the quantity and distribution. There are certain limitations on the composition of the diet in children, but within these limitations, composition is of little importance. The calories from protein in the diet of children should not be restricted below 12% of the total calories, or the child will not grow properly. Also, it is probably not wise to exceed 25% of the calories as protein calories because of palatability and economics. A diet of 20% of calories as protein calories is most commonly used and is a good diet for any growing child—diabetic or not. The fat content probably should vary between 30% and 35% of the calories. A fat content above 40% or below 30% is not very palatable. Diets varying the carbohydrate content between 35% and 65% of the calories have been used. If the insulin is adjusted properly, the total number of calories is correct, and the food distributed properly with the insulin and exercise patterns, control can be realized with diets of varying amounts of carbohydrate.

A rational approach to the problem of simple sugar is needed. It must first be realized that the sugar intake of western society, especially American and British society, far exceeds that of the rest of the world and probably far exceeds that which is wise or prudent. The diet of the diabetic child should be no different from the diet that any other healthy growing child *should* eat. Many feel that the small amounts of sugar commonly used in cooking can be allowed, and concentrated sweets should be allowed on special occasions. There are those who advocate no simple sugars[9,10]; however, there are those who have found that sugar is well tolerated under certain circumstances.[11-15] As the trend for lower fat consumption becomes prevalent, it is obvious

Table 13-9. Diabetic diets in terms of exchanges*

Diet number	Kcal	Milk	Vegetable	Fruit	Bread	Meat	Fat
1	1200	2	4	3	4	5	1
2	1500	2	4	3	6	6	4
3	1800	2	4	3	8	7	5
4	2200	2	4	4	10	8	8
5	1800†	4	4	3	6	5	3
6	2600†	4	4	10	7	11	
7	3500†	4	4	6	17	10	15
8	2600	2	4	4	12	10	12
9	3000	2	4	4	15	10	15

*Composition is shown in Table 13-10.
†For children.

that carbohydrate intake will increase. However, an increase of simple refined sugar is generally not recommended.

Tables 13-9 to 13-11 show examples of diets with various caloric levels and distributions. Some indicate 40% to 50% of caloric intake from carbohydrate and 30% to 40% from fats. Table 13-12 shows 60% of total caloric intake from carbohydrates according to the points system. The points system is explained in Section V.

Often obese non-insulin-dependent patients with diabetes can be given a calorie-restricted diet without too much concern for the ratio of carbohydrate, protein, and fat. If they eat an adequate diet that offers the essential nutrients except calories, they may or may not determine the fat or carbohydrate intake when controlling the calories.

Some professionals insist that the practice of considering only calories and ignoring carbohydrate, protein, and fat when making replacements, exchanges, or substitutions could result in tremendous variations in blood glucose levels (available glucose). Some professionals determine the available glucose contribution of food and meals. They make replacements for foods not eaten and/or require that meals offer a certain ratio of available glucose. This same result, with less calculation, can be

Table 13-10. Kilocalories and suggested carbohydrate, protein, and fat distribution
for diabetic diets*

Diet number	Kcal	Carbo-hydrate (gm)	Protein (gm)	Fat (gm)	Diet number	Kcal	Carbo-hydrate (gm)	Protein (gm)	Fat (gm)
1	1200	135	85	40	33	2000	205	100	90
2	1500	165	80	60	34	2000	255	100	65
3	1800	195	90	75	35	2100	215	105	95
4	2200	235	100	100	36	2100	270	105	65
5	1800	190	85	80	37	2200	220	115	95
6	2600	260	110	125	38	2200	280	115	70
7	3500	385	145	150	39	2300	235	115	100
8	2600	265	120	120	40	2300	295	115	75
9	3000	310	125	140	41	2400	240	120	105
10	500	50	40	15	42	2400	300	115	80
11	600	60	45	20	43	2500	250	125	110
12	700	70	55	25	44	2500	315	125	80
13	800	80	55	30	45	2600	260	130	115
14	900	90	65	35	46	2600	330	125	85
15	1000	105	65	35	47	2700	275	135	115
16	1100	110	65	45	48	2700	340	135	85
17	1200	120	70	50	49	2800	280	135	125
18	1200	150	65	40	50	2800	350	135	95
19	1300	130	70	60	51	2900	295	140	130
20	1300	165	65	40	52	2900	365	135	100
21	1400	135	70	65	53	3000	305	140	135
22	1400	175	75	45	54	3000	380	145	100
23	1500	150	70	70	55	3100	315	140	140
24	1500	190	75	50	56	3100	390	145	105
25	1600	160	70	75	57	3200	320	145	145
26	1600	200	85	55	58	3200	405	155	110
27	1700	170	80	80	59	3300	335	150	150
28	1700	215	85	55	60	3300	415	161	125
29	1800	180	85	80	61	3400	340	155	155
30	1800	225	85	60	62	3400	420	165	120
31	1900	190	85	90	63	3500	350	165	160
32	1900	240	90	65	64	3500	435	165	125

*Adapted from Kansas Dietetic Association: Kansas diet manual, Topeka, 1972, The Association.

Table 13-11. Suggested ways of using points for special diets

Calories		Carbohydrates		Proteins		Fats	
Content of label	Points	Content of label (gm)	Points	Content of label (gm)	Points	Content of label (gm)	Points
19-56	½	4-11	½	3-6	½	2-3	1
57-94	1	12-19	1	7-9	1	4-6	2
95-131	1½	20-26	1½	10-13	1½	7-9	3
132-169	2	27-34	2	14-17	2	9-11	4
170-206	2½	35-41	2½	18-21	2½	12-13	5
207-244	3	42-49	3	22-25	3	14-16	6
245-281	3½	50-56	3½	26-29	3½	17-18	7
282-319	4	57-64	4	30-33	4	19-21	8
320-356	4½	65-71	4½	34-37	4½	22-23	9
357-394	5	72-79	5	38-41	5	24-26	10
395-431	5½	80-86	5½	42-45	5½	27-28	11
432-469	6	87-94	6	46-49	6	29-31	12
470-506	6½	95-101	6½	50-53	6½	32-33	13
507-544	7	102-109	7	54-57	7	34-36	14
545-581	7½	110-116	7½	58-61	7½	37-38	15
582-619	8	117-124	8	62-65	8	39-41	16
620-656	8½	125-131	8½	66-69	8½	42-43	17
657-694	9	132-139	9	70-73	9	44-46	18
695-731	9½	140-146	9½	74-77	9½	47-48	19
732-769	10	147-154	10	78-81	10	49-51	20
770-806	10½						
807-844	11						

Table 13-12. Some sample diets—protein and fat fractions are ignored

KIND OF DIET (APPROX.) K CAL.**		MEAL I	Bread-Cereal	Fruit	Milk	Fat Points*	MEAL II	Bread Group	Vegetable-Fruit	Milk	Meat-Substitute	Fat Points*	SNACK	MEAL III	Bread Group	Vegetable-Fruit	Milk	Meat-Substitute	Fat Points*	SNACK	Bread Group	Vegetable-Fruit	Milk	Meat-Substitute	Fat Points*
3000 - MAN	♦ 29	6	4	1	1	7*	6	3	3		2	6*	4	7	3	4	3	3	15*	6	1	3	2	1	9*
	♥ 7	1					2						3	3						1					
	■ 40	7					6						3	15						9					
2100 - WOMAN	♦ 20	4	2	1	1	4*	4	1	2	2	1	4*	3	5	3	3	2	3	12*	4	1	2	1	1	6*
	♥ 6	1					1						2	3						1					
	■ 28	4					4						2	12						6					
2900 - BOY (10-18)	♦ 29	6	4	1	1	7*	6	1	3	3	1	6*	4	7	3	4	2	1 2	14*	6	1	3	2	1	9*
	♥ 6	1					3						3	3						1					
	■ 39	7					6						3	14						9					
2300 - GIRL (10-18)	♦ 22	4	2	1	1	4*	4	1	2	2	1	4*	4	5	3	2	2	1 2	12*	5	1	2	2	1	7*
	♥ 6	1					1						3	3						1					
	■ 30	4					4						3	12						7					
1500 - PRE-SCHOOL	♦ 15	3	1½	1	½	5*	3	½	2	1		½ 3*	3	3	1	1½	1	½ ½	6*	3	½	2	½	½	4*
	♥ 3	¼					½						½	1						½					
	■ 21	5					3						3	6						4					
2400 - SCHOOL AGE	♦ 24	5	3	1½	1	7*	5	1	3	1½ ½	½	5½*	4½	5	1½	2½	2	½ 1	8½*	4½	1	2½	1	1	6*
	♥ 4½	½					1						¼	1½						1					
	■ 32	7					5½						5	8½						6					
1200 - REDUCING	♦ 10	3	2		1	3*	3	2	2	1	2	4*	1	4	3	2		3	7*	2	1	1		1	2*
	♥ 7	1					2							3						1					
	■ 16	3					4							7						2					

* Fat Points are found in foods such as meat, used in cooking or used as spreads, salad dressings, etc. "Meat-Sub." = ♥ in foods.

** ♦ = to kcal. ÷ 100 = 60% of cal. as cho. cal.   ■ = to kcal. + $\frac{kcal}{3}$ ÷ 100 = 30% of cal. as fat cal.

From Stucky, V.: Kernel Beard says, Wichita, Kan., 1976, Diet Teaching Programs, Inc.

SOME DIET EXAMPLES *

Diet No.*	Kcal	CHO points	PRO points	FAT points		Diet No.*	Kcal	CHO points	PRO points	FAT points
13	800	5½	7	12	1 CHO point =	39	2300	15½	13	40
14	900	6	8	14		40	2300	19	12	30
15	1000	7	8	14	◇ =	41	2400	16	14	42
16	1100	7½	8	18		42	2400	19½	12	32
17	1200	8	8	20	12-18 grams	43	2500	16½	14	44
18	1200	10	7	16		44	2500	20½	13	32
19	1300	8½	8	24		45	2600	17	15	46
20	1300	11	7	16		46	2600	21½	13	34
21	1400	9	8	26		47	2700	18	15	46
22	1400	11½	8	18		48	2700	22½	14	34
23	1500	10	8	28		49	2800	18½	15	50
24	1500	12½	8	20	1 PRO point =	50	2800	23	14	38
25	1600	10½	8	30		51	2900	19½	15	52
26	1600	13	9	22	♡ =	52	2900	24	14	40
27	1700	11	9	32		53	3000	20	15	54
28	1700	14	9	22	7-9 grams	54	3000	25	15	40
29	1800	12	9	32		55	3100	20½	15	56
30	1800	14½	9	24		56	3100	25½	15	42
31	1900	12½	9	36		57	3200	21	16	58
32	1900	15½	10	26		58	3200	26½	16	44
33	2000	13½	11	36		59	3300	22½	16	60
34	2000	16½	11	26	1 FAT point =	60	3300	27	17	46
35	2100	14	12	38		61	3400	23	17	62
36	2100	17½	11	26	▭ =	62	3400	27½	17	48
37	2200	14½	13	38		63	3500	23	18	64
38	2200	18½	12	28	2-3 grams	64	3500	28½	17	50

$$\left(\text{CHO points} + \frac{\text{CHO points}}{2} \right) \times 10 \text{ grams of carbohydrate} = \text{grams of carbohydrate}$$

PRO points × 8 grams of protein = grams of protein $\left(\dfrac{\text{FAT points}}{4} \right) \times 10$ grams of fat = grams of fat

60% of kcal as CHO calories is equal to
kcal ÷ 100

30% of kcal as FAT calories is equal to
$$\left(\text{kcal} + \frac{\text{kcal}}{3} \right) \div 100$$

*Odd number diets—approximately 40% kcal as carbohydrate; 40% as fat. Even number diets—approximately 50% kcal as carbohydrate; 30% as fat.

*From Stucky, V.: Easy way diet, Wichita, Kan., 1976, Diet Teaching Programs, Inc.

Table 13-13. Composition of exchange lists in grams and points

Exchanges	Carbohydrate		Protein		Fat		Kcal	Calorie points
	Gm	Points	Gm	Points	Gm	Points		
Milk								
Nonfat	12	1	8	1	0	0	80	1
Whole	12	1	8	1	10	4	170	2
Vegetable (nonstarchy)	5	⅓	2	0	0	0	25	⅓
Fruit	10	⅔	0	0	0	0	40	½
Bread, cereal, pasta,								
starchy vegetables	15	1	2	0	0	0	70	1
Meat								
Lean	0	0	7	1	3	1	55	⅔
Medium fat	0	0	7	1	5	2	75	1
High fat	0	0	7	1	8	3	100	1¼
Fat	0	0	0	0	5	2	45	½

accomplished by controlling carbohydrate, protein, and fat.

A more liberal approach for the patient using insulin requires a control of only calories and carbohydrate and recommends that meals and snacks always contain some protein. Of course, if calories and carbohydrate intake are controlled, there will be an automatic control of fat intake. For the usual diabetic person, the Committee on Food and Nutrition of the American Diabetes Association accepts carbohydrate calories that are 45% or more of total caloric intake.[2]

• • •

Liberal amounts of carbohydrate are usually well tolerated if calorie intake is regulated appropriately.[7,8,16-18]

SECTION IV: MEAL DISTRIBUTION

Dr. Kelly M. West [7,8] says that it is generally agreed that well-spaced feedings of modest size are more desirable than large feedings. Most professionals agree that simple concentrated carbohydrates such as sucrose should usually be limited or avoided.[19] When initiating control, it is also generally accepted that the patient receiving insulin needs a day-to-day consistency in intake of calories and perhaps carbohydrate, protein, and fat. The calories would be changed with variations in exercise.

Not everyone agrees about the necessity for day-to-day consistency in the *ratio* of calories and/or carbohydrate, protein, and fat for each feeding. Many health professionals consider the individual patients, their activity or exercise, and the insulin dosage when determining meal distribution. One should not become too involved in changing diet when it affects the patient's life-style if insulin dosage could be changed with less affect on the life-style.

Non-insulin-dependent obese patients

The obese patient not requiring insulin who considers the total caloric intake does not need to be greatly concerned with meal distribution, or ratio distribution of calories. However, an increased number of small feedings that remain within the total calorie allowance has been shown to benefit some obese patients. Overeating, that is, consuming more than one third of the total calories at one meal, is not generally recommended. In general, it is best to eat three or more times a day, thereby avoiding feast or famine.

Insulin-dependent patients

One of the following alternatives may be used to regulate meal patterns for the insulin-dependent patient:

1. Divide calories throughout the day according to individual need, activity, and kind and

amount of insulin being taken. Research reveals that some health professionals recommend a distribution of calories as $2/10$, $3/10$, and $4/10$, respectively for the three meals, with a snack containing $1/10$; others advocate calorie distributions of $1/5$, $2/5$, $2/5$ or $1/3$, $1/3$, $1/3$, with calories for snacks and bedtime feedings taken from calories alloted for the meals. For the patient requiring long-acting insulin, some suggest using calorie divisions of $1/7$, $2/7$, $2/7$, and $2/7$. Jackson, Guthrie, and others[20] have observed good results with calorie divisions of $4/18$, $2/18$, $5/18$, $1/18$, $5/18$, and $1/18$ for children.

2. Use one of the above described ratios to divide carbohydrates for each meal in addition to (or rather than) calories because carbohydrate division more closely affects hypoglycemia and hyperglycemia. Distribute some protein and fat in each meal and snack according to the patient's desires.

3. Control the time of meals and snacks, but distribute the food according to individual food habits rather than adhering to a ratio. The physician then determines the insulin dosage to meet these individual circumstances. An acceptable daily meal pattern is planned for consistency but not divided according to a specific ratio. (Close supervision is required to determine a correct insulin dosage for the specific meal pattern.)

Most health professionals feel that the patient receiving insulin requires regularity of food intake and exercise. Most agree that the food intake should be spaced to consider the activity and kind and dosage of insulin in order to avoid hypoglycemia. Controversy occurs because not all agree to a fixed ratio of distribution of meals. It is important to consider the patient's lifestyle. Often the teenager and adult patient rebel at the "food division of meals" more than any other aspect of their diet. More consideration to food habits, with the physician adjusting the insulin dosage accordingly, may result in greater patient acceptance and eventually greater stability of blood glucose levels. For the rebellious person, perhaps a ratio distribution of carbohydrate, rather than calories, would be more acceptable. Such a person would continue controlling caloric intake, however, only carbohydrates would be distributed

according to a ratio based upon insulin dosage and blood glucose levels.

A more liberal approach would be a distribution of calories only and the suggestion of some protein at each meal and snack. Patients using insulin are required to have a bedtime feeding that consists of carbohydrate, protein, and generally some fat. The fat and protein are taken so that the supply of glucose extends over a longer period of time, thus impeding a very low blood glucose curve through the night.

It is crucial that meals and snacks are so distributed for the patient requiring insulin that intermittent hypoglycemia does not occur. The best program can be determined by observation and adjustment of the regimen best suited for each individual.

• • •

Some form of regularity of food intake appears to promote ease of metabolic management particularly in those patients receiving insulin therapy.

SECTION V: TOOLS

Effective nutritional care for the patient with diabetes demands accurate measuring or weighing of food. When patients are first learning the diet, weighing or measuring assists them in better recognizing correct size of servings and in realizing the importance of accuracy. Once they have learned the diet, estimations can be made. From time to time, patients should reevaluate their estimated serving size by again weighing or measuring. It is especially necessary to remeasure or weigh food if trouble develops or if the family has become careless.

Developing a planned diet

The planned diet becomes the tool that allows the professional to execute the appropriate nutritional care that meets the patient's individual needs. The methods for developing a meal pattern (diet) are as follows:

1. *Control calories only.* Foods containing re-

fined sugar can also be restricted. This method is most effective for the older obese non-insulin-dependent patient with diabetes. Diets A or B (below) can accomplish this objective.

2. *Control carbohydrate, protein, and fat as well as calories.* This method is effective for the patient requiring insulin. This diet controls the intake of carbohydrate, protein, and fat, thus allowing a specific amount of glucose to react with a specific amount of injected insulin. Diets A or B (below) can accomplish this objective.

3. *Control of calories and carbohydrates.* This method is also effective for the patient requiring insulin. Generally refined sugar is restricted or not allowed.

The following kinds of meal patterns (diets) can accomplish the above programs.

Diet A: "Exchange Lists for Meal Planning." This plan includes *six food groups.* The list of foods in one group contain somewhat similar amounts of carbohydrate, protein, fat, and nutrients. Patients are told to choose a food from a group if their diet plan indicates they may have a food from that group. They may exchange one food for another food within the same allowed group. Most foods that contain refined sugar are omitted. Exchange lists have been recommended since 1950 by the American Dietetic Association and the American Diabetes Association. (See Tables 13-9, 13-10, and 13-13.)

Diet B: Points system. This plan includes *three nutrient groups* and *one calorie group.* The protein, fat, carbohydrate and calorie composition of specific amounts of foods is considered. The most used plan allows for control of only 2 groups, calories and carbohydrates. Depending on the individual plan, the patient chooses any foods that will give the prescribed amount of calories and carbohydrates (and protein and fat if regulated). All refined sugar can be restricted if desired. Normal nutrition information for an adequate diet is acquired with this system. (See Tables 13-11 to 13-13 and boxed material on pp. 153-155 and pp. 157-158. Use the information in Section VIII to control the saturated fat and cholesterol in a diet.)

Calculating a diet prescription

This procedure for calculating a diet is used with the exchange list or points system and is based on 45% of calories from carbohydrate, 20% of calories from protein, and 35% of calories from fat. The same procedure could be developed for any ratio desired. The following steps are taken:

Step I

Patient's desirable weight:

$$\text{_____} \div 2.2 \text{ lb} = \text{_____ kg}$$

For a bed patient	25 kcal/kg
For light work	30 kcal/kg
For medium work	35 kcal/kg
For heavy work	40 kcal/kg
For weight loss (obese)	20-25 kcal/kg

To determine calories per kilogram according to activity of patient:

$$\text{_____ kcal} \times \text{_____ kg} = \text{_____ total kcal}$$

Step II

To convert calories to grams, divide calories by caloric values of each of nutrients.

To determine carbohydrate:

$$\text{Total kcal _____} \times 0.45 = \text{_____} \div 4 = \text{_____* gm carbohydrate}$$

To determine protein:

$$\text{Total kcal _____} \times 0.20 = \text{_____} \div 4 = \text{_____* gm protein}$$

To determine fat:

$$\text{Total kcal _____} \times 0.35 = \text{_____} \div 4 = \text{_____* gm fat}$$

Some interesting facts exist when one calculates the diet using the point system. If the number of fat points are the same as the number of calorie points, the fat calories are 30% of total calories. If the number of carbohydrate points are $\frac{1}{2}$ the number of calorie points, the carbohydrate calories supply 40% of the total calories. If the number of carbohydrate points is $\frac{1}{100}$ of the calories, the carbohydrate calories are 60% of the total calories. The health professional will find it necessary to decide which tools to use. (See p. 149.)

Using the exchange list. To calculate a diet prescription by using the exchange

---

*Round off to nearest 5.

POINT EQUIVALENTS OF THREE NUTRIENT GROUPS *
Protein, fat, and carbohydrate

Nutrition number rule

In the chart below find the number in the first column that corresponds with the serving size that equals ONE POINT as shown in this table.

Run your finger (or eye) to the right of the number until you come to the column that represents the *amount* of the food that was *eaten*. The number in the column representing the amount that you ate gives the number (or fraction) of points of a nutrient contained in the amount of the food that was consumed or is planned to be eaten.

(All amounts must be in the same household unit.)

Amount shown to equal one nutrient point	Amount eaten or planned to be eaten				Amount shown to equal one nutrient point	Amount eaten or planned to be eaten			
	¼	½	¾	1		¼	½	¾	1
¼	1.0	2.0	3.0	4.0	2	0.13	0.25	0.38	0.5
⅓	0.75	1.5	2.25	3.0	2½	0.1	0.2	0.3	0.4
½	0.5	1.0	1.5	2.0	3	0.08	0.17	0.25	0.33
¾	0.33	0.67	1.0	1.33	3½	0.07	0.14	0.21	0.29
1	0.25	0.5	0.75	1.0	4	0.06	0.13	0.19	0.25
1⅓	0.19	0.38	0.56	0.75	4½	0.06	0.11	0.17	0.22
1¼	0.2	0.4	0.6	0.8	5	0.05	0.1	0.15	0.2
1½	0.17	0.33	0.5	0.67					

One point of protein equals ♡

1 ounce
  Cheese (hard)
  Meat

1½ ounce
  Luncheon meat

¼ cup
  Cottage cheese

⅓ cup
  Nuts (almond, cashew, and
    walnut)
  Soybeans, cooked

½ cup
  X Custard
  Dry beans, cooked

1 cup
  Bulgur
  Milk
  X Pudding

1⅓ cup
  X Ice cream

Portions
  Bacon, 3 slices
  Bread, 2¼ to 4 slices

Egg, 1
Frankfurter, 1
Peanuts, 3 Tbs
Peanut butter, 2 Tbs
Pizza (⅛ of 14-inch d or a
  5½-inch piece), 1 piece
Pumpkin seeds, 1⅓ oz
Sunflower seeds, 1 oz
Tortillas, 5
Waffle (7-inch d), 1

One point of fat equals ▭

¼ cup
  Milk
  Potato, mashed
  X Pudding

¼ ounce
  Cheese (hard)
  X Chocolate candy

⅓ ounce
  Meat with fat

1 ounce
  Lean meat

Portions
  Avocado (3⅛-inch d), 1/12

Bacon, ½ slice
Bagel, 1
Biscuit, 1
Bread, 2½ slices
Butter or margarine, ½ tsp
Cream, 1 Tbs
X Doughnut, ½
Egg, ½
Frankfurter (⅛ lb), 1/6
Half and half, 1½ Tbs
X Ice cream, 1/6 cup
Mayonnaise, 1 tsp
Muffin, ½
Nuts, ½ Tbs
Oil, cooking fat, or lard,
  ½ tsp
Olives, 3 large
Peanut butter, 1 tsp
Pizza (⅛ of 14-inch d),
  ½ piece
Potato chips, 3
Potato, french fried (2 ×
  ½ × ½ inches), 4
Roll or bun, 1
Salad dressing, 1 tsp
Seeds, 1/5 oz
Soybeans, cooked, ¼ cup

From Stucky, V.: *Don't read this . . . unless*, Wichita, Kan., 1976, Diet Teaching Programs, Inc.   *Continued.*

POINT EQUIVALENTS OF THREE NUTRIENT GROUPS—cont'd
Protein, fat, and carbohydrate—cont'd

One point of carbohydrate equals ◇

BREAD, CEREAL, AND STARCHY FOODS

1 tablespoon
  X Honey
  X Jam, jelly, marmalade
  X Molasses
  X Sugar

¼ cup
  X Baked beans, no pork
  X Catsup

⅓ cup
  Dry beans, cooked
  Rice
  Split peas, dry or cooked

1 cup
  Milk

½ cup
  Bran flakes
  Cowpeas
  Grits, hominy
  X Ice cream
  Macaroni
  Noodles
  Peanuts
  Spaghetti
  X Sweetened gelatin
  Wheat flakes

¾ cup
  Cream of wheat
  Oatmeal

Portions
  Bagel, ½
  Biscuit (2-inch d), 1
  Bread, 1 slice
  X Chocolate candy, 1 oz
  X Cookie, vanilla wafer, 6
  Cornbread (3-inch d), 1
  Cracker, graham (2½-inch
    square), 3
  Cracker, round, thin, 7
  Cracker, saltine, 7
  X Doughnut, cake, 1
  Flour, 2½ Tbs
  Muffin (3-inch d), 1
  Pancakes (4-inch d), 1½
  Peanut butter, 5 Tbs
  X Pie, 2 crust, 1 oz

Pizza (14-inch d), ¹/₁₆
Popcorn, plain, 3 cups
Potato chips, 15
Pretzel, thin twist, 3
Roll or bun (1 oz), 1
Tortilla, 1
Waffle (7-inch d), ½

FRUITS AND VEGETABLES

⅛ cup (2 Tbs)
  Raisins

⅓ cup
  Corn, canned
  Grape juice
  Prune juice

½ cup
  Apple juice
  Apricot nectar juice
  Applesauce
  Cherries, red sour
  Orange juice
  Peach nectar juice
  Pineapple juice
  Potato, mashed
  Squash, winter

¾ cup
  Blackberries
  Blueberries
  Grapes, European type
  Green peas
  Pineapple

⅔ cup
  Parsnips

1 cup
  Beets
  Dandelion greens
  Grapes, American type
  Onion
  Papaya
  Pumpkin
  Raspberries
  Rutabagas

1¼ cup
  Strawberries

1½ cup
  Brussels sprouts

Carrots
Cranberries
Collards
Egg plant
Sauerkraut
Tomato, cooked
Tomato juice

2 cups
  Beans, green, wax
  Bean sprouts
  Broccoli
  Mushrooms
  Spinach
  Squash, summer
  Turnips

2½ cups
  Asparagus
  Cabbage, cooked
  Mustard greens

3 cups
  Beet greens
  Cabbage, raw, shredded
  Cauliflower
  Chard
  Turnip greens

4 cups
  Kale

½ medium
  Banana
  Cantaloupe (5-inch d)
  Grapefruit (3¾-inch d)
  Honeydew melons (5-inch d)
  Mango
  Pear (3 × 2½-inch d)
  Sweet potato (5 × 2 inches)

¾ medium
  Potato (⅓ lb) or 1 smaller

Portions
  Apricots, dried, 6 halves
  Celery (8-inch stalks), 8
  Cherries, sweet, 15 large,
    25 small
  Escarole, 12 large leaves
  Okra (⅝ × 3 inches), 24
  Onions, young green,
    18 small

POINT EQUIVALENTS OF THREE NUTRIENT GROUPS—cont'd
Protein, fat, and carbohydrate—cont'd

One point of carbohydrate equals ◇ —cont'd

Peppers, green, 4 shells
Radish, 60 medium
Watercress, 1 lb
Watermelon (4 × 8-
  inch wedge), ½ wedge

1 medium
  Apple (⅓ lb)
  Avocado (3⅛-inch d)
  Corn (5 × 1¾ inches)
  Lettuce, head (4¾-inch d)
  Orange (2⅝-inch d)

1½ medium
  Peach (2-inch d) (¼ lb)
  Tangerines (2⅜-inch d)
  Tomato (2¼ × 3-inch d)

2 medium
  Cucumbers (7½ × 2 inches)
  Nectarines
  Plums (2-inch d)

3 average
  Apricots (¹/₁₂ lb)

Carrots (1 × 5½ inches)
Dates

4 medium
Prunes

1 large
Fig

Table 13-14. The exchange list

Steps in calculation	Food group	Exchanges allowed per day	Carbohydrate (gm)	Protein (gm)	Fat (gm)
Step 1 —→	Nonfat milk	2	24	16	
	Vegetable	3	15	6	
	Fruit	4	40		
Step 2 — — — — — — — — — — — —→			79		
Step 3 — — — — — — — — — —→			(200* − 79 = 121)		
Step 4 —→	Bread, cereal, and starchy vegetables	8	120	16	
Step 5 — — — — — — — — — — —→			199 — — — —→	38	
Step 6 — — — — — — — — — — — — — — — —→				(70* − 38 = 32)	
Step 7 —→	Low-fat meat, protein rich	5		35	15
Step 8 — — — — — — — — — — — — — — —→				73 — — —→	15
Step 9 — — — — — — — — — — — — — — — —→					(50* − 15 = 35)
Step 10 —→	Fat	7			35
					50

*Total daily allowance: carbohydrate—200, protein—70, and fat—50.

list, take the following steps and refer to Table 13-14:

1. Determine needs for milk, fruit and vegetables. Calculate the carbohydrate, protein, and fat in the servings allowed.
2. Total the carbohydrate of items (milk, vegetable, fruit) in Step 1. (24+ 15 + 40 = 79)
3. Subtract the amount in Step 2 from the daily total allowance of carbohydrate grams. This is the remaining amount of carbohydrate that will be allowed in "bread exchanges." (200 − 79 = 121)
4. Divide the answer in Step 3 by 15 (carbohydrate grams in bread). This answer is the number of "bread exchanges" that will be allowed. (121 ÷ 15 = 8)

5. Add up the protein grams in all the above required foods that have carbohydrate (16 + 6 + 16 = 38)
6. Subtract the answer in Step 5 from the total grams of protein required. (70 − 38 = 32)
7. Divide the answer in Step 6 by 7 (protein grams in meat). This answer is the number of "meat exchanges" that will be allowed. (32 ÷ 7 = 4½ or 5)
8. Add up the fat grams in all of the above foods that are allowed. (15 + 0 = 15)
9. Subtract the answer in Step 8 from total grams of fat required. (50 − 15 = 35)
10. Divide the answer in Step 9 by 5 (fat grams in "fat exchanges"). This answer is the number of "fat exchanges" that will be allowed. (35 ÷ 5 = 7)

After total amounts of each food group are determined, arrange meal pattern in one of the following ways:

- Whenever possible arrange the meal pattern according to patient's food habit questionnaire (see pp. 163-166). The pattern should always provide an adequate diet.
- Use Table 13-13 to determine calories in each food group. Arrange food groups into meals and snacks that will provide the desired calorie ratio. Include protein in each meal and snack.
- Use Table 13-13 to determine grams of carbohydrate in each food group. Arrange food groups into meals and snacks that will provide the desired carbohydrate ratio. Arrangement of protein and fat foods should consider the patient's desires provided some protein and fat is in every meal and snack.

Using the points system. The points system is a simplified method, based on the calories, carbohydrate, protein, and fat content of food. It stresses the importance of calories, fat, carbohydrate, and protein points for each meal and snack, as included in the prescribed diet plan. Foods are not placed into the 6 food exchange groups. Instead, they are placed into four categories —calories, carbohydrate, protein, or fat, depending on the foods' actual composition. Each food is assigned a point value under these categories. Using the system

is similar to purchasing foods from a grocery store: As it is necessary to know the cost of food to be purchased, it is necessary to know point values of food to be consumed.

METHOD I. This method applies to patient's controlling calories, as well as carbohydrate, protein, and fat distribution.

1. Divide allowed grams of *carbohydrate* by 15 to obtain the total allowed carbohydrate points for the day. (200 ÷ 15 = 13 carbohydrate points)
2. Divide allowed grams of *protein* by 8 to obtain total allowed protein points for the day. (70 ÷ 8 = 9 protein points)
3. Divide allowed grams of *fat* by 2.5, or multiply by 0.4 to obtain total allowed fat points for the day. (50 × 0.4 = 20 fat points)

METHOD II. This method applies to patients who can ignore carbohydrate, protein, and fat distribution in their diets and are only concerned with the calories. Counting 20 calorie points is easier than counting 1500 calories. (See p. 157.)

Divide total allowed calories by 75 to obtain total allowed calorie points for the day.

This method can be used with Step 1 of Method I for those controlling calories and carbohydrates only. (See p. 158.)

After the total amount of points for each food is determined, arrange in meal pattern in one of the following ways:

- Use patient's food habit questionnaire (p. 163) and arrange a somewhat similar meal pattern that offers some carbohydrate, protein, and fat, or calorie points, at each meal and snack. Patterns should always provide adequate nutrition.
- Determine the distributions for meals and snacks. Multiply the allowed calorie points (or carbohydrate, protein, and fat points, depending on individual method of control) for the day by the fraction that represents the desired ratio. The answers are the number of points of each nutrient that will represent the desired ratio for each meal or snack. If only carbohydrate and calories are multiplied by the proper fraction and protein and fat are distributed in each meal and snack as desired,

CALORIE POINT DIET*

Counting calorie point foods is the secret of YOUR SUCCESS.

The Calorie Point Chart tells the total number of points that are right for you. (Notice: The total number of points corresponds with the total number of calories that you should eat during the day.)

Next—when you know the number of points that are right for you, choose your food for the day from the lists of foods with calorie points. These lists of foods are in the FOOD POINT CHART. To make this diet work for you—choose each food, add up the points for the foods you eat so you have the exact total number of points that the Calorie Point Chart said was right for you. It is like adding up the cost of food when you go to the grocery store.

1. EAT EVERYTHING ON THE DIET
2. KEEP A RECORD OF ALL FOODS EATEN
3. WEIGH ONLY ONCE A WEEK

Approximately 75 calories equal 1 calorie point.

$$\text{Calories in food} + \left(\frac{\text{Calories}}{3}\right) \div 100 = \frac{\text{Calorie}}{\text{Points}}$$

CALORIE POINT CHART

Conversion of Calories to Calorie Points

Calories in Diet Order	Calorie Points in Diet in One Day	Calories in Diet Order	Calorie Points in Diet in One Day
800	11	1900	25½
900	12	2000	26½
1000	13½	2100	28
1100	14½	2200	29½
1200	16	2300	31
1300	17½	2400	32
1400	18½	2500	33½
1500	20	2600	35
1600	21½	2700	36
1700	22½	2800	37½
1800	24	2900	38½
		3000	40

FOOD POINT CHART—**EXAMPLE**

Food	Amount	Calorie Points
Rolls:		
Cloverleaf. Pan commercial	1 (1 ounce)	1
X Danish Pastry	1 (1 ounce)	1½
Hard	1 (1½ ounces)	2
Sauces:		
X Barbecue	4 Tablespoons	1
X Chili	4 Tablespoons	1
X Chocolate	2 Tablespoons	1
X Soy	9 Tablespoons	1
Tartar	1 Tablespoon	1
X Tomato Catsup	4 Tablespoons	1
White. Medium	4 Tablespoons	1½
X Worcestershire	2 Tablespoons	½
Salad Dressing:		
Blue Cheese	2 Tablespoons	2
French	2 Tablespoons	1½
Italian	2 Tablespoons	2
Mayonnaise	2 Tablespoons	2½
Mayonnaise Type	2 Tablespoons	1½
Thousand Island	2 Tablespoons	2
Soup:		
Canned, condensed. ready-to-serve		
Prepared with equal amount of milk		
Cream of Chicken	1 cup	2½
Cream of Mushroom	1 cup	3
Tomato	1 cup	2½
Prepared with equal amount of water		
Bean with Pork	1 cup	2½
Beef Broth, Bouillon		
Consomme	1 cup	½
Beef Noodle	1 cup	1
Cream of Chicken	1 cup	1½
Cream of Mushroom	1 cup	2
Split Pea	1 cup	2
Tomato	1 cup	1
Vegetable Beef	1 cup	1
Vegetarian	1 cup	1
Dehydrated. dry form		
Chicken Noodle	1 package	3
Onion Mix	1 package	2
Spaghetti, Cooked	½ cup	1
Spaghetti, with		
Meat Balls. Tomato Sauce	1 cup	3½
Tomato Sauce, Cheese	1 cup	2½
Spanish Rice	½ cup	1
X Sherbet	½ cup	1½
Sugar:		
X Brown	2 Tablespoons	1½
X Powdered	1½ to 2 Tablespoons	1
X Lump, white	3 (1¼x¾x⅜)	1
X White	2 Tablespoons	1
Sunflower Seed Kernel	1 ounce	2
Syrup:		
X Chocolate	4 teaspoons	1
X Sorghum	1 Tablespoon	½
X Table	1 Tablespoon	1
Tomato Paste	1 ounce	½
Tomato Puree	6 Tablespoons (3½ ounces)	½
Tortilla. Plain	1 (6″ diam.)	1

*From Stucky, V.: Easy way diet, Wichita, Kan., 1976, Diet Teaching Programs, Inc.

the result will be only a specific carbohydrate and calorie ratio for each meal and snack.

Using exchange list and points system. Any food within a list can be substituted or exchanged for any other food in that list (see Appendix F). For example, in List 4 in Appendix F, Bread exchanges, 1 slice of bread, ½ cup of cooked cereal, ½ cup rice, ½ cup of mashed potato, and many other listed foods would contain 15 grams of carbohydrate. Persons told to eat from the bread list choose any food in the amount that the list states. Persons told to eat 2 exchanges from the bread list could choose any 2 foods in the amounts shown or 2 exchanges of one food. Two slices of bread would be the equivalent of 2 bread exchanges as would 1 slice of bread and ½ cup of mashed potato. This same procedure is followed for the fruit list, which is equivalent to 10 grams of carbohydrate. Persons may choose a food from their allowed list, but they cannot choose a food from other lists unless they are told to do so. For example, if an exchange from the fruit list is required they cannot decide to choose a food from the bread list.

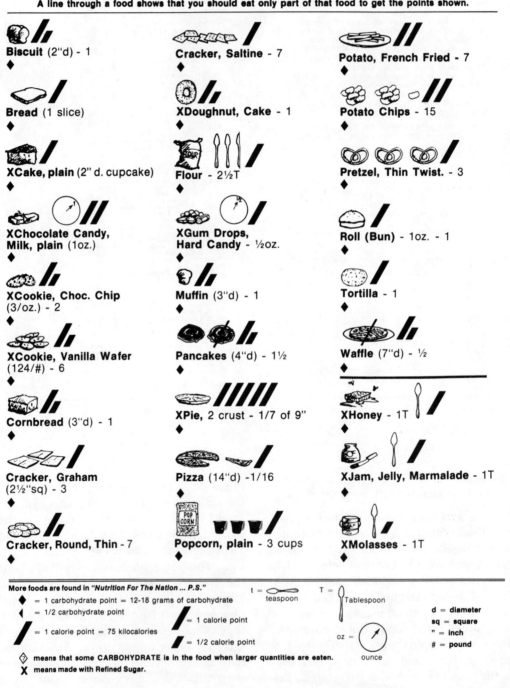

CALORIE POINTS / IN FOODS

Ask if you are to choose foods that **do not** have X's because foods with an X have refined sugar.
TOO MUCH SUGAR IS HARMFUL.
A line through a food shows that you should eat only part of that food to get the points shown.

Biscuit (2"d) - 1

Bread (1 slice)

XCake, plain (2" d. cupcake)

XChocolate Candy, Milk, plain (1oz.)

XCookie, Choc. Chip (3/oz.) - 2

XCookie, Vanilla Wafer (124/#) - 6

Cornbread (3"d) - 1

Cracker, Graham (2½"sq) - 3

Cracker, Round, Thin - 7

Cracker, Saltine - 7

XDoughnut, Cake - 1

Flour - 2½T

XGum Drops, Hard Candy - ½oz.

Muffin (3"d) - 1

Pancakes (4"d) - 1½

XPie, 2 crust - 1/7 of 9"

Pizza (14"d) -1/16

Popcorn, plain - 3 cups

Potato, French Fried - 7

Potato Chips - 15

Pretzel, Thin Twist. - 3

Roll (Bun) - 1oz. - 1

Tortilla - 1

Waffle (7"d) - ½

XHoney - 1T

XJam, Jelly, Marmalade - 1T

XMolasses - 1T

More foods are found in "Nutrition For The Nation ... P.S."

◆ = 1 carbohydrate point = 12-18 grams of carbohydrate

◀ = 1/2 carbohydrate point

／ = 1 calorie point = 75 kilocalories

／ = 1 calorie point

／ = 1/2 calorie point

◇ means that some CARBOHYDRATE is in the food when larger quantities are eaten.

X means made with Refined Sugar.

t = teaspoon

T = Tablespoon

oz = ounce

d = diameter
sq = square
" = inch
= pound

From Stucky, V.: Calorie point diet, Wichita, Kan., 1976, Diet Teaching Programs, Inc.

FOOD with Points Amount - Preparation	etc.	PT.

Date   Name   Total

MORE:	etc.	PT.

POINTS — I should have_____
POINTS — I did have_____
EVALUATION: Date_____

Circle the appropriate—
O.K.   Ate too much   Ate too little

MY SUCCESSES:

WHAT I PLAN TO DO:

MEAL PATTERN AND FOOD RECORD: EXCHANGE LIST*

Meal pattern completed by professional

Amount	Your meal plan

Amount   *Your meal plan*

BREAKFAST:
- 1 — Milk from list 1 (Kind skim)
- 1 — Fruit exchange from list 3
- 2 — Bread exchange from list 4
- 1 — Meat exchange from list 5
- 2 — Fat exchange from list 6
- ____ Coffee or tea (any amount)

MIDMORNING SNACK:
- ____ Milk from list 1 (Kind ___)
- 1 — Fruit exchange from list 3
- 1 — Bread exchange from list 4
- 1 med. fat — Meat exchange from list 5
- ____ Fat exchange from list 6

LUNCH OR SUPPER:
- 1 — Milk from list 1 (Kind skim)
- 1 — Vegetable exchange from list 2
- ____ Fruit exchange from list 3
- 2 — Bread exchanges from list 4
- 2 — Meat exchanges from list 5
- 3 — Fat exchanges from list 6
- ____ Coffee or tea (any amount)

AFTERNOON SNACK:
- ____ Milk from list 1 (Kind ___)
- ____ Fruit exchange from list 3
- ½ — Bread exchange from list 4
- 1 med. fat — Meat exchange from list 5
- ____ Fat exchange from list 6

DINNER OR MAIN MEAL:
- ½ — Milk from list 1 (Kind skim)
- 1 — Vegetable exchange
- 1 — Fruit exchange from list 3
- 2 — Bread exchange from list 4
- 3 — Meat exchanges from list 5
- 2 — Fat exchange from list 6
- ____ Coffee or tea (any amount)

BEDTIME SNACK:
- ½ — Milk from list 1 (Kind skim)
- ____ Fruit exchange from list 3
- ½ — Bread exchange from list 4
- ____ Meat exchange from list 5
- ½ — Fat exchange from list 6

Daily food intake recorded by patient

Amount and preparation

BREAKFAST:
- Nonfat milk, 1 cup
- Orange juice, ½ cup
- Bread, 2 slices
- Ham, 1 oz
- Margarine, 2 tsp

MIDMORNING SNACK:
- Apple, 1 small
- Bread, 1 slice
- Peanut butter, 2 Tbs

LUNCH:
- Nonfat milk, 1 cup
- Lettuce
- Tomatoes, ½ cup
- Bread, 2 slices
- Roast chicken, 2 oz
- Margarine, 3 tsp

AFTERNOON SNACK:
- Bread, ½ slice
- Cheese, 1 oz

DINNER:
- Nonfat milk, ½ cup
- Beets, ½ cup
- Peach, 1 medium
- Baked potato, 1 small
- Bread, 1 slice
- Roast beef, 3 oz
- Margarine, 2 tsp

BEDTIME:
- Nonfat milk, ½ cup
- Graham cracker square, 1
- Margarine, ½ tsp

*1800 calories, 45% carbohydrates, calories divided $\dfrac{4\text{-}2\text{-}5\text{-}1\text{-}5\text{-}1}{18}$.

MEAL PATTERN AND FOOD RECORD: POINTS SYSTEM*

Meal pattern completed by professional	Daily food intake recorded by patient

Total daily allowance: 24 calorie [CAL] points with 13½ carbohydrate [CHO] points. Milk, meat, and/or fat at each feeding.

Time of meal or snack	Points	Amount and preparation	CHO point	CAL point
1ST MEAL: 7 AM	= 5½ CAL	BREAKFAST:		
	= 3 CHO	Skim milk, 1 cup	1	1
		Orange juice, ½ cup	1	1
		Bread, 1 slice	1	1
		Poached egg, 1		1
		Margarine, 3 tsp	___	1½
			3	5½
SNACK: 10 AM	= 2½ CAL	MID-MORNING SNACK:		
	= 1½ CHO	Apple, 1 medium	1	1
		Bread, ½ slice	½	½
		Cheese, ⅔ oz	___	1
			1½	2½
2ND MEAL: NOON	= 7 CAL	LUNCH:		
	= 3½ CHO	Skim milk, 1 cup	1	1
		Bread, 2 slices	2	2
		Roast chicken, 4 oz		2
		Margarine, 3 tsp		1½
		Lettuce, Tomato, ¾ medium	½	½
			3½	7
SNACK: 2:30 PM	= 1 CAL	AFTERNOON SNACK:		
	= 1 CHO	Saltines, 3	½	½
		Skim milk, ½ cup	½	½
			1	1
3RD MEAL: 6 PM	= 7 CAL	DINNER:		
	= 3½ CHO	Skim milk, 1 cup	1	1
		Bread, 1 slice	1	1
		Peas, 6 Tbs	½	½
		Baked potato, 1 small	1	1
		Tossed salad, 1 Tbs French dr.		1
		Roast beef, 2 oz		2
		Margarine, 1 tsp	___	½
			3½	7
SNACK: 9 PM	= 1 CAL	BEDTIME:		
	= 1 CHO	Skim milk, ½ cup	½	½
		Graham crackers, 1½	½	½
			1	1

*1800 calories, 45% carbohydrates, calories and carbohydrates divided $\frac{4\text{-}2\text{-}5\text{-}1\text{-}5\text{-}1}{18}$.

It is the responsibility of the health professional to develop a meal pattern that offers foods that meet the diabetic person's requirements of vitamins and minerals as discussed in Section I. (An additional 3 to 4 cups of milk are required for children and pregnant and lactating mothers.)

If the point system is used, the patient chooses any foods that will not give more or less than the required points. When they have consumed the foods that contain the correct number of points, they cannot have any more food that has that kind of point. The amount of food that is eaten tells how many points one gets from the food and the patients are told never to eat foods with more or less than their required points. It is similar to buying food at a grocery store: When the money is gone, no more food can be purchased. For example, 1 slice of bread or 1 cup of skim milk gives 1 calorie point. If the person is required to eat foods that give 2 calorie points, both of these foods could be eaten. One ounce of meat or 1½ tomatoes are other foods that each have one calorie point. The list of equivalents is endless and can include the foods that have nutrition labeling. (Detailed exchange lists appear in Appendix F, and points lists are available from the Kansas Wheat Commission.) Patients are also told to always obtain adequate vitamins and minerals, as discussed in Section I.

ADVANTAGES OF TEACHING ABOUT NUTRIENTS

Because diabetes is an error in metabolism, it is desirable to teach diabetic individuals about nutrients. If persons with diabetes are to receive any benefits from the nutrition labeling of purchased food, they should learn to interpret the information in terms of their individual diets. Moreover, if they are to be considered as near normal as possible, they should receive the same nutrition information given to normal children or adults.

In accepting persons with diabetes as human beings with psychological and social needs, health professionals must consider their life-style and obtain their food history (see questionnaire on p. 166). Food questionnaires are easier to consider for developing meal patterns when teaching about nutrients. If persons with diabetes are beset with economic problems or other unavoidable situations and cannot afford a specific food group, they must have the opportunity to learn how to choose other available foods with the same nutrients.

If persons with diabetes are to recognize fads and fallacies, it is essential that they become intelligent about nutrients. Nutrients can be taught with the exchange list system, but the emphasis is less on "nutrients" than on "food groups." If one decides to teach nutrients by points, the material is offered at no cost.[20] Books are available for anyone requiring larger print, pictures of food, and a simplified diet. The books offer possibilities for the older person who needs a less rigid diet with little control or the person who has severe diabetes and needs the most accurate control. The intelligent person who does not have a sight problem may prefer to carry the free, pocket-size editions. Even if one decides that the points system is not superior to the exchange list system for all patients, the points system can be used for certain patients. Moreover, a new technique sometimes gives a patient a "new lease on life." The public continually responds to new diets for obesity; they may respond accordingly to new diets for diabetes, especially if these new programs are approached with enthusiasm by the professionals.

The "Exchange Lists for Meal Planning" is available at a reasonable cost from the American Diabetes Association or American Dietetic Association. Other versions that are more sophisticated and expensive are also available.[21] The diets explaining the point system are available free of charge from the Kansas Wheat Commission.[20] Tools, other than the diet booklet, that are used for nutritional care include posters, charts, booklets, cook books,

FOOD HABIT QUESTIONNAIRE*

Phone: _____ Physician: _____

Name: _____ Birthdate: _____ Date: _____

Address: _____ Spouse: _____

How much milk do you drink a day? _____

What type? Regular _____ Low fat (2%) _____ Skim _____

Do you use butter? _____ or margarine? _____

If margarine, what brand? _____

How many times a week do you eat the following foods?

Name of food	Never	Less than once a week	1 to 3 times a week	3 to 5 times a week	5 or more a week	How much is a serving?
Hard cheese						Slices
Eggs						Whole
Steak, hamburger, porkchops, etc.						Ounces
Liver or other organ meats						Ounces
Cold cuts, hot dogs, sausage, or luncheon meats						Pieces or ounces
Pizza						Pieces
Sweet rolls, doughnuts						Whole pieces
Cookies, cakes, pies, pastries, etc.						Pieces
Deep-fat fried foods—french fries, etc.						
Soda pop, cola, etc.						Cups
Alcoholic beverages—beer wine, whiskey, etc.						Cups or ounces
Milk shakes, ice cream, etc.						Cups
Candy						Pieces
Potato chips						Whole pieces

*Developed with assistance from the American Heart Association, Kansas Chapter, Wichita.

Continued.

FOOD HABIT QUESTIONNAIRE—cont'd

Name of food	Never	Less than once a week	1 to 3 times a week	3 to 5 times a week	5 or more a week	How much is a serving?
Crackers						Whole pieces
Hot breads						Whole pieces
Vegetables—dark green or deep yellow						Cups
Citrus fruits or tomato						Cups
Potato						Whole
Sweet potato, yam						Whole
Corn, hominy						Cups
Other fruits and vegetables						Cups
Fish (including tuna)						Ounces
Chicken, turkey, birds						Ounces
Lean meat						Ounces
Cottage cheese or yogurt						Cups
Macaroni, noodles, spaghetti						Cups
Cereal cooked						Cups
Cereal, dry						Cups
Corn bread, biscuits, muffins, waffles, pancakes						Whole pieces
Breads, buns, tortillas						Slices
Jelly, honey, jam, syrup						Tbs*

*Tablespoons.

FOOD HABIT QUESTIONNAIRE—cont'd

Name of food	Never	Less than once a week	1 to 3 times a week	3 to 5 times a week	5 or more a week	How much is a serving?
Bacon, salt pork						Slices
Peanut butter						Tbs
Baked or cooked beans—pinto, navy, butter, lima						Cups
Salad dressing, mayonnaise						Tbs
Rice, grits						Cups
Popcorn						Cups
Catsup						Tbs
Molasses, sorghum						Tbs
Chili						Cups
Sweetened gelatin or popsicles						Cups
Cream						Tbs
Soup						Cups
Soup with milk						Cups
Olives, pickles						Pieces

slides, filmstrips, cassette tapes, and workbooks. Most of these help the patient understand the dietary treatment. It is desirable that the patients be seen individually and that they also attend classes. Materials that allow the patients to become involved in self-learning at their own pace are usually very effective. The health profes-

sional using these materials can spend the time with the patients in more valuable and constructive ways. (See Section VII for further explanations on teaching.)

It is essential that some of the self-learning tools force the patients to become involved with their diet booklets. It is necessary that they use the booklets as they learn

DIET HISTORY

Name: _____

Please record all foods you have eaten during the last 24 hours. It may be easier if you try to work back from your last meal. Thank you.

Food	How cooked	Amount (Specify portion, size, and amount.)	Place (Specify home or type of restaurant.)
Morning			
Afternoon			
Evening			

so that they will become accustomed to the diet booklet, which is their most important tool for survival. It is vital that they discover that the diet booklets are indispensible for finding answers as they are learning and when they are home. Using the books when learning makes diet control easier at home. (At the end of this chapter is a partial list of where materials for learning may be obtained.)

• • •

Use a meal pattern that is accurate, acceptable, and understood.

SECTION VI: INDIVIDUALIZATION

"How much would you like to eat?" This is a good question to ask patients from time to time. It is easy for health professionals to maintain that they are individualizing the dietary treatment of diabetic patients: their activities, insulin needs, age, and height are usually taken into account. However, it is not uncommon to ignore their individuality and life-styles. There is no one else like the specific person being treated, and if one ignores the psychosocial needs of that particular person, there may be repercussions. Thus, it is necessary to ask oneself, "How much of this unique person is it essential to change—and perhaps destroy?"

To determine the patients' life-style and cultural background one must determine their food habits and customs, their economic status, their likes, dislikes, and other food idiosyncrasies, and their facilities for obtaining and preparing food. After one obtains this history, it is essential to use it effectively. It should be used for a greater knowledge of the patient and for a point of reference when discussing food habits. Moreover, it should be used to the fullest extent for developing "that person's" daily meal pattern. Health professionals should actually compute their patients' nutritional intakes and make only the changes that are necessary for their vitamin and mineral requirements (as discussed in Section I). This means more than requiring all patients to

eat the Basic-4 food groups. For example, it is necessary to determine whether the patient is getting the same amount of B vitamins, protein, and iron from other foods before one forces the addition of meat. In other words, changes should be made only when vital.

Health professionals have pretended that they "adjust the diet to suit the patient"; at the same time, they are saying, "If we tell you to eat a fruit and 3 ounces of meat, we intend for you to do just that." The patient may quietly think, "I can't afford those foods and did not have them in the house every day last week." Too often when one obtains a patient food questionnaire (history) it becomes an exercise in futility. On the other hand, it is unforgiveable that occasionally a history is not obtained. Too often meal patterns are developed or given to the patient without determining the patient's pattern of living because there "isn't time" to acquire a food questionnaire. Time can be saved if the history is self-administered. For example, a 55-year-old patient with poor eyesight was given a food questionnaire to be completed before her first visit with the nutritionist. She said that her grandchild would help her at home. She returned with a many-folded paper in her purse. It had been completed with a purple crayon. Her grandchild took several days to help her because the grandmother kept recalling more information that she thought "we needed to know." This same self-administered questionnaire was given to another patient who remained in the hospital for 1 day of tests. Because he left before the questionnaire was obtained, he mailed it to the hospital saying, "I think you might want this about me." Many repetitions of such incidents substantiate the fact that a self-administered questionnaire is better than none. However, a history is not worthwhile if it is not used effectively by the health professional. (See Food habit questionnaire on p. 163-166.)

If we are to be effective, it is necessary to ask the following questions:

1. Are the dietary restrictions that we demand a necessity? Treatment and demands placed on the patient should vary, depending on many individual factors, such as kind and amount of insulin, time of injection, patient's blood glucose level, and other symptoms.
2. Is the blood glucose level stable, moderately labile, or severely labile?
3. What planned exercise can be executed?
4. Which patients can control their diabetes by eating foods that will not supply more than their allowed calories?
5. Is it necessary to give the patient the exchange list when an easy and flexible calorie point diet will meet the patient's needs?
6. Which patients require a control of carbohydrate only?

Some patients may require control of only calories and carbohydrate. The young patient and the patient with severe diabetes may be required to control calories as well as carbohydrate, protein, and fat intake with a rigid meal distribution. It is critical that the health professionals, as a team, determine which type of control is necessary. Economic situations should be considered. If the questionnaire reveals an adequate diet that supplies all the essential amino acids, vitamins, and minerals, it seems unnecessary to require *more* of an expensive food such as meat.

• • •

Meal pattern changes are made if they are necessary.

SECTION VII: DIET COUNSELING

Etzwiler[3] has said that 6 to 12 hours of diet instruction are necessary to continue diet counseling at the level of the patient's understanding. The National Health Survey found that 50% of the patients were below the 9th grade educational level.[1]

The salesmen who sell the most cars believe that their cars are the best. The health professionals who counsel their patients must believe a diet is necessary if they are to be effective in diet counseling. Dr. Joslin once said that the first person who sees the patient is "master of the patient's fate" because this person will convey an attitude toward diet that the patient will accept as his own. Health professionals are qualified to become valuable components in motivating the patient to follow a diet providing they place emphasis on the person and *not* the person's diet. For example, the nurse can help the patient succeed because the nurse's education is people oriented not diet oriented.

Frustrations are many! However, the trend toward higher carbohydrate diets can make it easier to develop habits that are continued forever. Using a diet that gives many choices usually results in more success. A meal pattern that is easy and simple and that closely matches the patient's lifestyle may bring more success.

Health professionals should attempt to develop a relationship with a patient that allows honesty. Problems should be discussed before they occur. It is better for the patient to say, "I am going to a party, I wonder what I will do" rather than go to the party, cheat, and inform no one. The teenagers who continually eat candy and know how to increase their insulin before an office visit have not developed an honest relationship with the health professionals. If the rigid authority that directed children in their earlier years is continued through the teen years, it may be directly responsible for later nonconformity. The adolescent should be considered as a young adult. Extreme authority from professionals should be replaced with encouragement and guidance toward acceptance of increased responsibility as young adults. An ideal relationship can develop more easily after the patient receives the facts. It is important to remember that teaching begins when telling stops.[22] Learning and motivation will result when the health professionals:

1. Help the patients to *obtain facts.*
2. Help the patients to *use facts.*
3. Help the patients to *assume responsibility.*

Guiding patients

To obtain facts. Patients can acquire facts from books and pamphlets, hospital tray service, movies, filmstrips, slides, posters and other visuals, cassette tapes, teaching machines, workbooks, and the educator/counselor. Usually greater learning occurs when the patients become involved in acquiring facts. When a cassette tape gives the facts and the patients use the facts at the same time to answer questions in a workbook, the professionals can use their time to consider each patient's invididual needs. The professional in a health setting motivates the patients by listening to them, helping them solve their own problems, and maintaining an adult-to-adult relationship. This helps the patients accept their own responsibility after they receive the basic facts. This kind of professional relationship is more easily maintained if the patient receives the facts from *other sources*. Cassette tapes can give the facts as well as involve the patient in answering questions. The professionals use their time to add the human element, which is based on each patient's individual needs. Nutritional interviews become much more exciting and fun when this type of education is used.

To use facts. If the patient is allowed to go home, keep records of food intake, and return with these records, the health professional can effectively evaluate the patient's ability to use facts. The records of the patient's food consumption at home serves as an effective feedback tool similar to a test. (See boxed material on p. 159.) Tests and questions can also be administered from time to time for evaluation of the patient's learning.

To assume responsibility. Cassette tapes can be effective in giving facts. Table 13-15 shows the scores of individuals with diabetes: the experimental group were instructed by cassette tape and then tested; the control group were instructed by a dietitian and then tested. The individuals instructed by tape had consistently higher scores than those instructed by a dietitian without a tape.

Motivating the patient

Perhaps it is easier to motivate the patients if the professional has not also played the role of a "tape recorder." One helps the patients to make their own plans and asks them to consider these plans as a contract.

Briefly, the individual encounter with patients consist of the following:

1. Give nutritional (dietary) facts. Use self-study tapes so that patients become involved in learning the facts, or use other media for teaching facts.
2. Immediately after the patients hear the tape or receive the facts, ask them: Can you follow the diet? What do you think of the diet? Will you keep records of your daily food intake and *return* in one week?
3. When patients return, ask: How did you get along with your diet? How well did you follow the diet? May I see your food records? What are you going to do after today?
4. Upon examining food records, you will note the errors by asking: Do you understand this part of the diet? Should you hear the tape again? What can you change to improve the next weeks' food records?
5. On all returns ask for food records. Speak about these records and about patient's successes with diet and patient's plans for future dieting. Accept patients *and* their records. Discuss plans (contracts).
6. Help patients decide to attend group sessions.

Table 13-15. Mean scores (number correct, possible 50) for pretest and posttest made by control and experimental patients with diabetes

Individuals with diabetes	Experimental group		Control group*	
	Pretest	Posttest	Pretest	Posttest
Newly diagnosed	17.0	46.71	19.0	33.0
Diabetes for over a year	41.5	48.25	40.63	45.5

*Taught by a dietitian. Experimental group saw dietitian after posttest.

Listening. To be a good counselor one needs to be a good listener. Patients may want more information, but they do not want advice. Usually people want to talk and do not want to listen. As a counselor one must listen skillfully and successfully. The art of listening can be learned. If patients do not follow their diets, one must find out why. The principle goal should be to find all of the reasons for their lapses and to know what is implied by their "excuses." It is important to ask how they feel about the diet.

Forming adult-to-adult relationships. If counseling is to be effective, the professional must speak as an adult conversing with another adult. The professional who speaks down to, or tells the patients what to do, is talking as a parent to a child. If a parental role is taken, the patients are likely to react as children and will probably not tell the counselor what they are doing wrong. Instead they will let the counselor try to find out their secrets. (This becomes a good game of hide-and-seek.)

Solving problems. Health professionals can help the patients determine their problems but cannot solve them. It is important that patients do not settle for a solution only because they felt that they should. It must be *their* solution, and if they and the health team (or counselor) investigate a number of solutions, they must choose the one that is most desirable for them.

Involving the family. Group sessions seem to be effective for most patients, not only for instructional purposes but for sharing experiences. Weinsier and others[23] report success with an effective multifaced educational group in Boston. After the initial visit, their group, which involved the family, was seen for a series of 14 visits (generally at 2-week intervals).

It is important that the family be included in the counseling. The family should offer support to the patient and adequately understand the patient's condition and treatment.

It is surprising that some families refuse to offer support to the patient. Some continually tempt the patient with large amounts of inappropriate food. Others let the patient know that the diet is a burden to them. Some parents refuse to learn the methods of offering a variety of foods for different situations. They refuse to make the extra effort that would help a child feel "less different" and more able to "cope." Often at a diet counseling session with parents of a child who has diabetes, one hears a member of the family blaming the spouse who has "diabetes in his family." A discussion of true facts and the many feelings that the family have is necessary before positive reinforcement toward diet is available from the family.

Modifying behavior and changing habits. Emphasis on behavior modification in groups has shown good results both for obese patients and for some patients having a great amount of difficulty adhering to a diet.

When clients plan their diet with the health professional and say, "This is the way I will eat," it may be possible to adjust insulin dosage and time to meet the demands of such a diet. If not, then it is essential that the counselor and the client make the necessary dietary changes. Some motivational techniques may have to be employed. The client may become more flexible and able to adjust to a diet in a behavior modification group. Many behavior modification groups that are successful focus less on diet and more on actions. This could be easy to accomplish with the "point system,"[24] which focuses on the person, not on diets.

Fear motivates only a few. The reasons for following a diet should be the patient's reasons. They should verbalize *all* of their reasons. Every visit with the patient should focus on actions that affect eating. It is imperative that the patients participate in activities other than eating and change their exposure, susceptibility, and response to food. Alternate actions should be enjoyable and readily available. Reading, watching television, and other activities should never accompany eating. Change in activities should be developed in small steps at a time to become habits. It is very helpful to discuss the patient's reasons for eating and determine the antecedent that brings on the desire to overeat. The health professional can better help patients by asking them to keep records of their actions related to eating, their successful actions related to change, the food they ate, and their plans (contracts) for new actions. Success is more readily attainable to the patient who recognizes the three R's—Responsibility, Record keeping, and Replacing undesirable eating behaviors with other behaviors that can become habits.

• • •

The patients assist in the development of a meal pattern and favorable actions that are appropriate to their life-style. Patients are members of the team.

SECTION VIII: PROBLEMS

When patients feel that they are considered as individuals, one may hear them make the following comments: "I can't afford the diet. I have a garden with vegetables, and we always have bread; but we do not always have fruit or meat." Others may say, "I want to go with my friends on a canoe trip in the North Woods, and we will have staples such as flour and beans." "As editor of a large city newspaper, I want to travel all over the world. On the African safari, my food was different." "I'm tired of my diet because it is the same old thing." "I want to use nutrition labeling found on food packages." "I can't see the diet very well, because the print is too small." "I don't read well." Problems like those expressed demand that the health professionals collaborate closely with all members of the team, including the patient. They must know where to go to get answers to problems and teach the patient where to go to get questions answered.

The above statements from patients do not always require the same response. Children, pregnant women, and persons with severe diabetes on accurately controlled diets will get different responses from the professional than persons with mild diabetes or obesity. More professionals are saying that for the less rigid diet the points system allows for flexibility and easily considers the patient's economic situation or temporary changes in life-style. The traveler, using the exchange list first, can determine the carbohydrate, protein, and fat content in foods and then attempt to place the food within one or more of the six food groups. The points in the foods are determined when one uses the points system. A similar situation occurs when one is using the nutrition labeling found on packages of food.

When using the points system with nutrition labeling, one calculates according to Methods I and II on p. 156. (See Table 13-11.)

$$\text{Calorie points} = \left(\text{calories} + \frac{\text{calories}}{3}\right) \div 100,$$
$$\text{or calories} \div 75$$

$$\text{Carbohydrate points} =$$
$$\left(\text{grams of CHO} - \frac{\text{grams of CHO}}{3}\right) \div 10,$$
$$\text{or grams of CHO} \div 15$$

$$\text{Protein points} = \text{percentage of protein}$$
$$\times 0.08, \text{ or grams of protein} \div 8$$

$$\text{Fat points} = \text{grams of fat} \times 0.4, \text{ or grams of fat} \div 2.5$$

Some companies or industries offer lists showing the exchanges represented in their food products. Other organizations have compiled lists of a variety of foods offered on the market. Cultural foods from the South are included in the food exchanges in a publication by Davidson and Goldsmith.[21] If one uses points, companies also have lists showing the calories, as well as grams of carbohydrate, protein, and fat in their products. Consumer Guide has developed a book showing the carbohydrate, protein, fat, and calories of many foods.[25] The procedures using nutrition labeling also apply to special dietetic foods. Labeling may help people discover that some special foods are less desirable in nutrient content than the less expensive regular foods. Dietetic foods can be unnecessarily expensive and misleading. It is essential to calculate into the diet all of the flour, sorbitol, and other forms of carbohydrate in the special diet food. Often waterpacked fruits are cheaper than the dietetic fruits.

The person who has poor eyesight, lacks education, or reads English poorly, may find the pictures and large bold print of the point system an advantage.[20]

Eating away from home becomes a problem for some patients. This, like all the other problems, is solved differently, depending on the individuals and the severity of their disease. When eating out, those patients not receiving insulin can omit foods from previous meals to allow for additional food with equivalent calories. Those receiving insulin cannot delay meals or exchange food from one meal to another because of the potential threat of hypoglycemia. When an invitation is issued for dinner, patients can tell the hostess of their special needs. When ordering food at a restaurant, patients may patronize those establishments that cater to their needs and who are willing to disclose the composition of some of their foods. One large pizza establishment informs their customers of the calories, carbohydrate, protein, and fat in their pizzas. This practice is becoming more prevalent. Often a cafeteria may be an easier place to choose the food that meets the patient's needs. Many diets and cookbooks give suggestions for food preparation or selection, such as: the steak should be prepared without fat or oil; meats and vegetables should not be fried and should be prepared without fat, gravy, or cream sauce or other sauces; it is best to eat fruit for dessert.

When ill or lacking an appetite, patients are reminded of the necessity of always eating food that supplies glucose. Tolerated foods may be found that contain appropriate carbohydrate, protein, or fat. The composition of foods such as eggnog (see Table 13-16) and cream soup can be determined for inclusion in the diet or meal pattern. Some pediatricians restrict fat for gastroenteritis.[6] If insulin has been taken, the carbo-

Table 13-16. Point and exchange method of calculating a recipe to use with illness

Eggnog	CAL points	CHO points	Exchanges
1 egg	1		1 Meat, medium fat
1 cup whole milk	2	1	1 Milk + 2 Fat
4 Tbs sugar	2+	3	5 Fruit
TOTAL	5+	4	

Table 13-17. Emergency foods equal to approximately 15 gm of carbohydrate*

Food	Amount	Weight (gm)
Fruit	1½ exchanges from fruit exchange	
Cola beverage	⅔ cup	155
Gingerale	¾ cup	185
Ice cream	½ cup	65
Gelatin dessert (sweetened)	½ cup	120
Orange juice (all varieties)	½ cup	125
Other carbonated beverages	¼ cup	125
Sugar	4 tsp	15

*Very approximate. Use this information when food is being refused by a person receiving insulin.

hydrate or calorie equivalent of the diet should be consumed. In an emergency, the carbohydrate can be obtained from foods such as sweetened beverages. Health professionals should impress upon patients who use insulin the necessity of a daily supply of glucose even though they may be vomiting or have diarrhea. Under circumstances of illness, there is continued metabolism of endogenous carbohydrate. They should not omit their insulin or some form of food but should seek professional assistance if they have not been told the essential emergency measures or they cannot control the problems alone.

When the points system is used, any food or ingredient may be exchanged for another food that has the same points (for composition of ingredients, refer to the booklet published by the Kansas Wheat Commission[20]). Points may also be exchanged for food groups in the exchange list (see Table 13-13).

Patients with diabetes who require sodium restriction or control of saturated fat usually need the same advice given to patients who require these restrictions and do not have diabetes. The American Heart Association* and the Nation Heart and Lung Institute† offer information for restricting sodium and/or controlling saturated fat or cholesterol. Diet Teaching Programs, Inc.‡ offers cassette tapes and worksheets for modifying the sodium, fat, and cholesterol.‡ The Kansas Wheat Commission offers free points system diets with large print and pictures.[20] A very excellent cookbook for using the exchange list system is available from the American Diabetes Association. Many good nutrition textbooks teach the modifications of diets.

Some scientists advocate less fat, especially the fat that comes from animals, such as whole milk, butter, cream, egg yolk, and fatty meats and products made from these foods. Skim milk with less than 0.5% butter fat is recommended. Lean meat, especially fish, veal and poultry without skin or fat is preferred. Also preferred are oils that are not hydrogenated such as safflower oil, corn oil, and cottonseed oil. The food (e.g. margarine) that has a P/S ratio of 2 to 1 is desirable. P/S ratio means the percent of polyunsaturated fatty acids to saturated fatty acid content in a food. Vegetable oils or vegetable fat does not necessarily mean the oil has the correct P/S ratio unless the nutrition label indicates the desired P/S ratio.[20]

When using the new exchange list, one should choose nonfat milk and foods in bold type in the meat and fat exchanges, of "Exchange Lists for Meal Planning."

SUMMARY

As was said in the beginning of this chapter, much remains to be discovered about the nutritional care of patients, and new research often brings confusion and controversy. There is an explosion of knowledge that has been available and more becomes available with each new day.

At this point in our knowledge of research and planning, it is necessary to make decisions with the rest of the team, including the patient, about the nutritional care of the patient. The following are general regimes suggested for a particular group of patients:

- *Calorie restriction* (counting calories) is for those obese patients *not* required to use insulin.
- *"Exchange Lists for Meal Planning"* is for obese patients and for those requiring insulin. It offers a choice of foods from the allowed six food groups.
- *Points system* offers a choice of foods; individuals with diabetes learn to choose foods depending upon their calories and/or carbohydrate, protein and/or fat values. It is for the obese patient and for those requiring insulin. Professionals have found that counting calorie points and carbohydrate points and limiting animal fat are simple and effective for the patient using insulin.

• • •

More important than the regimen is the patient. Ignore unfounded theories, ancient philosophies, and prejudices. Apply imagination and creativity to nutritional counseling.

REFERENCES

1. National Center for Health Statistics: Characteristics of persons with diabetes, July 1964-June 1965, Series **10**, No. 10, October, 1967.
2. Bierman, E. L., Albrink, M. J., and Connor, W. E.: Principles of nutrition and dietary recommendations for patients with diabetes mellitus, Diabetes **20:**633, 1971.
3. Etzwiler, D. D.: The patient is a member of the medical team, J. Am. Diet. Assoc. **61:**421, 1972.
4. Food and Nutrition Board, National Academy of Sciences, National Research Council: Recommended dietary allowances, ed. 7, Washington, D.C., 1968, U.S. Government Printing Office.
5. Food and Nutrition Board, National Academy of Sciences, National Research Coun-

---

*American Heart Association, Dallas, Tex.
†National Heart and Lung Institute, Bethesda, Md.
‡Diet teaching programs, Inc., PO Box 18014, Wichita, Kan., 67518.

cil: Recommended dietary allowances, ed. 8, Washington, D.C., 1974, U.S. Government Printing Office.

6. Jackson, R. L., and Guthrie, R. A.: The child with diabetes, Current Concepts, Kalamazoo, Mich., 1975, The Upjohn Co.

7. West, K. M.: Diet therapy of diabetes: an analysis of failure Ann. Intern. Med. **79:**425, 1973.

8. West, K. M.: Prevention and therapy of diabetes, Nutr. Rev. **33:**193, 1975.

9. Antar, M. A., Little, J. A., Lucas, C., and others: Interrelationship between the kinds of dietary carbohydrate and fat in hyperlipoproteinemic patients. III. Synergistic effect of sucrose and animal fat on serum lipid, Atherosclerosis **11:**191, 1970.

10. Cohen, A. M., Teitelbaum, A., Balogh, M., and Groen, J. J.: Effect of interchanging bread and sucrose as main source of carbohydrate in low fat diet on the glucose tolerance curve of healthy volunteer subjects, Am. J. Clin. Nutr. **19:**59, 1966.

11. Rodger, N. W., Squires, B. P., and Du, E.: Improved glucose tolerance in asymptomatic diabetics on diets high in simple sugar content, Diabetes **19:**399, 1970.

12. Burnzell, J. D., Lerner, R. L., Hazzard, W. R., and others: Improved glucose tolerance with high carbohydrate feeding in mild diabetes, New Engl. J. Med. **284:**521, 1971.

13. Lerner, R. L., Burnzell, J. D., Hazzard, W. R., and others: Mechanism of improved glucose tolerance on high carbohydrate diets in normals and mild diabetics (abstract), Diabetes, **20:**342, 1971.

14. Birchwood, B. L., Little, J. A., Antar, M. A., and others: Interrelationship between the kinds of dietary carbohydrate and fat in hyperlipoproteinemic patients. II. Sucrose and starch with mixed saturated and polyunsaturated fats, Atherosclerosis **11:**183, 1970.

15. Anderson, J. W., Herman, R. H., and Zakin, D.: Glucose tolerance and insulin response

to prolonged high carbohydrate feeding in normal men, Am. J. Clin. Nutr. **21:**529, 1968.

16. Weinsier, R. L., Seeman, A., Guillermo. H., and others: High-and-low carbohydrate diets in diabetes mellitus: study of effects on diabetic control, insulin secretion, and blood lipids, Ann. Intern. Med. **80:**332, 1974.

17. Brunzell, J. D., Lerner, R. L., Hazzard, W. R., and others: Improved glucose tolerance with high carbohydrate feeding in mild diabetes, New Engl. J. Med. **284:**521, 1971.

18. Brunzell, J. D., Lerner R. L., Porte, D., Jr., and Bierman, E. L.: Effect of a fat free, high carbohydrate diet on diabetic subjects with fasting hyperglycemia, Diabetes **23:**138, 1974.

19. Wood, F. C., Jr., and Bierman, E. L.: New concepts in diabetic dietetics, Nutr. Today **7:**(3):4, 1972.

20. Stucky, V.: Don't read this . . . unless, Easy way diet, Series III and IV, Calorie point diet, Nutrition for the Nation and Nutrition for the Nation, P. S., Wichita, Kan., 1976, Diet Teaching Programs, Inc. (Kansas Wheat Commission, 1021 North Main Street, Huchinson, Kan., 67501.)

21. David, J. K., and Goldsmith, M. P.: Diabetes guidebook: diet section, Columbus, Ga., 1974, The Litho-Krome Co.

22. Hatch, W. R.: Approach to teaching. Washington, D.C., 1966, U.S. Bureau of Research, Superintendent of Documents, U.S. Government Printing Office.

23. Weinsier, R. L., Seeman, A., Guillermo, M. H., and others: Diet therapy of diabetes, Diabetes **23:**699, 1974.

24. Orkow, B. M., and Ross, J. L.: Weight reduction through nutrition education and personal counseling, J. Nutr. Educ. **7:**65, 1975.

25. Consumer Guide: The brand name food game, New York, 1974, New American Library.

SECTION FOUR
Special problems

14

Pregnancy and diabetes

Colleen Sheets

Before the use of insulin, very few insulin-dependent diabetic women were able to become pregnant. With the discovery and use of insulin, more diabetic women became pregnant, but the mortality of mother and infant was high. There has been a drastic decrease in maternal mortality as our knowledge of the use of insulin has improved. However, perinatal mortality of infants is still a very significant problem. In 1940, the perinatal mortality of infants of diabetic mothers was 40%. By 1960 this rate had dropped only to 15%.[1] With the treatment method used at the University of Missouri over the last few years, perinatal mortality has dropped to less than 2% when the team of obstetricians, endocrinologists, and the diabetes nurse practioner closely follow the pregnant diabetic woman.[2]

Ideally, the pregnant diabetic woman should have a thorough knowledge and understanding of diabetes. If her diabetes has been well controlled before pregnancy, the woman has less chance of having severe complications of diabetes that would pose additional problems for the pregnancy. The 2% mortality at the University of Missouri, while a marked improvement from the past, is still not ideal. It represents the entire spectrum from the woman in an ideal situation to one who is seen late in pregnancy with minimal prenatal as well as diabetic care. Careful prenatal care and diabetic control throughout pregnancy can decrease the infant mortality to that resulting from nondiabetic pregnancies.

CHANGES IN PHYSIOLOGY

Pregnancy causes some very important changes in physiology. Two of these important changes that affect the control of diabetes are: (1) increased need for calories as the fetus develops and (2) increased need for insulin during the latter half of pregnancy because of the secretion of hormones from the placenta.

These changes in physiology during pregnancy call for very close observation of the woman with diabetes. The pregnant diabetic woman should be seen frequently in the outpatient clinic, perhaps as often as every 1 to 2 weeks during the first and second trimester. At the beginning of the third trimester, she is usually seen at least at weekly intervals. If problems arise, more frequent visits may be needed. As the need arises, but usually by the beginning of the third trimester, all insulin-dependent women may be started on a regimen of multiple doses of insulin each day. (Recommended regimens are discussed on p. 178.) Changes in the prepregnancy dietary and insulin regimens are almost always needed to maintain control, especially in late pregnancy, and the pregnant diabetic woman should be closely followed in order to effect these changes.

IMPORTANCE OF CONTROL

A discussion of the need for diabetic control is in order at this point. In the early days of insulin therapy, only regular insulin was available. Most diabetic persons received four doses of regular insulin per day. Pregnant diabetic women had few problems. Deliveries were often accomplished at home, at term, and the infants had few difficulties. In the 1930's, the intermediate-acting and long-acting insulins were introduced, and compromises of therapy became the rule. By the late 1930's and early 1940's, almost all diabetic women were receiving one or at most two injections of insulin per day, and perinatal morbidity and mortality rose steadily. In recent years, the relationship between control and perinatal problems has been better understood and mortality has begun to fall. Significant morbidity and mortality continues, however, because the known facts are often poorly implemented.

In the classical pregnancy of a diabetic woman, the infant may die in utero or in late pregnancy; if born alive, the infant has significant neonatal problems. The infants classically are large, fat, and plethoric (flushed red). They usually suffer from significant and often refractory hypoglycemia. Because of the high incidence of intrauterine deaths in late pregnancy, these infants are often delivered prematurely and are then subject to all the problems of prematurity, including respiratory distress, hypocalcemia, and jaundice, to name a few.

Many of the problems of the infant are now understood and are related to the metabolic fiery furnace in which the fetus has dwelt. Glucose from the mother is readily passed across the placenta to the fetus. Persistent fetal hyperglycemia results in an increased fetal insulin output with deposits of the excess glucose as fat and glycogen in the tissues, thus the overgrown, fat appearance of the fetus. The persistent hyperglycemia resulting in fetal hyperinsulinism eventually leads to hypertrophy of the beta cells. Hyperinsulinism, which continues after delivery, and beta cell hypertrophy account for the hypoglycemia that occurs after birth. Maternal ketosis should be avoided at all costs. It is especially devastating to the infant and often results in fetal death, even when the mother had only mild ketosis of short duration.

The important implication from the above facts is that hyperglycemia must be controlled and prevented. In order to prevent hyperglycemia, the pregnant diabetic woman must be followed closely, the diet controlled carefully, and the insulin given in small frequent doses. During the first two trimesters, two daily doses of mixtures of regular and NPH insulins work well. During the third trimester, four doses of regular insulin per day are highly desirable for the insulin-dependent diabetic woman to effect the level of control needed to prevent fetal and neonatal problems. In the woman with gestational diabetes, insulin therapy should often be instituted and careful dietary control should be exercised.

DIET AND INSULIN MANAGEMENT

It is important that each diabetic woman have an individual diet plan with the correct number of calories adjusted as needed throughout pregnancy. The diet should be divided into three meals and three snacks. The composition is usually 40% to 50% carbohydrate, 30% to 40% fat, and 20% protein. A frequently used distribution is $\frac{2\text{-}1\text{-}2\text{-}1\text{-}2\text{-}1}{9}$; that is, $2/9$ of the total daily calories at each meal and $1/9$ at each snack. A pregnant diabetic woman who has normal weight is usually given an increase of 200 to 500 calories over her prepregnancy level. Most obstetricians do not recommend a reducing diet during pregnancy because the needs of the growing and developing fetus must be met. Because there is much concern that the diet be as exact as possible, it is recommended that the woman use a gram scale and weigh all the food eaten during the pregnancy.

The following four-dose distribution of regular insulin has proved to be a good regimen for late pregnancy[2]:

Percentage of total daily insulin	Time
35%	30 minutes before breakfast
25%	30 minutes before lunch
30%	30 minutes before supper
10%	At midnight

This four-dose program keeps the blood glucose at a lower level for a longer period of time without significant hypoglycemia.

In early pregnancy, a two-dose insulin schedule is recommended. If the diabetic woman has not been using two doses of insulin, one can determine a two-dose insulin schedule by taking the total amount of insulin and dividing it as follows: $^2/_3$ of the total dose 30 minutes before breakfast, as 2 parts intermediate-acting insulin with 1 part short-acting (regular) insulin; and $^1/_3$ of the total dose 30 minutes before supper, as 1 part intermediate-acting insulin with 1 part short-acting insulin. An example follows:

Total daily insulin = 40 units

$^2/_3$ before breakfast = 18 units intermediate-acting insulin
   8 units short-acting insulin
26 units

$^1/_3$ before supper = 7 units intermediate-acting insulin
   7 units short-acting insulin
14 units

The pregnant diabetic woman checks the level of diabetes control and modifies the insulin dose accordingly by keeping urine test records at home. The 2-drop Clinitest is recommended because strip tests are extremely sensitive to small amounts of glucose in the urine, which may normally be present in the urine of any pregnant woman. (The renal threshold decreases in pregnancy, allowing glucose to spill even into the urine of nondiabetic women.) The urine tests are done before each meal and at bedtime. If there is 2% (4+), 3%, or 5% glycosuria, the urine is checked for acetone. (A check for acetone should also be made during any illness.) Anytime there is a positive test for ketones, the diabetic woman must notify her physician or nurse practitioner at once because of the grave danger to the fetus if ketoacidosis develops during the pregnancy, and supplementary regular insulin should be given immediately.

Aglycosuria is the goal; however, this is very difficult to attain with some women. Light insulin reactions during pregnancy are tolerated more than during the nonpregnant state. Hypoglycemia is *less* dangerous to the fetus than ketosis or prolonged hyperglycemia.

Diabetic women who have had previous difficulty in conception and in carrying the fetus may be assured of better results if the control of the disease is as optimal as possible. If complications develop prior to pregnancy, serious consideration needs to be given to the choice of becoming pregnant or not. If the woman has heart disease or retinopathy, serious thought should be given to avoiding pregnancy. It is possible that retinopathy may worsen during the pregnancy and may even be a cause for terminating the pregnancy. Bypass surgery for heart disease has been followed by safe and successful pregnancy.

GESTATIONAL DIABETES

A woman with gestational diabetes (non-insulin-dependent diabetes during pregnancy) should be educated about the necessity of control and follow-up care during and after her 9 months of pregnancy. Often, insulin therapy needs to be begun in these women during the pregnancy, and dietary control must be carefully maintained because the infants often have as much difficulty as those of the insulin-dependent diabetic woman. Each time the woman comes for a clinic visit, a random blood sample for glucose testing should be obtained. The blood glucose level should be kept preferably at 120 mg/dl or less. Of course, the test results of a random blood sample do not reveal what kind of overall control a particular woman achieved; however, with the addition of urine records, two parameters are available for comparison.

Many physicians choose to deliver the infant 2 to 4 weeks before the expected date of confinement, although infants of woman with well-controlled diabetes may safely be delivered at or near term. Vaginal delivery is becoming increasingly more common over caesarean sections as the preferred method of delivery, especially if the diabetes is well controlled and the pregnancy carried to term.

TIME AND METHOD OF DELIVERY
Using laboratory tests

Estriol determinations. Various laboratory tests may be of help to the physician in the decision regarding the time and method of delivery. Some centers use serial testing of urine or plasma to determine estriol levels and choose to deliver when a rapid fall in these levels is observed. To be meaningful, estriol determinations should be frequent (daily or at least every other day) and should be plasma determinations. Urine estriol levels are of limited value. If the plasma estriol levels remain normal by serial testing, the infant is kept in utero until the lecithin-sphingomyelin (L/S) ratio indicates maturity and the oxytocin test confirms maturity and indicates that an induced vaginal delivery is possible (see discussion below). If the estriol level falls before these latter two events, immediate cesarean section is indicated.

L/S ratio and oxytocin test. The use of amniocentesis is becoming increasingly more popular; the amniotic fluid is tested for lecithin-sphingomyelin ratio,[3] which indicates fetal lung maturity. An L/S ratio with a predominance of sphingomyelin (a complex lipid containing chemical) indicates an immature lung and an infant likely to develop respiratory distress if delivered. An L/S ratio with a predominance of lecithin indicates an infant who can be safely delivered. Beginning at about the 36th week of gestation, an amniocentesis is performed

to obtain the amniotic fluid for the L/S ratio. Whenever the L/S ratio reaches 2:1 or greater, the infant can be delivered. The method of delivery depends on whether or not the obstetrician feels he can induce labor. An oxytocin stimulation test is also performed. The oxytocin test also determines maturity of the fetus and the readiness of the woman for vaginal delivery.[4,5] However, if labor cannot be induced, then a cesarean section is scheduled.

Maintaining metabolic control

Regardless of the method of delivery chosen, a very high level of metabolic control must be maintained. Insulin must be given until delivery is accomplished and calories normally received must be calculated and given intravenously. If labor is prolonged and intravenous glucose therapy is constant, the insulin should be given in equal doses subcutaneously. Care should be taken not to give large doses of glucose to the mother immediately before delivery because this will induce hyperglycemia and insulin release in the fetus. There will then be a rebound hypoglycemia in the newborn.

Summary

With careful monitoring of the blood and urine glucose levels, careful adjustment of the diet and insulin, serial testing of plasma estriol levels, use of oxytocin tests and L/S ratios, and hospitalization, if necessary, the proper time for delivery can be accurately determined and a good result obtained.

POSTPARTUM PERIOD

Soon after the baby is delivered, the mother's blood glucose level may noticeably drop if the insulin dosage is not decreased. Often the postpartum insulin dose is returned to the woman's usual dose, if there are no postpartum complications, such as infection. The woman with gestational diabetes will often have blood glucose levels return to normal by 4 to 6 weeks after delivery.

Table 14-1. White classification*

Class†	Onset age	Duration	Insulin or oral agents	Chronic complications
A	Any	Any	None	None
B‡	Over 20 years of age	Under 10 years	Insulin or oral agents	None
C‡	10-19 years	10-19 years	Insulin or oral agents	None
D‡	Under 10 years	Over 20 years	+	Calcified arteries in legs or nonproliferative retinopathy
E‡	Any	Any	+	Calcified arteries in pelvis or nonproliferative retinopathy
F‡	Any	Any	+	Calcified arteries, nonproliferative retinopathy, or nephropathy
R	Any	Any	+	Calcified arteries or proliferative retinopathy
FR	Any	Any	+	Calcified arteries, proliferative retinopathy, or nephropathy
H	Any	Any	+	Calcified arteries, proliferative retinopathy, or nephropathy

*Data from Dr. Priscilla White, Joslin Clinic, Boston, Mass.
†Fetal loss: A = 0, B = 35%, C = 55%, D = 67%, E = 87%, F, R, and FR = very slim chance for viable infant; H = Heart.
‡Represents the whole period of pregnancy. Includes both early and late losses.

CLASSIFICATION OF DIABETES AND PREGNANCY

Dr. Priscilla White has worked out a classification for the pregnant diabetic woman (Table 14-1). The White classification is useful in helping the team working with the pregnant diabetic woman. It gives some idea of what can be anticipated for each woman and helps in predicting the outcome of the pregnancy. Too much emphasis should not be placed on the classification, but it can be useful.[6,7]

GENETICS AND COUNSELING

Pregnancy in the diabetic woman should be carefully considered long before it occurs. Education may begin in the home, at camp, in classes, in school, in diabetes centers, or in the physician's office. Counseling needs to include genetic information, cost, control of the disease, and the need for cooperation during the prepartum and postpartum periods as well as during the pregnancy, in order to have a viable, healthy infant. At some point, preferably long before pregnancy occurs, it is very important to talk about genetics and birth control for the diabetic woman. Most people know that "diabetes runs in families." Although there seem to be several factors involved, up to this time, the means or method of inheritance is not fully understood. One problem that must be faced is that no method of predicting who will become diabetic has as yet been found. At the present time, there is no way of detecting diabetes until the abnormality of carbohydrate metabolism can be shown or measured. Thus there is no way of determining whether the father is or is not a carrier of the diabetic gene and whether the infant will develop diabetes.

When a young couple is counseled either before or after marriage, it is very important that the problems of living with a person who has a chronic disease be considered. The marriage of two known diabetic persons should usually be discouraged, especially if they desire to conceive children. Theoretically, all of their children would develop diabetes. Table 14-2 can be used to inform diabetic women of the prob-

Table 14-2. Probability of developing diabetes*

Diabetic relatives	Percent
Both parents	100
Identical twins	100
1 parent on one side and a grandparent and an aunt or uncle on the other side	80
1 parent on one side and 1 grandparent or an aunt or uncle on other side	60
1 parent and 1 sibling	50
1 parent and first cousin on other side	40
Grandparent from each side	35
One sibling	25
One parent	22
Both grandparents (spouses)	14
Uncle or aunt	12
None	5

*From Steinberg, A. G.: Heredity and diabetes, Eugenics Quarterly (now Social Biology) **2:**26, 1955.

ability of their children developing diabetes sometime during their lives.[8]

As already discussed, a diabetic woman needs to face the fact that there is an increased chance of having a stillborn infant, although one 4-year study reports fetal loss of only 2% if the mother's diabetes is controlled. A diabetic woman should also realize that congenital defects, usually minor but sometimes severe, are more common in the children born to mothers with diabetes.

In genetic counseling, the couple should have all the information possible, both pro and con, so that they are able to make an educated decision regarding whether or not they want to have children. Providing this information and supporting the couple in whatever decision they finally make are the responsibilities of the health care team.

In the past, many couples decided to adopt children rather than have biological children. The couple should be made aware that this is not always an easy answer. In many areas, babies are very hard to obtain unless the couple is willing to take children that are racial mixtures or that have some type of medical problem that makes them difficult for the adoption agency to place. At any rate, the waiting period may range from months to years before the couple may become parents through adoption.

What about birth control? If the man is diabetic and wishes permanent sterilization, a vasectomy should be performed. When the woman is the diabetic, the method of contraception needs to be no different from that for any other woman. Any contraceptive device or surgical procedure desired by the individual woman and her gynecologist is usually acceptable to the physician responsible for her diabetes.

SUMMARY

Medical science has come a long way in developing methods of caring for the pregnant diabetic woman. At the present time, the most important factor that seems to relate to a successful pregnancy is how closely the diabetes is able to be controlled.

Members of the health care team working with a woman with diabetes must consider a number of factors as part of the control of the disease. Proper care and adjustment of food and insulin are important considerations during prepartum and postpartum periods as well as during delivery. In the prepartum period, the diabetic woman needs a balanced nutritional intake to meet her needs and the needs of the developing fetus. Food intake must be regulated by the woman's life-style and the action of the insulin. The woman needs to understand what high blood glucose levels do to the fetus she is carrying and why she is asked to restrict concentrated sweets, eliminate excess salt in her diet, and perhaps self-administer insulin. Toxemia and polyhydramnios are more prevalent in the woman with diabetes, and control of blood glucose levels is the best prevention of these problems.

Oral agents should be discontinued before pregnancy and insulin therapy begun. Oral agents are contraindicated during pregnancy because of the greater incidence of congenital abnormalities with oral agents and the beta cell hypertrophy effect of the oral agents.

The woman with gestational diabetes should be carefully controlled and insulin therapy instituted if control by diet alone is not satisfactory.

In the insulin-dependent diabetic woman, a rise in insulin requirements should be expected until after delivery, and multiple-dose regimen is almost always required to provide the kind of control needed for a satisfactory outcome to the pregnancy.

Maternal and infant mortality can and should be reduced to nearly that of nondiabetic women. A high level of metabolic control before, during, and after the pregnancy will accomplish this desirable goal.

REFERENCES

1. Kahn, C., White, P., and Younger, D.: Laboratory assessment of diabetic pregnancy, Diabetes **21**:31, 1972.
2. James, R.: Rational approach to the treatment of insulin dependent diabetes mellitus, Mo. Med. **70**:650, 1973.
3. Dunn, L. J., and Bhalngar, A. S.: Use of lecithin/sphingomyelin ratio management of the problem obstetric patient, Am. J. Obstet. Gynecol. **115**:687, 1973.
4. Gluck, L.: Diagnosis of respiratory distress syndrome by anmiocentesis, Am. J. Obstet. Gynecol. **109**:440, 1971.
5. Merkus, J. M. W., Koch, H. C. L. V., Merkus, E. W. H. W., and others: Evaluation of the amniotic fluid test and its relationship to the respiratory distress syndrome, Am. J. Obstet. Gynecol. **115**:859, 1973.
6. White, P.: Pregnancy complicating diabetes, Am. J. Med. **7**:609, 1949.
7. White, P.: Diabetes mellitus in pregnancy, Clin. Perinatol. **1**:311, 1974.
8. Steinberg, A. G.: Heredity and diabetes, Eugenics Quarterly **2**:26, 1955.

15

Infant of the diabetic mother

Diana W. and Richard A. Guthrie

Problems of the infant of the diabetic mother (IDM) are of great significance, especially when one considers that the death rate of these infants may be very high when special care is not available. Moreover, mortality is higher in IDMs than in infants of nondiabetic mothers, even when special care is available.[1] The IDM must therefore be classed as a high-risk infant who needs specific attention in nursing and medical care.

A number of factors, a major one being hypoglycemia, contribute to the high morbidity and mortality of the IDM. Other causes of fetal death are congenital anomalies and early delivery. Early delivery causes a multitude of problems, such as respiratory distress, prematurity, hypoglycemia, hypocalcemia, and hyperbilirubinemia. Control of the mother's diabetes during pregnancy significantly reduces the incidence of mortality and morbidity in the infant during the neonatal period of life, particularly the morbidity associated with hypoglycemia.

FETAL AND NEONATAL (PERINATAL) METABOLISM

Shaw and Moriarty[2] recognized neonatal hypoglycemia and described it as an important entity in 1924. Since their recognition of this important problem, much knowledge regarding the pathophysiology of the IDM has evolved. There are a number of complex mechanisms involved in carbohydrate metabolism in the perinatal period (prebirth to 1 month after delivery).

Different organs have differing energy requirements and differing ability to utilize glucose and other substrates. The brain needs a constant supply of energy, which is provided by circulating glucose in normal circumstances. The brain however is unable to make or store glucose and is thus dependent on the maintenance of a normal circulating blood glucose level. Under certain circumstances, the brain can use glycerol, beta-hydroxybutyrate, and acetoacetate (ketone bodies) when glucose is unavailable; however, under normal circumstances, these substances supply minimal amounts of energy to the brain. The liver's function is almost opposite to that of the brain; it may both store glucose as glycogen (glycogenesis) or make new glucose (gluconeogenesis) from amino acids. Therefore, in the liver there is a dynamic equilibrium between the uptake, storage, and release of glucose and gluconeogenesis. A complex set of enzymatic reactions control this equilibrium and serve to maintain the blood glucose level within narrow limits.

The energy sources of the fetus are maternal amino acids, free fatty acids, and glucose. Glucose is the main source of energy for the fetus. Some of the glucose is used for energy, and most of it is stored as glycogen. The energy needs of the fetus are supplied by the mother. The blood glucose level in the fetus is usually about one third less than that of the mother. If the placenta is affected by disease, such as in toxemia, there may be less glucose trans-

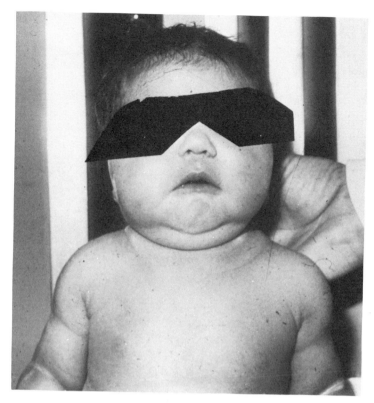

Fig. 15-1. Infant of the diabetic mother (IDM).

ferred to the fetus and less glucose available to the fetus to store as glycogen for use in early neonatal life. Hypoglycemia may result.

Glycogen concentrations in the fetus at term compare with adult levels as follows[3]:

Liver	2 × adult level
Heart	10 × adult level
Skeletal muscles	3 to 5 × adult level

Once the newborn is delivered, the stored glycogen is released to provide energy for the maintenance of body temperature, brain metabolism, respiration, and muscle activity until supported by outside sources. The carbohydrate reserve is only adequate for a few hours after birth, and then fat is increasingly used for energy production. There is, therefore, a need for early feeding, especially in the premature infant where glycogen and fat stores are inadequate to meet energy needs for very long.

HYPOGLYCEMIA IN THE NEWBORN

Hypoglycemia in the newborn is loosely defined as a blood glucose level of less than 30 mg/dl,[4] though some authors believe a level of 40 to 45 mg/dl should be considered minimal. Hypoglycemia in most infants is usually thought to be caused by inadequate stores of glycogen, such as may be found in the infant of the toxemic mother, the premature infant, the erythroblastotic infant, or the asphyxiated infant.

In the IDM, the mechanism of hypoglycemia is different from that observed in most infants. As has been previously noted, glucose is readily transferred across the placenta, and the fetus reflects about one third less glucose than that observed in the mother. When the maternal glucose is elevated beyond normal levels, it is believed that the fetus also becomes hyperglycemic. The fetal pancreas responds to these elevated blood glucose levels by increasing the output of insulin from the beta cells. The pancreatic beta cells then become hyperplastic from constant and prolonged stimulation in order to produce this "extra" insulin. Although the maternal glucose is transferred to the fetus, the fetal insulin is not transferred to the mother. As more glucose is available from the mother and the fetal secretion of insulin increases, the glucose that is not utilized for energy is deposited as glycogen or fat into the liver or other tissues. This explains why diabetic women so often deliver large, fat, puffy infants.

At delivery, the excess supply of glucose is suddenly interrupted, though the excess insulin production is not. Overproduction of insulin by the neonate causes an increased utilization rate of the available glucose, most of which is stored. With the fall in the blood glucose level, many counterregulatory mechanisms (such as the release of glucagon, growth hormone, glucocorticoids, and epinephrine) are activated. However, the effect of these hormones is not sufficient to counterbalance the effect of the excess insulin production. In many cases, the blood glucose level may become stabilized within a few days of birth, but in some cases hypoglycemia may persist for weeks. If the blood glucose level becomes erratic enough, as it often does, glucose deficiency to the brain will develop and may become manifest by shakiness or convulsions. Hypoglycemia in the IDM may become recurrent over the first few days of life.

Detection and treatment

Death in utero may be caused by fetal hyperglycemia and after birth by hypoglycemia caused by lack of glucose to the brain. Untreated hypoglycemic infants have extensive degeneration of nerve cells throughout the central nervous system. It is of utmost importance to prevent hypoglycemia in the neonate. If hypoglycemia is suspected, then prompt treatment may prevent further consequences.[5]

A simple test to detect hypoglycemia may be carried out with the Dextrostix-Reflectance meter system. This test requires only capillary blood and can be performed in about 2 minutes. It should be performed frequently, beginning at about $1/2$ hour of age in any IDM. This test should be repeated every 3 to 4 hours or more frequently, as indicated by the rate of fall in blood glucose levels. Testing can usually cease when the infant has shown blood glucose levels above 40 mg/dl for a period of 12 hours or longer. If the values are below 40 mg/dl, as indicated by Dextrostix, then definitive laboratory tests are warranted and glucose should be administered parenterally.

Signs and symptoms of neonatal hypoglycemia are:

Jittery or lethargic disposition	Seizures
	Respiratory distress
High-pitched cry	Apnea or tachypnea
Rolling eyes	

If the infant is asymptomatic, early feeding, close observation, and frequent monitoring of blood glucose levels may be all that is needed unless hypoglycemia is persistent.

Glucose therapy. If the infant has symptoms of hypoglycemia, therapy should certainly be initiated. Glucose solutions must be administered carefully because the hypertrophied pancreas is highly sensitive to glucose. Small amounts of glucose may cause release of insulin and result in rebound hypoglycemia. Ten percent to 20% glucose solutions are administered by slow continuous perfusion, usually with an infusion pump. Appropriate electrolytes may be added as needed. Glucose therapy is then slowly withdrawn over several days.

Slow and constant perfusion is a necessity in order to prevent the overstimulation of excess insulin release. These infusions need to be maintained until the suck reflex and eating pattern have become normal. Glucagon as well as a 50% glucose solution, elevates glucose levels, thus stimulating insulin release and causing rebound hypoglycemia. Therefore, these agents should rarely be used.

Epinephrine administration. More recently, epinephrine has been used to treat hypoglycemia in the IDM. Epinephrine has been found to raise the blood glucose levels and to inhibit the release of insulin.[6] Some studies suggest that hyperinsulinism may have resulted from or been influenced by decreased release of epinephrine from the adrenal medulla in some IDMs who have been profoundly hyperglycemic in utero. Replacement of this depleted counterregulatory hormone can be important in certain infants. The untoward effect of a lack of epinephrine may be heart failure resulting from a lack of appropriate beta-adrenergic action and fatty acid release. Fatty acids act as a basic fuel supply to the heart. Without an adequate fuel supply, the IDM's heart may fail during delivery. Intramuscular epinephrine is used in a 1:10,000 solution to decrease the amount of insulin released by the beta cells as well as to promote glycogenolysis and fatty acid release. The epinephrine is diluted from a 1:1000 to a 1:10,000 solution by the addition of sterile water for injection. There is a greater incidence of tissue necrosis when epinephrine is given in the more concentrated form.

A more popular method of epinephrine administration is the use of a long-acting preparation called Sus-phrine (epinephrine hydrochloride). This medication is injected intramuscularly (0.01 ml/kg every 8 hours), and its use results in normal glucose levels and a reduction of insulin output.[7] Sus-phrine is diluted from a 1:200 to a 1:1000 solution before injection.

RESPIRATORY DISTRESS SYNDROME IN THE IDM

The problem of respiratory distress in the IDM deserves some consideration. There is no doubt that the IDM has a several times' greater chance of developing the respiratory distress syndrome (RDS) with all of its attendent morbidity and mortality, than does the average infant. Because the IDM is usually delivered prematurely, many medical professionals have said that the respiratory distress of the IDM results exclusively from the premature delivery. However, some recent data have begun to change this belief. Recent studies in animals reveal that insulin will inhibit the maturation of the fetal lung while adrenal corticosteroids will mature them.[7] This finding, if also true in the human fetus, would explain the increased respiratory distress observed in the IDM, even in fairly mature infants. Maternal hyperglycemia induces fetal hyperglycemia, which would in turn both stimulate insulin secretion and suppress adrenocorticosteroid production. The result would be a marked retardation of fetal maturation and RDS observed in infants with immature lungs. These new data provide further evidence of the need for a high level of control of the maternal diabetes.

RDS is a serious complication in the IDM and must be carefully managed. Meticulous attention must be paid to proper oxygenation, fluid and electrolyte management, bicarbonate administration, and temperature control. An umbilical artery catheter should be placed both for the administration of bicarbonate and concentrated glucose solutions and for the measurement of blood gases.

On the first day of life, fluids should be administered at a rate of 65 to 85 cc/kg/day as a 10% glucose solution. If the blood glucose level cannot be maintained, the rate of infusion should be increased but should not exceed 100 cc/kg/day. If administration of 10% glucose solution at the maximum rate does not maintain the blood glucose level, the concentration should be gradually increased to a 20% solution. If the blood glucose level still cannot be maintained at maximal concentration and flow rate, consideration should be given to epinephrine therapy, though it is rarely necessary.

Administration of environmental oxygen is controlled by measuring the serum pH, P_{CO_2}, and P_{O_2} at frequent intervals via the umbilical artery. If the blood oxygen concentration cannot be maintained within the normal range (50 to 70 mm Hg partial pressure of O_2) with an environmental oxygen of 50% to 60%, continuous positive airway pressure (CPAP) should be started and the expiratory pressure increased as needed to raise the arterial oxygen concentration. The ventilatory assistance and rate are increased as needed to lower the P_{CO_2} if it becomes elevated.

Bicarbonate is administered as needed to control the serum arterial pH but should not exceed a dose of 10 mEq/kg/day, or the sodium in the solution will exceed the amount that the infant can tolerate. If more alkali is needed, THAM (tromethamine, an alkalyzing agent) should be substituted for bicarbonate.

OTHER PROBLEMS OF THE IDM
Hypocalcemia

Hypocalcemia is a common problem in the IDM. The infant is often fairly refractory to calcium therapy but responds reasonably well to correction of the hypoglycemia. The hypocalcemia is somehow related to the hypoglycemia, possibly through the glucagon-thyrocalcitonin axis. Hypoglycemia causes glucagon secretion. Glucagon stimulates thyrocalcitonin, which lowers blood calcium levels. Correction of the hyperglycemia lowers the blood glucagon level, which in turn ceases to stimulate thyrocalcitonin, and calcium levels increase. The IDM with hypocalcemia should nonetheless be treated with calcium as would any infant with hypocalcemia.

Signs and symptoms of neonatal hypocalcemia are:

Tremors	Thready, rapid pulse
Leg cramps	Arrhythmia
Muscle spasms	Nausea and vomiting
Muscular weakness	Abdominal cramps

Hyperbilirubinemia

Hyperbilirubinemia is another common problem in the IDM, probably related to prematurity. Hyperbilirubinemia should be carefully watched for and treated as in any infant, especially the premature infant.

PREVENTION OF DEATH IN UTERO AND PREMATURITY

Death in utero frequently occurs at 36 to 38 weeks in the IDM. To prevent intrauterine death, the physician often chooses to deliver the high-risk infant at approximately 35 to 36 weeks. Although early delivery may prompt earlier treatment and prevent death in utero, the problems related to premature delivery may cause the complications of respiratory distress, hypoglycemia, hyperbilirubinemia, and hypocalcemia. Certainly if delivery is delayed to 37 to 38 weeks, the problems related to prematurity would be decreased. Even more importantly, if the maternal blood glucose levels are kept to normal limits thoughout pregnancy, the baby may safely be delivered closer to term with fewer consequences resulting. Therefore, it is of utmost importance to recognize that the best preventive of intrauterine death and prematurity is control of the maternal glucose levels.

NURSING CARE: OBSERVATION AND PREVENTIVE MONITORING

Nursing care of the IDM involves meticulous observation, whether the infant is suspect, high-risk, or actually symptomatic. If the infant is high-risk or suspect, monitoring will involve frequent blood glucose determinations and measurements of neurologic functioning, such as the suck reflex, Moro's reflex, or seizurelike activity. Respiratory difficulty will also need to be noted and heat maintenance rigidly adhered to. Monitoring of vital signs and glucose levels are important in detecting early hypoglycemic problems. If preventive monitoring has not been successful or adequately performed, symptoms of hypogly-

Grading: O(absent)
+1 (fair) +2(good
—(moderate) —2 (severe)

INFANT OF DIABETIC

Flowsheet

Name: _____

Date: _____

Time	Respiratory Rate	Retraction	Nasal Flare	Grunt	Cyanosis	Pulse	Precordial Bound	Moro	Toe Grasp	Stimulated Cry	Spontaneous Cry	Suck	Muscle Tone	Tremors	Dextrostix	Other Blood Spec.	% of O_2	Gms of Glucose in 20% conc.	Type and Dosage Sub Q, IM, IV Medications
7—3																			
3—11																			
11—7																			

Time	Temp	Pulse		8 hr. IV Fluids	8 hr. Oral Fluids	8 hr Urine	Stool Output	Remarks
7-3: 10 A.M				Fluid:	Kind:	Vol:	Time(s):	
2 P.M.				Vol:	Time(s)		Comment:	
	Wt.	H.C	Abd.c		Vol: / Est. Loss			
3-11 6 P.M.				Fluid:	Kind:	Vol:	Time(s):	
10 P.M.				Vol:	Time(s)		Comment:	
					Vol: / Est. Loss:			
11-7 2 A.M.				Fluid:	Kind:	Vol:	Time(s):	
6 A.M.				Vol:	Time(s)		Comment:	
					Vol: / Est. Loss:			

Fig. 15-2. Flow sheet for monitoring IDM. (From Guthrie, D. W., and Guthrie, R. A., editors: Syllabus for the 7th Allied Health Conference on Diabetes, New York, 1975. Used with permission of the American Diabetes Association.)

cemia may develop. The fat, floppy babies, even though large, should be monitored in the same manner as premature infants.

Frequent positioning and maintenance of oxygen levels. If difficulties progress, the infants become more lethargic. As they become more lethargic, frequent positioning will assist in circulatory response. When respiratory distress is first noted, supportive measures are correct positioning in the incubator (see below) and maintenance of adequate oxygen levels. Monitoring of the blood oxygen level is of utmost importance. The infant with respiratory distress should be positioned as follows:

1. Flat on back
2. Shoulders slightly elevated
3. Head back
4. Chest and neck in a straight line
5. Head of bed slightly elevated

Monitoring hydration. Hydration may be monitored by determining intake and output. Perfusion of intravenous fluids with an infusion pump lessens the danger of inadequate or excess levels of fluid therapy. Any oral feeding should be carefully recorded. Emesis should be monitored as closely as possible. If a small Chux is placed under the head, emesis can be noted by weight of the Chux before and after emesis. Output is also noted by number of stools (and weight of stools if needed). Urine output may be determined by bagging the infant (especially recommended are urine collection units that contain tubing as well as bag). Excoriation of tissue is less if bags are attached for 24 to 48 hours.

Keeping a flow sheet. A flow sheet to display the infant's condition at a glance should be kept at the bedside (Fig. 15-2). This flow sheet demonstrates the 24-hour monitoring of the newborn.[8] At each hour, a notation that summarizes the response during the last 60 minutes may be made. If any laboratory tests have been completed, vital signs taken, intake and output observed, such must be clearly noted. Vital signs will probably be noted more fre-

quently, every 5 to 15 minutes, when the infant is in crisis. The area for hourly determination on the flow sheet should display the highest and lowest response of each temperature, pulse rate, and/or respirations. Of course, a supplementary sheet or graph placed on the back of the flow sheet may be used for results of the frequent vital signs.

Administering epinephrine. If epinephrine is given, care must be taken that it is injected deeply into the muscle, otherwise noticeable necrosis will occur (Fig. 15-3).

Oral feeding. Once the infant is able to tolerate oral feedings, other problems may occur. Aspiration of emesis is one such problem. To prevent this occurrence, one should place the infant on its side with the head elevated when feeding in the incubator. The newborn should be burped in the side or abdominal position. Observation of the suck reflex should be noted; if the infant has a decreased suck, feeding should be delayed because swallowing is usually also impaired. Lavage feeding may be needed for several days and should be carefully administered. Burping should be attempted with ingestion of every ½ to 1 ounce of formula. Once fed and finally burped, the infant should be positioned on the abdomen or side and not on the back, unless other problems (such as respiratory distress) warrant such positioning. All of these measures may lessen the possibility of aspiration.

Placement in an open crib. After the infant has become stabilized, the next course of management is placement in an open crib. As with all premature infants, it is wise to acclimatize the infant gradually before final placement in the open crib. Gradual acclimatization assists in closer observation. Temperature maintenance should be most carefully observed as the external source of heat is gradually decreased. One accomplishes a gradual transition by moving the infant from a heated to a partially heated incubator with intermittently opened port holes or moving a bundled in-

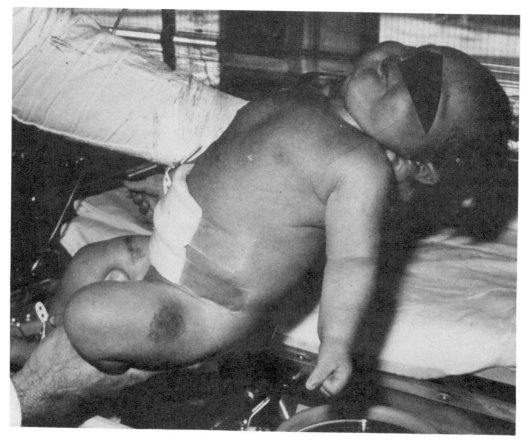

Fig. 15-3. Necrosis caused by improper injection of epinephrine.

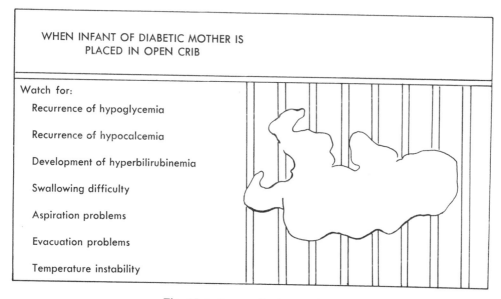

WHEN INFANT OF DIABETIC MOTHER IS
PLACED IN OPEN CRIB

Watch for:

Recurrence of hypoglycemia

Recurrence of hypocalcemia

Development of hyperbilirubinemia

Swallowing difficulty

Aspiration problems

Evacuation problems

Temperature instability

Fig. 15-4. Open crib observations.

fant to a nonheated incubator with opened port holes.

Even after the infant is placed in the open crib, monitoring should be maintained for signs of temperature changes and respiratory or reflex deterioration. Hyperbilirubinemia (observable jaundice) may be noted, and hypoglycemia (seizures, irritability) and hypocalcemia (tremors of extremities) may recur. Although these infants may weigh 9 pounds or more, they are still of a decreased gestational age. If they are delivered 4 weeks prematurely, they will respond as a 36-week premature infant. Continual monitoring of sucking and evacuation should be continued in the open crib, as well as at home, until all danger has passed.

GOALS OF THERAPY

Restoration and control of physiologic and pathologic responses results in a normal neonate. If a mother has insulin-dependent, non-insulin-dependent, or gestational diabetes, the goals should all be the same[9]:

1. Delivery of an infant of normal weight
2. Prevention of both hyperglycemia and hypoglycemia in the mother
3. Prevention of both hyperglycemia and hypoglycemia in the infant

If it is impossible to support the mother adequately at home, hospitalization may be necessary in order to maintain normoglycemia up to the time of delivery and thereafter (see Chapter 14, Pregnancy and diabetes). Once the infant is born, the parents should be aware that the infant is somewhat more likely to develop diabetes than is an infant of a nondiabetic mother. Fetal hyperinsulinism may cause beta cell exhaustion and therefore lead to chemical diabetes or an overt diabetic state within a few weeks, months, or years, especially if the genetic makeup is that of diabetes mellitus. Retrospective studies are lacking to determine the percentage of hypoglycemic infants that later develop insulin-dependent or non-insulin-dependent diabetes, but it is thought to be higher than normal.

Parents should be encouraged to give the high-risk child adequate nutrition, restricting concentrated sweets as a part of good nutrition, and to have a 3- or 5-hour oral glucose tolerance test administered during growth spurts (at 2 to 3, 5 to 6, and 10 to 15 years of age) and 4 to 6 weeks after any severe illness, surgery, or emotional trauma. With close observation, the deteriorating carbohydrate metabolism may be detected at an early stage so that closer observation and treatment may begin.

SUMMARY

There has been much progress in decreasing maternal mortality in the pregnant diabetic woman, but there is still much room for improvement in fetal death rates. Fetal mortality is thought to be influenced by:

1. Poor maternal control of diabetes
2. Congenital defects
3. Degree of maternal vascular disease
4. Prematurity
5. Duration of maternal diabetes mellitus
6. Age at inception of diabetes mellitus
7. Imbalance of sex hormones

Some of these factors are easier to control than others. Prematurity is one area that has been researched to a great extent in recent years. Before the development of the lecithin-sphinogomyelin test, it was very difficult for the obstetrician to calculate just when to deliver the baby. If the infant was delivered too early, there was always the chance of RDS developing. On the other hand, if not delivered in time, the infant would die in utero. With the advent of the L/S ratio, one is able to tell the level of fetal pulmonary maturity[5,6,7] and to time the moment of delivery with more certainty. Control of the maternal diabetes is still the best preventive to the problems of the IDM. When control is not possible, premature delivery may be inevitable and careful nursing and medical care will be needed.

Careful surveillance of environmental factors (such as oxygen and temperature) and control will reduce infant mortality even when hypoglycemia and RDS develop.

Intensive nursing care is nowhere needed more than in the care of the IDM. Cooperation between the various members of the health care team caring for the mother and her newborn will significantly reduce morbidity and mortality for the pregnant woman with diabetes and her infant.

REFERENCES

1. Warner, R. W., and Cornblath, M.: Infants of gestational diabetic mother, Am. J. Dis. Child. **117:**678, 1969.
2. Shaw, E. B., and Moriarty, M.: Hypoglycemia and acidosis in fasting children with idiopathic epilepsy, Am. J. Dis. Child. **28:**553, 1924.
3. Guthrie, R. A.: Hypoglycemia of the newborn. *In* Van Leeuwen, G., editor: A manual of newborn medicine, Chicago, 1973, Yearbook Publishers, pp. 147-161.
4. Cornblath, M., and Schwartz, R.: Disorders of carbohydrate metabolism in infancy, Major problems of clinical surgery, vol. 7, Philadelphia, 1966, W. B. Saunders Co., Chapter 4, p. 2.
5. Finberg, L.: Infant of the diabetic mother. *In* Ellenberg, M., and Rifkin, H., editors: Diabetes mellitus: theory and practice, New York, 1970, McGraw-Hill Book Co., pp. 724-731.
6. McCann, L., Miyazaki, Y., Guthrie, R. A., and Jackson, R. L.: Infant of the diabetic mother, Mod. Med. **65:**275, 1968.
7. Robert, M. F., Neff, R. K., Hubbell, J. P., and others: Maternal diabetes and the respiratory distress syndrome, New Engl. J. Med. **294:**357, 1976.
8. Guthrie, D. W.: Flow sheet for infant of a diabetic mother. *In* Guthrie, D. W. and Guthrie, R. A., editors: Syllabus for the 7th Allied Health conference on Diabetes, New York, 1975, American Diabetes Association, p. 105.
9. Guthrie, D. W., and Guthrie, R. A.: Infant of the diabetic mother, Am. J. Nurs. **74**(11):2008, 1974.

16

Surgery and diabetes

Liddy Dye

At any time, persons with diabetes mellitus may be in need of a surgical procedure. The diabetic person may have an accident, an infection, or any other disease that a nondiabetic individual may have. Additionally, the complications associated with diabetes may require surgical correction.

A number of the complications of diabetes can be alleviated by surgical procedures. However, physicians disagree in their evaluation of the surgical risk of the diabetic person. Some surgeons believe that the diabetic patient encounters a surgical risk no greater than that of the general population. Such an evaluation is probably true of the well-controlled diabetic patient in particular. However, most surgeons would not agree with this evaluation, which is certainly not true for the poorly controlled diabetic person. In the diabetic patient, even one who is well-controlled, care is twofold: it includes care for the surgical procedure as well as care for the diabetic conditon.

CARDIOVASCULAR STATUS AND SURGERY

Diabetes mellitus is a condition that most frequently occurs in middle-aged and elderly individuals. Cardiovascular changes, not only associated with advancing age but also associated with diabetes mellitus, cannot be overlooked when the patient is considered for surgery.[1,2] In order to more accurately assess the vascular age of the diabetic individual, one adds together the number of years the individual has had diabetes plus the chronologic age.[3,4] This total best indicates the physiologic age of the cardiovascular system.

The outcome of any surgery in the individual with diabetes mellitus may be influenced by the probable existence of premature arteriosclerosis with resulting cardiac, renal, and cerebral complications. Whether the cardiovascular problems are associated with the state of the diabetes control is controversial. Although control can be maintained over the metabolic derangement of diabetes mellitus, little as yet has been accomplished to alter the progress of the macrovascular changes associated with diabetes in the older population. Insulin and vigilance, however, remain the best hope for the diabetic individual.

The following situation illustrates the higher-risk factors in the patient with diabetes mellitus: The patient is admitted to the hospital with the primary diagnosis of cholecystitis. Additional conditions on the problem list are diabetes mellitus, obesity, and cardiovascular disease. The latter are three conditions that would not likely affect nondiabetic patients who develop cholecystitis.

SURGICAL PROCEDURES IN THE DIABETIC PERSON

A number of surgical procedures are performed more frequently for the diabetic than the nondiabetic patient. The surgery most often performed is the amputation of a part or all of a limb because of gangrene.[1] The cause of the gangrene or ulcers of the lower extremities is the peripheral vascular disease.[3] Neuropathy involving the lower extremities may also result in problems that require surgical intervention. Sophisticated surgical procedures such as vascular grafts can benefit the diabetic person with peripheral vascular disease.

Abscesses, such as furuncles and carbuncles, are not observed in diabetic persons as often as they were in past years. The use of antibiotics has brought about the decline in the occurrence of this once serious problem. When abscesses do occur, however, some of them require extensive surgical incisions to promote drainage and healing.

Acute and chronic cholelithiasis must be mentioned in association with the diabetic person. The progression of cholelithiasis to necrosis and sepsis increases the indications for early surgery in the diabetic person. Controversy exists only over when the surgical procedure should be done, not if it needs to be done.[5]

PHYSIOLOGIC CONSIDERATIONS

The diabetic person has faulty metabolism of carbohydrate, fat, and protein because of an absolute or relative lack of insulin. In addition, diabetic control is affected by stress, which may be caused by both emotional or physiologic upheavals.

Surgery itself and the anesthetic agents are physiologic stresses. The body reacts to these stresses in order to maintain homeostasis. The homeostatic reaction involves the release of at least two hormones, epinephrine and the glucocorticoids, which cause a rise in the blood glucose level, an increase in free fatty acids, and a fall in the serum insulin levels in diabetic persons with endogenous insulin-secreting ability. Epinephrine raises the glucose level in the blood by breaking down glycogen in the liver; the glycogen is converted to glucose. Epinephrine also decreases the uptake of glucose by muscle tissue and inhibits the release of endogenous insulin. The glucocorticoids raise the blood glucose level by increasing the production of glucose from protein (gluconeogenesis) and by inhibiting

the uptake of glucose by fat tissue.[3,6]

A decrease in glucose tolerance has been observed in most people undergoing a surgical procedure. The greatest degree of glucose intolerance was noted on the third postoperative day. By the eighth postoperative day, the glucose tolerance returned to normal. Endogenous insulin secretion is initially depressed and later enhanced by surgery in nondiabetic individuals.[7]

PREOPERATIVE PREPARATION

The outcome of any surgery is a result of the combined effort in planning, execution, and follow-up by three key medical professionals: the internist, or pediatrician in the case of children, the surgeon, and the anesthesiologist.[4]

Preoperative preparation of the diabetic person includes careful consideration of the choice of the anesthetic agent to be used. Some anesthetizing agents cause an increase in blood glucose levels. However, the ability of a drug to raise or lower the blood glucose level is not the sole criterion in choosing or rejecting the drug. The type of surgery to be performed is a definite determinant in the choice of anesthesia. The age of the patient is another. The physiologic state of the individual is yet another factor to be considered. Spinal anesthetics are often chosen for diabetic persons because fewer complications are noted and aspiration is not as common with these agents.[8] Because the most common surgery in the diabetic individual involves the lower extremities, spinal anesthesia is ideal.

The following is a brief summary of anesthetizing agents and their effect on blood glucose level[6]:

Effect on blood glucose levels	Anesthetizing agent
Least increase	Halothane (Fluothane) and trichlorethylene (Chlorylen, Trethylene, Trilene)
Moderate increase	Cyclopropane and halothane (Fluothane)
Greatest increase	Ether, chloroform, and ethyl chloride

Preoperative preparation must proceed with detail. Preferably, most surgery should be performed on an elective rather than an emergency basis. Preparing the patient for elective surgery should allow adequate time to ensure that the diabetes is under reasonable control. Reasonable control means the absence of symptoms of hyperglycemia (polydypsia and polyuria) and a blood glucose level of less than 300 mg/dl. Though not financially sound for some patients, it is advisiable for the diabetic patient to spend at least one full day in the hospital before the day of surgery.[4]

The medical workup should include, but is not limited to, all of the following:

1. Detailed diabetic history
   Number of years' duration of the diabetes
   Method of control now and in the past
   Number of times of ketoacidosis and hypoglycemia
   Diet and dietary habits
   Weight control
2. Evaluation of the vascular status and complications of diabetes mellitus
   Renal status
   Cardiovascular status
   Peripheral vascular status
   Cerebral vascular status
3. Previous illnesses, accidents, and infections
4. General history and physical examination
5. Diagnostic tests, particularly those whose results reflect the diabetes control and the absence or presence of complications
   Fasting, postprandial, and PM blood glucose samples in the insulin-controlled patient
   Electrolytes, sodium, potassium, HCO_3^-
   Blood urea nitrogen
   Creatinine
   Serum cholesterol
   Hemoglobin, white blood cell count
   Urinalysis
   Electrocardiogram
6. Drug therapy, excluding diabetic medication but including over-the-counter drugs; drug allergies

MANAGEMENT

Understanding the management and care of the diabetic patient undergoing surgery is facilitated if one knows the patient's needs, which are based on the method of control: diet control, oral agent control, and/or insulin control. However, this classification neglects the presence or absence of vascular complications, which must be considered as a serious complicating factor.

The diet-controlled diabetic patient

The diet-controlled diabetic patient requires little more preoperative preparation than does the nondiabetic individual. Some physicians prefer to admit this patient a day or two before surgery to ensure stabilization before surgery. Hospitalization at an early date may be unneccessary if an extensive workup has been previously done in the physician's office and the individual is in optimal control.

On the day of surgery, the fasting blood glucose level is obtained. It serves as a baseline for later in the day when subsequent blood glucose values are obtained during surgery or postoperatively. Testing the urine for glucose and acetone levels at the same time that the blood is drawn gives a rough indication of the renal threshold. A second-voided specimen must be used for this urine test. As stated previously, most diabetic patients are 40 years of age and over. It is expected that a patient within this age range, would have a higher than normal renal threshold. Results of urine tests are not indicative of diabetic control if the patient has a high renal threshold. The urine test results will usually be positive when the blood glucose concentration ranges between 160 to 180 mg/dl. Renal thresholds of 200 to 300 mg/dl are not uncommon in older diabetic patients. It is therefore appropriate to know the renal threshold for a particular patient in order to determine the value of urine tests in the postoperative regulation.

During the postoperative period, the

complications one watches for are hyperglycemia, ketoacidosis, and hyperosmolar coma. The latter is a particular danger in the very elderly. Surgery, physiologic stress, and fluid and electrolyte losses may hasten the onset of the complications mentioned.

Oral agent–controlled diabetic patient

The diabetic patient taking oral hypoglycemic agents should be admitted to the hospital 1 to 2 days before surgery. If the person's control of diabetes is poor, it may be advisable to institute insulin therapy during the surgical period. On the day of surgery, the oral agents should be withheld. Cholorpropamide should be discontinued 3 days before surgery. Close observation for signs and symptoms of hypoglycemia during and after surgery is necessary with all patients whose control was achieved with chlorpropamide because the hypoglycemic effect of this drug has a half-life of 36 hours. There is less danger of a significant drop in the blood glucose levels with other oral agents such as tolbutamide, acetohexamide, and tolazamide.

A fasting blood glucose value must be obtained on the day of surgery as a baseline. Intravenous feedings with a solution of 5% dextrose in water should be started in the morning on the day of surgery. Except in those patients who had been taking chlorpropamide, hypoglycemia during surgery in this group is rare. On the other hand, hyperglycemia could occur secondary to the administration of dextrose solution in combination with loss of fluids and electrolytes.

In the postoperative period, it may be necessary to administer small amounts of insulin at regular intervals to maintain control. As soon as the patient is able to eat, oral hypoglycemic agents are reinstituted. A blood glucose value should be obtained in the afternoon of the day of surgery.

Insulin-controlled diabetic patient

The diabetic patient who depends on insulin for control requires close observation and careful monitoring of the diabetic status. Such patients should enter the hospital at least 1 or 2 days before surgery. If control is less than reasonable, that is, if blood glucose levels are greater than 300 mg/dl, these patients should enter the hospital several days before surgery and receive regular crystalline zinc insulin at frequent intervals in addition to or in place of the intermediate- or long-acting insulin. Insulin-dependent diabetic patients should be free of the symptoms of hyperglycemia (polydipsia and polyuria).

Ketoacidosis must be brought under control before any consideration for surgery, except in the most extreme, life-threatening emergencies. Dehydration and electrolyte imbalance secondary to glycosuria and ketoacidosis can be expected to develop within a 24-hour period during which the insulin-dependent diabetic person is without exogenous insulin. Surgery is extremely hazardous in the presence of these complications and should almost always be deferred for 24 hours in order to bring ketoacidosis and electrolyte imbalance under control.

During surgery, both hypoglycemia and hyperglycemia should be prevented. It is most important to prevent hypoglycemia because this condition is most immediately damaging. However, extreme hyperglycemia results in dehydration, electrolyte imbalance, and ketoacidosis, which can also be devastating and life threatening. The balance lies in determining the most appropriate amount of insulin to prevent both hypoglycemia and hyperglycemia. It is advisable to question the dosage of insulin that the patient takes at home on a regular basis. Dietary indiscretion requires larger amounts of insulin. However, upon entering the hospital, the patient receives a concise, calorie-counted diet, and insulin requirements may drop drastically. If the home insulin dosage is not appropriately altered, hypoglycemia during or after surgery may result.

On the morning of the surgery, a fasting

blood glucose value should be obtained. Intravenous feedings are started with a solution of 5% dextrose in water.

There is some disagreement among surgeons and diabetologists regarding how much insulin, what kind of insulin, and at what time insulin should be administered during and after surgery. This disagreement suggests that the ideal system of management has not yet been devised and that research in this vital area is needed. Since there is no ideal method, flexibility and sensitivity to the patient's changing needs is required. The following are alternative regimens:

1. No intermediate- or long-acting insulin is given on the day of surgery. At the beginning or shortly before surgery, regular crystalline insulin is given in the amount of 1 unit for every 2 gm of dextrose to be given. Additonal insulin can always be given as indicated by blood glucose determinations.[9]

2. One half of the usual dosage of intermediate- or long-action insulin is administered before surgery. The remaining half is given in the recovery room after surgery. The infusion of dextrose solution must be continuous to cover the insulin.[9]

3. One third of the usual dosage of intermediate- or long-acting insulin is administered before surgery. An additional third of the usual dosage is given after surgery.[3]

4. In children and insulin-dependent young people, insulin administration is best accomplished in the following manner: No intermediate- or long-acting insulin is given on the day of surgery. The total daily insulin dose is divided into four equal doses of regular insulin, which are given subcutaneously at approximately 6-hour intervals. The initial dose is reduced by approximately one third to one half of the calculated dose and given before surgery. A solution of 5% dextrose in water is administered in appropriate doses for maintenance and replacement fluids. During surgery, Ringer's lactate is usually given for fluid loss; following surgery, a 1/4- to 1/2-normal multiple electrolyte solution is given. If 5% dextrose solutions do not maintain the blood glucose levels at normal infusion rates, 10% solutions may be used. Postoperatively, fractional or block urine specimens

are collected, and the insulin dosage adjusted as needed, based on the urine and blood glucose determinations. The Dextrostix-Reflectance meter system is an excellent way to rapidly monitor the blood glucose levels in such patients. Postoperatively, a four-dose regular insulin regimen should be continued until oral intake is well established and the child is ambulatory; then intermediate-acting insulin can be resumed. Small, frequent doses of short-acting insulin are always safer than larger doses of longer-acting insulin. The insulin should be given subcutaneously. It should not be put in the bottle for intravenous infusion, because the dosage is too small and infusion is too slow. Moreover, insulin is electrostatically precipitated onto glass and plastic. Such sticking of insulin to the container reduces the available insulin to such negligible amounts as to be ineffective.

The greatest danger for the insulin-dependent diabetic patient is hypoglycemia. Unrecognized and untreated hypoglycemia will endanger the patient's life. In the already anesthetized, unconscious individual, the danger signal for hypoglycemia cannot be observed. Any drop in the blood pressure during and after surgery must be recognized as a potential sign of hypoglycemia.[6] If an error in the diabetic control is inevitable, the error should occur on the side of hyperglycemia rather than hypoglycemia. Consistent and close observation of the blood pressure, testing of the urine for glucose and acetone levels, and frequent blood glucose determinations from patients with extremely brittle diabetes may assist in the early recognition of hypoglycemia. The Dextrostix-Reflectance meter system is a fairly reliable and convenient way to monitor blood glucose levels during and immediately after surgery.

During and after surgery, as long as there is no food intake, dextrose solution should be administered intravenously. In the adult, 150 to 200 gm of dextrose, or 50 gm for every missed meal, evenly distributed throughout the 24-hour period, should be adminstered. Insulin is best administered during this period in four equal doses of regular crystalline insulin given at approximately 6-hour intervals. The dosage can be altered as needed, based on blood and urine glucose determinations. It should be pointed out that while calorie intake is decreased postoperatively, thus decreasing insulin needs, stress may counteract this effect and elevate insulin requirements. The net effect of these counteracting forces may be an immediate postoperative insulin requirement that is similar to the preoperative requirement.

Complications directly related to diabetes mellitus are, on one hand, the undertreatment of hyperglycemia with resulting ketoacidosis and, on the other hand, the overtreatment of hyperglycemia with resulting hypoglycemia. Nausea and vomiting, anorexia, and the possible use of nasogastric suctioning during the surgery period influences the stability of the metabolic state. Diabetic control can very well fluctuate, requiring varying amounts of insulin. For each patient, the dosage of insulin must be determined on an individual basis. The use of frequent small doses of regular crystalline insulin are always safer in a changing situation.

NURSING CARE

The diabetic patient undergoing surgery presents a challenge to the nurse. In order to provide care for this patient, the nurse must be familiar with the needs of the surgical patient in addition to being knowledgeable of the specific needs of the diabetic patient. Basic to care are all of the following:

1. Assessment of the physical, emotional and psychologic needs preoperatively
2. Care and observation during surgery and the immediate postoperative period
3. Maintenance of optimal blood glucose levels throughout hospitalization
4. Care during the postoperative period, with emphasis on control of infection and promotion of wound healing
5. Preventive health care, which includes diabetes teaching

Assessment of the physical, emotional, and psychologic needs preoperatively

The day before surgery is used to prepare the patient for surgery. Reasonable control of the diabetes must be obtained that day. The nurse must know the normal ranges for blood glucose and electrolyte values. Urine specimens to test for glucose and acetone levels are obtained at least every 4 hours. Urine tests may be obtained more frequently if the patient was admitted with signs of polyuria and polydypsia and is receiving emergency insulin injections in addition to the regular dosage of insulin.

A review of the patient's medical history will provide a sketch of the medical background. Assessment of the needs should include a complete diabetic history. The North Carolina "Diabetes Mellitus Patient Assessment Guides"[10] are of definite help (see Chapter 18). These guides systematize the assessment, leaving less to chance. The benefit of these guides to the patient is threefold: First, they are helpful in obtaining necessary information about the patient to assist in the care to be given during hospitalization. Second, they help to establish a baseline for the initial teaching or for additional teaching before discharge. Third, assessment guides help to establish a baseline to correct previous misinterpretation of information.

With some patients, the diagnosis of diabetes mellitus is made at the time of admission for surgery. These patients will not only have to be prepared for the forthcoming surgery but will also require in-depth knowledge regarding diabetic self-care before discharge.

It is beneficial to share with the patients the plans for their care. They should be told what to expect before, during, and after surgery. Such procedures as the hours for the collection of urine samples, the frequency of blood sampling, meal times, insulin administration, and how the insulin will be "covered" with glucose if they are receiving intravenous fluids should be discussed.

Diabetic patients need preparation specific to the surgical procedure they are to receive. Friends may have to be restricted from bringing food of any kind. Likes and dislikes for foods must be listed on the Kardex. This information should be shared with the dietitian.

Care and observation during surgery and the immediate postoperative period

The nurses in surgery and in the postoperative recovery room must be familiar with the fact that the patient has diabetes mellitus. These nurses must know the signs of hypoglycemia and be constantly observant of the possibility of lowering the blood glucose level with the administration of insulin. Records are reviewed for any diabetic medication the patient had received before surgery. The kind, the amount, and the time must be known. Signs and symptoms that require action are diaphoresis, increased restlessness, and a drop in blood pressure, which could be the only significant indication of hypoglycemia in the semiconscious or drowsy patient. Convulsions observed during this time are almost certainly a sign of hypoglycemia. A blood sample for the blood glucose level should be drawn and a solution of 50% dextrose in water should be intravenously administered immediately.

In the absence of a Foley catheter and during the semiconscious state postoperatively, blood samples should be obtained every 2 to 4 hours from the patients who receive insulin. Careful recording of body fluid loss, through bleeding, emesis, and urinary output, is essential. With fluid loss, there is also an electrolyte loss. Thus an insulin-controlled diabetic patient may develop hyperglycemia quickly, and additional insulin may be required. In the absence of insulin, osmotic diuresis occurs, and increased urinary output results. Adequate replacement of fluids, electrolytes, and insulin should be based on the laboratory results. Monitoring of vital signs and intake and output and testing of urine for glucose and acetone levels is mandatory when the patient has hyperglycemia.

Maintenance of optimal blood glucose levels throughout hospitalization

The convenient method for maintaining control of diabetes is the testing of urine for glucose and acetone levels. As stated earlier, the use of this method for control is flawed if the renal threshold of the patient is not known. Second-voided urine specimens, which are commonly used for urine testing, may be difficult to obtain from patients after surgery. The fractional or block specimen, in which all the urine is collected in four 6-hour segments (see pp. 44 and 110), may be more practical to use postoperatively in the ill diabetic patient. The patient is encouraged to ambulate if permitted to do so. Ambulation will help the patient to comply with the requests for urine specimens.

Easiest for the patient and for the nurse is the insertion of a Foley catheter. Continuous drainage of the bladder will assist in the accuracy of test results. The danger of a bladder infection with the retention catheter might, however, outweigh the need for accuracy of urine testing. A bladder infection is a frequent cause of hyperglycemia and acidosis. Thus a Foley catheter should be used only when the patient has difficulty in diabetes control or the surgical procedure indicates its use.

In most cases, it is acceptable for the insulin-dependent diabetic to spill some glucose into the urine during the postoperative period. Test results of $1/2\%$ (1+) to 1% (2+) by the 5-drop Clinitest ($1/2\%$ to 1% by the 2-drop Clinitest) are acceptable. With these elevations hypoglycemia will not occur and serious hyperglycemia is prevented.

If there is acetone in the urine, the cause must be determined immediately. The cause may possibly be inaccuracy in the reading of test results if urine test sticks, paper strips, or the 5-drop Clinitest methods are used, because these methods often underestimate the amount of glucose in the urine. This is especially true in the presence of acetone. The 2-drop Clinitest is recommended as the most accurate urine test available. Laboratory values for blood glucose and carbon dioxide content should be obtained to verify the presence of acidosis. In the presence of acidosis, increased regular crystalline insulin should be quickly administered.

During the period in which healing is taking place, the insulin-controlled patient may have a drastically reduced need for insulin with the decrease of physiologic stress. Careful observation for hypoglycemia is needed. It is not only the commonly observed "before supper insulin reaction" noted with the use of intermediate-acting insulin that will give the nurse a clue to the decreasing need for insulin. Early morning diaphoresis can also be a sign of too large a dose of insulin and must be differentiated from diaphoresis secondary to fever or the administration of an antipyretic. Confusion or headache in the morning or other behavioral changes are also important indications of hypoglycemia. In the elderly, already fluctuating in their behavior and compliance, a blood glucose value must be obtained before the administration of the morning dose of insulin. The patient with infection will require the most careful observation for hypoglycemia during the postoperative course of his hospital stay. The patient who did not require insulin before his hospitalization and surgery may also become hypoglycemic as the surgical stress declines. After healing has taken place, these patients can probably return to the prehospital state of control. Discharge preparation must include the need for control and the possible reduction or removal of insulin.

Maintenance of the blood glucose within acceptable levels is necessary to promote healing, decrease infection, and prevent secondary diabetic complications. Control of blood glucose levels decreases the length of hospitalization and promotes a feeling of well being. It is difficult to achieve and maintain control while the patient is bedfast and is not on the regular prescribed diet. The sooner the patient can return to both full activity and a supervised meal plan, the easier it will be to control the diabetes.

Using the urine test results for glucose and acetone levels as the sole criterion for the administration of insulin can be hazardous, especially if the urine tests are improperly performed. The "rainbow coverage," or sliding scale, must be used with care or not at all, because this method may result in treating the patient retroactively. Using the sliding scale, one may administer insulin to a patient who is already hypoglycemic, or insulin may be skipped when it is needed. If the sliding scale is to be used, one should always obtain results from a second-voided urine specimen before the injection of insulin. This will assure the administration of insulin based on results from a fresh urine specimen that roughly has the same value as a blood glucose sample obtained at that moment. A better method of control is the collection of fractional, or block, urine specimens and the administration of insulin on a proportional basis, as outlined on pp. 35-37. The insulin dose can then be increased or decreased on a daily basis, with the proportions remaining the same during the 24-hour period, rather than changed every 6 hours as is done with the traditional sliding scale.

Care during postoperative period: control of infection and promotion of wound healing

The diabetic patient is more susceptible to infection than the nondiabetic patient. This is especially true of the poorly controlled diabetic patient. Postoperative care should include: (1) scrupulous care of the wound, (2) careful observation and recording of the patient's temperature, (3) inspection of the wound daily to note the healing process, and (4) recording and reporting of any signs of inflammation.

The diabetic patient who is hospitalized because of an abscess, such as carbuncles or boils, is best cared for in a private room to prevent cross-infection. Depending on the location of the abscess, patients are encouraged to participate in their own wound care. Irrigation of the incised area frequently has to be continued after discharge. The nurse should describe to the patient how a clean wound looks with healing taking place.

Generally, wound healing is not adversely affected in the presence of diabetes mellitus, provided optimal control is maintained. Persistent hyperglycemia can prolong the healing time of the incision and facilitate infection. Healing time will be increased if wounds are dirty and if the circulation to the affected part is diminished. Meticulous care of the incision is indicated.

Preventive health care and diabetes teaching

A number of surgical problems that bring the patient to the hospital should alert the nurse to include health teaching in the patient's care. Frequently foot problems are caused by the individuals themselves, either because of ignoring previous teachings or because of not knowing what is involved in self-care.

The signs and symptoms of infection, which includes both visual signs, such as redness and edema, and sensory signs, such as pain and heat, must be explained. Emphasis is placed on the visual signs because a patient with a long-standing diagnosis of diabetes mellitus may have sensory deprivation in the lower extremities.

Continued observation and care of the surgical incision should be explained before discharge. Appointments to the physician's office or clinic must be made and the importance of follow-up care emphasized.

Instruction in diabetes self-care is part of the total care for the patient, though it was not the primary reason for the patient's hospitalization. The nurse of the unit may decide to provide this phase of teaching or may consult with the diabetes teaching nurse.

REFERENCES

1. Brunner, L. S., Emerson, C. P., Jr., Ferguson, L. K., and Suddarth, D. S.: Textbook of medical-surgical nursing, New York, 1970, J. B. Lippincott C., pp. 99-154 and pp. 683-715.
2. Postel, A. H.: A surgeons' view, Surg. Med. **1:**11, 1973.
3. Steinke, J.: Management of diabetes in the surgical patient, Med. Clin. North Am. **55:**939, 1971.
4. Marble, A., White, P., Bradley, R. F., and Krall, L., editors: Joslin's diabetes mellitus, Philadelphia, 1971, Lea & Febiger, pp. 599-620.
5. Ellenberg, M., and Rifkin, H., editors: Diabetes mellitus; theory and practice, New York, 1970, McGraw-Hill Book Co. pp. 746-759.
6. Schwartz, S. I. M., editor: Principles of surgery, New York, 1969, McGraw-Hill Book Co., pp. 371-373.
7. Wright, P. D., and Johnston, I. D. A.: Insulin secretion and glucose tolerance during and after surgical operations, Br. J. Surg. **60:**309, 1973.
8. Maloney, M., moderator: Managing the diabetic during surgery and pregnancy, Patient Care **4:**93, 1970.
9. Gershberg, D.: An internist's view, Surg. Med. **1:**5, 1973.
10. Watkins, J. D., Moss, F. T., Lawrence, P. A., and others: Diabetes Mellitus patient assessment guides, North Carolina Regional Medical Program and North Carolina Diabetes Association, 1971.

Education and research

17

Developing an education program

Rita Nemchik

DIABETES: A "MODEL DISEASE" FOR HEALTH EDUCATION

Historically, diabetes control was probably one of the earliest subjects for client health education. Even before the discovery of insulin a little over 50 years ago, diabetic individuals calculated and weighed their food, a task that presupposed knowledge about a dietary regimen. Because of its chronicity and treatment complexity, diabetes has often been referred to as a model for developing programs for teaching clients about disease self-management. With few exceptions, it does indeed serve as a "model disease" for client health education, because control of acute and chronic complications of diabetes are to a large degree controllable if the client understands and follows adequate treatment.

Because diabetes has been and will continue to be a model subject for client health education, it behooves us, as educators in the field, to continually attempt to improve our teaching programs in terms of efficiency and innovation. If one were to survey most community hospitals for the types of client health education programs being offered, undoubtedly the diabetes program would constitute a major percentage. Why? The numbers of diabetic persons in the population have increased since the advent of insulin therapy; moreover, there has been an increasing recognition by health professionals of the need for and benefits from teaching programs. These factors have contributed to the increased development of diabetes client education programs around the country. Health professionals realize that medical treatment must be combined with "educational treatment," which includes the patients' acquisition of knowledge and skills and their development of positive attitudes toward health and purposeful yet correct behavior.

Another reason for improving existing programs as well as developing innovative effective ones is the current concern with third-party reimbursement for client health education in hospitals. Although subjective, it is apparent that the more knowledge, skills, and positive behavior changes clients demonstrate with regard to diabetes, the better their chances of avoiding the acute complications, especially those that necessitate hospitalization. However, there are only a few documented programs that indicate a direct cost-benefit ratio as a result of client diabetes education. If we are to expect third-party payers to reimburse clients for the expense of health education in hospitals and if we expect our clients to change their behavior as a result of our teaching efforts, then it is especially crucial at this time for us to demonstrate, document, and evaluate the effectiveness of educational programs.

Within the past few years, discussion regarding third-party reimbursement for client health education, and specifically diabetes education, has been increasing within concerned professional groups. Why? It is fairly easy to understand how effective teaching programs for diabetic persons would eventually serve to decrease health care costs. However, it is unrealistic to think that if most of our current efforts were evaluated we would be able to demonstrate lower health care costs.

It is especially relevant at this point to review some of the criteria currently being proposed for client health education programs within hospitals. According to Simonds,[1] the term patient (client) education

particularly as it is applied to hospitals and other organized services for patient care, refers to the educational experiences planned for the patient by professional personnel as a component of his care and differentiates these experiences from unplanned learning experiences in the hospital and from other organizational or environmental factors which influence his behavior.

As defined, patient (client) health education can be a reimbursable element of cost under the Blue Cross system, provided that the guidelines for programs in patient education contained in the Blue Cross Association's 1974 *White Paper on Patient Health Education* are followed. However, it is important to realize that the Blue Cross Association on a national scale is composed of individual local plans that may or may not totally agree with this concept of reimbursement for patient education. It is important to determine the interpretation of the paper in your particular geographical area.

The guidelines that are proposed—to designate a coordinator, program goals, objectives, etc.—should be the major elements in any good program. A copy of the *White Paper* can be obtained by writing to any Blue Cross Association office.

WHY ORGANIZE A PROGRAM FOR THE CLIENT WITH DIABETES

Why the concern about an organized program under the direction of a professional? Generally health professionals realize that random, haphazard teaching can be incomplete and ineffective. If the third-party carriers are agreeable to the points listed above and if there are a few organized diabetes educational programs that do demonstrate lower health care costs,[2] then it is quite apparent that we should be striving toward such criteria.

The 1974 Policy Statement on Provision of Health Services of the American Hospital Association (AHA) encourages hospitals to develop, conduct, evaluate, and maintain client health education programs in order to teach clients how to best care for their personal health responsibilities. This is another good reason for developing organized programs.

Present legislation of the Health Maintenance Organization (HMO) includes health education as a distinct component of health services delivery.

The Joint Commission on Accreditation of Hospitals (JCAH) has no formal criteria regarding client health education at the present time. However, it could probably become an essential agency in accreditation in the near future.

Hospitals currently developing criteria for medical-nursing audits are incorporating client health education as an identifiable component of quality care.

Third-party carriers, AHA, HMO, JCAH, and Peer Services Review Organization (PSRO) either by their philosophy or statements about the importance and necessity for health education are pointing the way to a more structured approach.

With the trend toward organized teaching programs, there has been an increasing recognition of the role and responsibility of the nurse in health education. Many states are currently in the process of revising their Nursing Practice Act to specifically state that health teaching directed to the client and family is a recognized nursing responsibility.

As health professionals and organizations are recognizing and assuming their teaching responsibilities to their clients, the rights of the consumer are also being realized. The American Hospital Association's Patient Bill of Rights guarantees the client a right to knowledge about his disease in understandable terms.

GENERAL OUTLINE FOR DEVELOPING A PROGRAM

If your hospital has an organized diabetes teaching program, review its efficacy in terms of fulfilling its objectives (behavioral) and documentation. If your hospital provides incidental teaching for diabetic clients, perhaps now is the time to develop your program goals, objectives, and evaluation and examine your target population, teaching personnel, and resources. If the latter is true, you are probably wondering, "How do I develop an organized teaching program for my clients? Where do I begin?"

Listed below are the steps generally applicable in planning a teaching program for diabetes client health education.

1. Assess program need.
2. Obtain administrative and professional support.
3. Determine potential clients, sources of referral, and subsequent follow-up.
4. Plan program content with an interdisciplinary team (committee).
5. Determine program goals, objectives, and evaluation procedures.
6. Select learning strategies.
7. Determine and utilize available resources.
8. Recruit, motivate, train, and retrain teaching personnel.
9. Implement the program.
10. Document teaching.
11. Follow-up.
12. Evaluate teaching and program.
13. Revise program.

These steps are offered as a general outline for developing a program for diabetic clients in a variety of settings—in community hospitals, university medical centers, and public and voluntary health agencies. Each point is discussed at length in this chapter from a practical point of view. Although the emphasis is on developing a diabetes teaching program in a hospital setting, it is realized that the need for diabetes education exists in outpatient (ambulatory) and community settings as well. Much of the following information can be applied or adapted to these other settings. The success or failure of a viable program depends on several important factors: staff time, interested personnel, teaching materials, space, patient referrals, administrative and professional support, and funding.

PROBLEMS INVOLVED IN ORGANIZING A TEACHING PROGRAM

Problems may arise when you organize a teaching program because of professional resistance or a lack of administrative support, space, teaching material, teaching personnel, or funding.

Lack of administrative support

Support from administration is essential to both the short- and long-term success of the program. Because of increasing financial demands being made on hospitals today in terms of services, plus the effects of inflation, providing client health education may be initially viewed as a potential for added cost with little apparent benefit. However, if diabetes client education were completely effective in reducing hospital readmissions, then bed utilization would conceivably be lowered, creating lower incomes for hospitals. These two facts can be used quite effectively by adminstrators to argue against the need for client health education.

On the other hand, data today indicate that many patients seen by physicians fail to follow their prescribed therapy, a fact that seems to indicate a need for more health education.

It now seems that the greatest potential for improving the health of the American people is probably not to be found in increasing the number of physicians or hospital beds, but rather in what people can be taught and motivated to do for themselves, in influencing personal behavior and attitudes.[3]

More and more administrators are beginning to realize the value of client education and therefore are becoming more receptive. However, in the present state of the economy, they are not as generous in initiating new areas of client service, nor should they be, if they are seriously concerned with maintaining or at least not escalating health care costs. If program directors are not able to prove the validity of their programs and are not frugal with their expenditures, then someone else will control the costs—third-party carriers who reimburse for hospital costs.

Part of the commitment for client education involves time and personnel, both of which translates into money. The remainder of the commitment is to the concept of education itself. From the onset, the success of the program demands the involvement and cooperation of administration. If full administrative support is available, a large segment of the groundwork will have been laid. However, partial support from the administration can be temporarily adequate, at least until the program is off the ground and success seems eminent. It hardly seems conceivable that no support would be a choice. However, if that appears to be the case, several alternatives seem likely: Proceed with planning and gather support along the way; investigate positive feelings toward the program among other administrative personnel; or find support from a physician (particularly an influential staff member or chief), from diabetic persons who are convinced of the benefits of a teaching program, someone on the medical staff, or an influential, contributing member of the community. Begin to build your base of support, but be prepared for arguments for and against the program. Be familiar with the latest legislation and hospital regulations as they relate to client health education; better yet, get involved yourself in current efforts to support the concept.

Questions that you should be prepared to answer are:

1. Is a program needed and/or worthwhile? Why?
2. How will hospital costs be affected with and without the program?
3. What resources are available?
4. What support or opposition exists among professionals and clients in the hospital and in the community?
5. How long will it take to develop and become operational?
6. Will it be a success or failure? Will it create new problems or solve old ones?
7. What will be the reaction of the community?
8. What could possibly happen if the program is not offered?

Part of the hospital's role includes educating the patient, health team, paramedical personnel, and community that the teaching program can lead to better compliance to medical treatment, thereby promoting better health care. The role of the program planner is to demonstrate to the hospital administrators how this can be accomplished. The efforts we exert now in this area will no doubt bear fruit in the future.

Professional resistance

Resistance to the program from professional colleagues is at first glance, surprising. Statements such as the following are common: "I can teach it all." "You won't teach it my way." "You're stealing my patients." "You won't get near my patients with a 10-foot pole." "My patient doesn't want to know." These comments may be heard from nurses, dietitians, and pharmacists as well as from physicians.

Invariably many who are bombarded with such comments find that those who initially did not want their patients in a teaching program will eventually discover that diabetes education is an integral part of good health care and become one of the program's strongest supporters. How does it happen? *The client as the consumer* is the key. Clients have been heard asking the following question: "Why does my hospital roommate, who also has diabetes and is basically on the same treatment schedule, receive information about diabetes self-management, while I don't?" After similar questions from other patients, physicians will seek out the program and want to know just what it has to offer and when. A staunch opponent may be converted into a firm believer if asked to either help plan the program or actively participate in it.

A common source of professional resistance to teaching is a lack of communication with other members of the health team. They feel they are uninvolved and not needed in the planning, or that they did not "agree" with the content to be covered. Often physicians feel that too much extraneous, detailed information will be given or that a client will learn too much and seek the services of perhaps a colleague specializing in diabetes.

In general, a real lack of understanding regarding the basic goal of the program can be unmasked if you explore in depth the following questions and comments:

The program represents an overstepping of my territorial rights.

How will the program interfere with my individual relationship with those people with diabetes?

If my clients participate in the program, does it mean I have failed in my professional responsibility to educate them in their self-care?

What right have you to tell me that my client "needs" to be taught?

My clients have never learned, have no desire to learn, and probably never will learn.

They will never be any different, I have already tried, and the only thing that will improve the diabetics' health is good medicine.

The preceding statements are a few examples of how program goals can be misunderstood by your colleagues. Often a promising program and enthusiastic planner are defeated before beginning if these comments are passively accepted and not defended.

Another key word in attempting to resolve the problem of professional resistance is *activity* rather than passivity. Before beginning the battle to overcome resistance to the program, it is imperative to ask yourself the question, "How firmly do I believe in client health education?" If the answer is in the slightest degree doubtful, convince yourself first of its merits, otherwise your opponents will easily sway or confuse you. Search the literature, talk to professionals who have already organized education programs, and critically quiz the client who has benefitted from an educational process. Arm yourself with the facts, and as an exercise, ask a colleague to pose to you the questions and statements above, and counter them with a convincing argument. If you rush ahead and try to convince an opponent and lose, it may harm the program's development and will necessitate a lot of backtracking.

If the professionals involved either directly or indirectly in the program understand exactly what it is you are hoping to accomplish (objectives) and have participated in planning, generally, less resistance will be encountered. However, if these suggestions have been attempted and have failed, another possibility mentioned earlier is available but often overlooked—the client.

Begin the program with as many supporters as possible. The following technique is often used in convincing an opponent to support a program: "accidentally" arrange for a client or his family to become aware of the program. This can be accomplished by such simple tactics as announcing the beginning of the program over the public address system, choosing a time to teach when the "other" diabetic patient (the one who is not in the teaching program) is in the room (some nurses have been known to place the slide-tape or videocassette between beds making it almost impossible for the other diabetic person to ignore the message), and leaving posters or pamphlets describing various aspects of the disease (or program) in full view of all (staff, visitors, and clients). Remember people do talk to each other, especially if one client is benefitting from an educational experience. The clients who are not receiving the information will often be motivated to request it for themselves or at least wonder why they have not been asked to participate. These suggestions, of course, presuppose that there is no real reason—physical, mental, or psychologic—for not teaching a particular client.

Often the attitude of the staff will be neither strongly positive nor strongly negative but rather indifferent to client health education. This attitude can stem from a lack of authoritative or peer support, a lack of knowledge about diabetes, a lack of understanding of the possible benefits of the learning experience for the client, a lack of time to teach, or a real or imagined lack of teaching ability. Each of these can be found singly or in clusters among professional personnel.

At times, the task of trying to convert everyone to the cause of health education can appear overwhelming. However, if you believe in the concept and are persistent, success will eventually come. Approach your colleagues enthusiastically and with a positive attitude. If the problem is a lack of peer support, encourage involvement, and create an atmosphere where teaching clients about their health maintenance is the norm rather than the exception. Urge those in authority to support this concept among the staff, and convince them to reward (verbally or otherwise, but not necessarily financially) their staff members who incorporate teaching as a routine part of care. Remind professionals that it is their responsibility to educate their clients.

If the problem is a lack of knowledge about diabetes, a misunderstanding of the benefits of self-management for the diabetic person, a lack of time to teach, or a lack of teaching skills, it is imperative that these deficiencies be corrected. This can be accomplished through regularly scheduled in-service programs endorsed by the administration.

Often professionals are reluctant to admit a lack of teaching skills. It must be noted that many practicing health professionals have never been exposed to courses in education or the principles of learning and teaching. However, more and more they are realizing the necessity for preparation in the basics of educational methodology. Such courses are available at local colleges and universities. Some hospitals with organized health education programs have felt the need to develop such courses for their staff and offer them on a routine basis.

It will never be possible for every health professional to become an expert teacher. However, all who deal with clients' health care are expected to teach in some way, and some states have already delineated health teaching and counseling as a defined responsibility of current nursing practice.

Professional schools that prepare basic students would be wise to include client health education in their curriculum, as a necessary component of the educational process, along with the principles of learning and teaching.

Another practical approach to motivate professionals to teach is through the use of nonprofessional personnel. The following example is offered as a suggestion. During orientation of professionals within a hospital to an inpatient teaching program, an invitation was also extended to nonprofessional groups, such as ward clerks, unit secretaries, and nurses' aides. The sessions were fairly well attended on all shifts, perhaps partly because of administrative support. However, the professional group at first glance appeared aloof and solemn. As the orientation progressed, the nonprofessionals (who were invited so that they could become familiar with the program) began to ask questions and eventually created so much enthusiasm that all those present became actively involved in the discussion. Afterwards a nurse commented that she was not going to allow the nonprofessionals to surpass her in her efforts in promoting health teaching.

If you can show your staff that educating the clients about their own health care is a satisfying experience that can easily become (with a little practice) a routine part of quality health care, the success of your program, insofar as personnel are involved, is almost guaranteed.

Lack of space

The availability of space in which to teach can pose either real or imaginary problems in the implementation of a teaching program.

If the program is group centered rather than on a one-to-one basis, a classroom setting would probably be most commonly available and utilized. In a hospital, such a room would ideally be centrally located, especially if patients are referred from various areas throughout the hospital. An exception would be locating within an area devoted entirely to metabolic diseases, or specifically to diabetes. The latter is becoming increasingly popular in proportion to the number of beds (usually over 500). Other areas that are commonly available include the visitor-patient lounge areas, a sun porch, or unit conference rooms. Other less obvious areas that are sometimes available include a hospital cafeteria, board room, nursing school classrooms, auditorium or gymnasium, clinic waiting areas, or even an empty hallway that might be adapted into an area for teaching.

Providing a relaxed atmosphere conducive to learning, however, is not exclusively dependent on space but also on the personality and attitude of the teaching personnel. If the interest in developing a program is genuine, any area may be adapted for use. However, if either administrative or professional support is questionable or weak, a space problem can easily become an excuse for delaying the program. In such a situation, a suggested approach might be to find an area that could be used for group teaching, find furniture and equipment that is not in use, and work out details regarding the class (such as referrals methods, and teachers). Next, present the program package, including who, what, where, and why to the appropriate personnel or committee for approval. Be prepared for any and all questions and roadblocks.

Lack of teaching materials

Teaching materials do not necessarily entail a great expense, although it is convenient and timesaving if finances are available for purchasing. Good, basic, professionally prepared teaching materials and literature can be obtained without cost from the various pharmaceutical companies that manufacture products for use by diabetics. Other resource areas include county agricultural extension services, dairy councils, local city and state departments of health, and companies that produce or distribute dietetic products. There are also some food companies that will provide exchange equivalents of their products. Your local and state diabetes association should also be contacted for teaching materials.

In general, there is a superabundance of material available. However, be cautious and discriminating in choosing such materials. It is far better to have a few quality items than too many of a mediocre quality. All too often professionals tend to become impressed with some of the printed materials or audiovisual aids and sacrifice good teaching strategies to a handful of artistically perfect pamphlets that unfortunately are soon laid aside by the client. Too much material will overwhelm and confuse your client. It is important to remember that the chief function of an audiovisual aid is to enhance or emphasize your teaching by stimulating the various senses. Choose your materials carefully.

When selecting teaching materials, be mindful of your client's socioeconomic and cultural backgrounds. The effectiveness of your teaching aids can be totally negated if your clients do not read, if they cannot see well enough to read, if they cannot understand your medical jargon or slang, or if they do not understand or read English.

Occasionally you might find clients who appear to comprehend a particular concept and answer your queries correctly during a teaching session. However, it becomes apparent during their next medical or teaching visit that they either did not learn what was previously taught or were not motivated to follow through on the teaching. Be patient and investigate the cause. You might find some clients who are masters at nodding or smiling their approval to correspond with the tone of your voice or the expression on your face.

A valuable yet inexpensive resource is yourself. You do not need a degree in art to create teaching aids for your clients. However, your own resources are of questionable value if they entail too much time, detail, or money. Simple, inexpensive, non-artistic aids that might be used in teaching your diabetic client are a complete set of empty soda or food cans that can be used to teach how to read a label when buying dietetic or sugar-free foods locally. Even if your clients are unable to read or if they read at a lower grade level than the label, they will remember the can by its shape, size, color, and label. It can be fun and effective.

Teaching good foot care involves a few basins, soap, water, and towels. Demonstrate proper daily technique either on yourself or another patient, and then allow time for your clients to not only demonstrate what they have learned but also to criticize one another.

One of the most pointless tasks performed by nurses or their assistants in hospitals today is testing urine for the client. With few exceptions, the daily task of urine testing can be a dual learning experience for both the recently diagnosed and more knowledgeable diabetic patients. It allows the experienced patients to demonstrate the proper urine-testing procedure as well as provides them with an opportunity to learn to interpret the results of their tests under supervision (assuming that those who are assisting them know the correct procedure and can interpret the significance of the tests).

Recruit students to provide materials and create games that help clients learn. Students will learn while creating. There are virtually no limits to the resources available to help your clients learn.

Lack of teaching personnel

The following personnel should probably be considered as teachers for your program: physicians, nurses, dietitians, podiatrists, students, social workers, dentists, physiotherapists, and knowledgeable diabetics. It is more important to have the best possible teacher regardless of credentials than a poor teacher with the proper accreditation.

If you have been successful in promoting your program, your teaching personnel will probably already be recruited. If not, look to the various disciplines and ask for help—or, do it yourself at first.

The following points are offered for consideration when you select teaching personnel. If the same person, or team, teaches, a certain level of consistency might be achieved. If you select a member of a specific discipline, be sure that the member's colleagues do not want to teach. If they do want to be involved in the program and have not been asked, you may find a lack of referrals or support as a result. Occasionally you will find professionals who are willing and eager but really cannot teach. If a diplomatic solution cannot be found, consider eliminating the discipline of that particular teacher and substitute other teachers to offer their content. If the program is held during off-duty hours but on a regularly scheduled basis, seriously consider paying for teaching time either financially or with compensation time. Even though teachers are willing to volunteer their time, it has been noted that if some reimbursement is given for teaching, there is a stronger commitment to the program and therefore less teacher absenteeism. Plan from the beginning of the program to have substitutes on hand in case of teacher absence.

Lack of funding

Funding for the program may or may not be a problem depending on the institution's commitment, capability, and interest in client health education. The following items should be included in the budget for the program: salaries and administration, space, instructional personnel, instructional materials, and food.

Funds for salaries and administration might cover a program coordinator's salary, part-time secretarial help, fringe benefits, travel expenses to meetings, office supplies and stationery, costs for duplicating material, telephone, and postage.

Funds for instructional personnel might cover fees for teachers, speakers, consultants, artists, or editors.

Funds for instructional material might cover books and periodicals, permanent equipment, audiovisual hardware and software, and supplies.

If a meal or snack is used as a part of the educational process, an allowance for food should also be made.

It is certainly not beyond the realm of possibility to conduct a program with little or no apparent funding in hand. However, remember that personnel and their time will constitute the greatest portion of the budget. The other most expensive budget item is audiovisual equipment. Examine all the possible offerings on the market and make your selection based on your type of program, clients, teaching personnel, and equipment already available. Beware of buying a piece of equipment that includes software for a limited audience or topic.

Logical sources of funding include grants, gifts or donations from former clients, service clubs or hospital auxiliaries, and class fees. Check your local diabetes association for financial assistance or perhaps make a collaborative effort.

ORGANIZING THE PROGRAM
Assess the need for a program

Occasionally, in an effort to justify the development of a program, you may find it necessary to research the need for an organized program for diabetes client education. This assessment may be accomplished through questionnaires or interviews with health professionals and clients, the medical records department, and various community health agencies (such as visiting nurse or diabetes associations). When requesting the medical records department to furnish statistics, it might be worthwhile to ask for the top five or ten admission diagnoses. Include both primary and secondary diagnoses. Although you may find diabetes within the top ten primary diagnoses, it might be wise to add the number of persons with diabetes who were admitted for non-diabetes-related problems. These clients as well as those experiencing complications of the disease process are likely candidates for an educational program. It has been shown that the longer the duration of the disease, the more likely errors in either medication or self-management are likely to occur; thus there is a need for reviewing and redemonstrating certain techniques while the diabetic person is hospitalized.

Determine and obtain available resources for the program

Most of the preceding information has alluded to sources of either materials or personnel for the teaching program. Additional resources for personnel include trained and knowledgeable diabetic persons, hospital auxiliaries, public health nurses, faculty of nursing schools, and retired nurses and dietitians.

Plan the program

Probably the best and definitely the most successful program planning is accomplished by a committee composed of the various disciplines that have some relationship to the future program. The committee can be used in many ways, including assessing the need for a program, brainstorming for ideas, and devising, supporting, and finalizing plans. It is timesaving to prepare in advance for the first meeting and to have available statistics supporting the need for the program, the various resources (personnel and materials) that are available for the program, an outline of course content, and a list of the possible problems that may be encountered. (The course outline in Appendix C is an excellent starting point.) It is also well to meet individually with each committee member and discuss what he or she feels needs to be included. During the meeting give a copy of the suggested outline to each member for revisions. Much time, energy, and discussion will be saved by this method. It appears that starting without a written guide often creates confusion and makes the task ahead seem insurmountable.

Implement the program

After the course outline has been developed and approved by the appropriate personnel, teaching personnel recruited and trained, a patient referral system developed, and teaching materials selected, the program should be implemented within a reasonable period of time. Delay in implementation because of a small number of patients or other reasons can quickly lead to a decrease in interest and enthusiasm for the program.

Publicity is an important factor in implementing the program. Circulate information about the program approximately a month in advance of its commencement to allow for adequate coverage. Numerous methods are available for disseminating information. Generally, these include announcements in newspapers, radio and television, posters, fliers, and letters. Keep the announcement short, simple, and to the point. Include an easy method for potential clients or their physicians to obtain more detailed information. If you have a public relations person in the institution, keep him or her well informed about the program, especially in the period immediately before the program begins. The choice of media to advertise or announce the program will probably be determined by the type of community in which your institution is located (urban or rural), its population mix, socioeconomic and cultural backgrounds of clients, and timing. Regardless of the medium, remember to include in the announcement: the intended audience, place, time, frequency, length, and cost of the program and a method for obtaining more information (such as a telephone number).

While proceeding in the initial stages of the program, the teaching personnel may find it worthwhile to follow each session with a brief critique and suggest more efficient methods for teaching or improving the overall functioning of the program.

Evaluate the program

Most nurses are overwhelmed or confused when the term evaluation is mentioned. Stated quite simply, it is the process of determining the worth of something. In client health education programs, you can evaluate either the client's learning or the program, or both. An easy mistake is to evaluate the program itself, conclude that it is functioning well, and then assume that the client has learned.

Evaluation can be subjective or objective. For the most part, subjective evaluation is fast and simple but generally inadequate. It can only describe the subject's (observer's) view of the learning process.

Perhaps the most difficult thing for those conducting inpatient programs to understand is that a pretest and posttest, or a return demonstration during the program, is not a guarantee that a change of behavior on the client's part has taken place. As defined, learning is a behavior change and for many reasons cannot occur spontaneously and oftentimes not even within the period of hospitalization or length of the program. It is extremely important to realize that changing a client's behavior takes time. Habits that have taken years to establish cannot be unlearned in a few weeks. This is especially true of eating patterns and habits.

The matter of evaluation is clarified if the

objectives for the client are written properly. There are many excellent texts available to aid in writing objectives in terms of changes expected in a client's behavior toward his or her own health care. Be realistic about the objectives you write. Can they be accomplished within a reasonable amount of time with your clients? Are they clearly stated with no ambiguity? If the objectives are well written, they will provide a guide for planning the teaching, an idea of what the learner should be able to accomplish at the end of the program, and also serve as a basis for evaluation of the client's learning.

Although there are obvious methods for evaluating or measuring learning—testing knowledge (cognitive) with an oral or written quiz before and/or after the program, demonstrating a skill such as urine testing, or interpreting the meaning of the results—there is the possibility that only short-term effectiveness can be measured. For example, the client may be able to explain in a written test the reasons for urine testing and describe the appropriate action to be taken if the results are positive. He or she may also demonstrate the correct method of urine testing. However, the skill and knowledge demonstrated in writing may not be adaptable to the home situation. Even if the patient *can* perform the skill, will he or she change behavior patterns that impede the habitual performance of this skill? Long-term effectiveness of learning, which is extremely important in terms of the client's health, is more complex and not always convenient to measure, especially if you are conducting the program within an institution. There are, however, community agencies and professional groups (visiting nurse associations, public health nurses, private physicians' offices, clinics, and schools) that may be consulted for guidance in evaluating the long-term effectiveness of teaching and learning. (See also Chapter 18.)

For evaluation to be worthwhile, it should be continuous. The results of the evaluation should be used to improve, revise, and update your program for maximum efficiency.

Document teaching

In view of the current status of client health education, documentation is important. Points to be documented on the hospital chart or record should include an assessment of the diabetic person's knowledge and skills before the program, the plan for teaching, what teaching was actually accomplished, barriers to learning, the client's response, and areas for reinforcement and follow-up.

Some programs incorporate this information in the nurse's notes or on a separate sheet developed specifically for teaching. The latter is convenient and could be used by the various disciplines involved in the program. Beware of having too many places for documentation; you might find none are being utilized.

Occasionally a checklist for teaching is found to be convenient for documenting; however, it does not allow for recording observed behavior or responses to teaching.

Because education is an ongoing process, it would be helpful if a copy (preferably carbon) of the documentation were sent to the client's private physician or clinic as a means of sharing information as well as obtaining further reinforcement. It is also beneficial to give the client a copy of the discharge instructions (such as activity, medication dosage and time, and diet). Clients find this useful because during discharge they usually find themselves excited or nervous and are apt to forget the exact instructions.

Revise the program and retrain personnel

Both program revision and in-service education of teaching personnel are crucial at regularly scheduled intervals. If either is omitted, the program and its potential benefits to the clients will be lost. Keep abreast of recent developments in diabetes research through reading and conferences as well as close contact with your local diabetes association. (See Appendix B for a list of resources and services.)

SUMMARY

The preceding discussion hopefully gave some practical suggestions and approaches that might be used in developing a teaching program for your client with diabetes. It is intended to serve as a springboard for further reading and research. The following bibliography, which complements the information presented in this chapter, may be helpful if you are beginning to plan a program or revising one that is already functioning.

REFERENCES

1. Simonds, S. K.: Focusing on the issues. Strategies for patient education, Chicago, American Hospital Association, 1969.
2. Miller, L. V., and Goldstein, J.: More efficient care of diabetic patients in a county-hospital setting, N. Engl. J. Med. **286:**1388, 1972.
3. Somers, H. M.: Health and public policy, Inquiry **12:**95, June 1975.

BIBLIOGRAPHY

American Association of Diabetes Educators: Guidelines for program evaluation, The Diabetes Educator **2**(1):5, 1976.
American Hospital Association Conference: Strategies for patient education, Part II. An agenda for the hospital, October 1969, Chicago, The Association.
Balas, M.: Learning and teaching principles, The diabetes educator, Part I, Winter 1975; Part II, Spring, 1976.
Education and management of the patient with diabetes mellitus, Elkhart, Ind., 1973, Ames Co.
Fylling, C. P., and Etzwiler, D. D.: Health Education, Hospitals **49:**95, 1975.
Gronlund, N. E.: Stating behavioral objectives for classroom instruction, New York, 1970, The Macmillan Co.
Knowles, S.: The modern practice of adult education, New York, 1975, Association Press.
Krosnick, A.: Guidelines for a teaching program, The diabetes educator **1**(4):16, 1975.
Mager, R. T.: Preparing instructional objective, Palo Alto, Calif., 1962, Fearon Publishers, p. 62.
Pohl, M.: Teaching function of the nursing practitioner, Dubuque, 1975, William C. Brown Co., Publishers
Richards, R. F., and Kalmer, H., guest editors: Patient education, Health Educ. Monog. **2**(1): 30, 1974.
Simonds, S. K.: Current issues in patient education, American Association of Medical Clinics, New York, 1974, Core Communications in Health, Inc.
Symth, Sister Kathleen, guest editor: Teaching patients, Nurs. Clin. North Am. **6**(4):571, 1971.

18

Assessment

Elizabeth L. Burke

Education of individuals with diabetes is a necessary adjunct to management. When beginning to teach persons with diabetes, one should know what to teach, how to teach, who in the family needs to be taught, and how soon to allow them to be on their own. Nurses, dietitians, physicians, and others involved in the care and education of patients find that they need a method of gathering the kind of information that will assist them in the patient's education and management. The formal term for information gathering is assessment or evaluation. Applied to the diabetic patient, assessment is a method of identifying physical, social, or emotional needs that may influence educational abilities and long-term management of the disease. Lawrence points out that "the potential volume of material to be taught [diabetic] patients makes it all the more crucial that the teaching be individualized according to carefully assessed needs."[1] The use of a guide to assess needs will establish priorities and eliminate needless repetition of material. Although some repetition is desirable, much time can be wasted in teaching patients something they already know and do well. On the other hand, some concepts need to be emphasized and reemphasized to be learned. Assessment and reassessment is then needed to determine the material to be taught, material to be retaught, and material to be eliminated in order to individualize the learning process.

TIME OF ASSESSMENT

Assessment is desirable and should be used in a variety of situations and settings. Assessment should be used when the patient first enters the hospital or outpatient clinic in order to determine the current status. Assessment also needs to be used near the end of the hospitalization to reassess learning. It can be used in the home by the visiting nurse and in the physician's office during follow-up visits. In other words, any time the diabetic patient is seen by the health professional, some type of assessment or reassessment of needs should be carried out.

Assessment of a patients' understanding of their disease can be used in several ways. While an evaluation that deals entirely with diabetes management practices is not applicable to the newly diagnosed diabetic person, this type of assessment certainly is helpful for the newly admitted previously diagnosed diabetic patient. According to Donna Nickerson, "Many patients with diabetes may be overlooked as candidates for teaching because they have had diabetes for a number of years."[2] It has been found that these patients need almost as much teaching as newly diagnosed diabetic individuals, and the use of an initial assessment specifies the knowledge they need.

In addition to learning the patient's past management practices, it is just as important to find out certain physical, social, and emotional needs of the patient. These factors can be evaluated in any patient, previously or recently diagnosed, and should be used as a reference point throughout the teaching program and after the patient returns home. The following patient situations are examples of the kind of factors that cannot be ignored. *Example:* The patient is color-blind, which inhibits his ability to accurately read the urine test color chart. Changing to a different test method may solve that difficulty. *Example:* The patient lives in a room-and-board situation, which makes a weighed or measured diet impractical. It might be better to teach him to estimate his food, have the cook attend the diet classes, or have him cook his own meals. *Example:* The patient is a newly diagnosed diabetic who has an uncle who has had diabetes and an amputation as the result of diabetes-related arteriosclerosis. She is terrified that the same thing will happen to her, and is therefore unable to concentrate and learn. She needs to be given time to accept the idea of having diabetes and have someone available to answer her questions. "Real learning" may have to wait. All of these factors, physical problems, social needs, and emotional responses need to be known early in the teaching process; however, many times, because of an absence of formal assessment guidelines, these factors are either overlooked or ignored.

ASSESSMENT METHODOLOGY

There are various methods of evaluation: questionnaire (written or verbal), demonstration, and interview. A combination of these three types of assessment is the most useful (unless the patient does not read or write). Ideally, the evaluation should also have a built-in mechanism for teaching the patients as well as gathering information about them.

A questionnaire form might include a detailed social history, information about how the patient has managed the diabetes in the past, and some general knowledge questions about diabetes. Patients can fill this out at their leisure. If they do not read, someone can ask them the questions. The questionnaire type of form saves much time for the instructor especially when working with a large number of patients at one time.

Patients should always have an opportunity to demonstrate that they can perform the various tasks they will have to do at home. The Assessment Guide of the North Carolina Regional Medical Program[3] follows this concept (p. 219). The assessment guide is set up with a page of questions to ask the patient and directions to the patient to demonstrate various testing techniques. There is a corresponding space for written observations about the technique and teaching carried out. There is a matching page of guidelines for the instructor (see p. 220). These instructions state what the patient is to know and do as a result of learning the information. Urine testing, insulin measurement and injection, and weighing or measuring of food are all included in the list of activities the patient should be able to perform before discharge from the educational program. Patients need not feel threatened by the demonstration. They should always understand that the staff wants to help them and to find out the reasons for any problems with control of the diabetes. This type of assessment can also be used in the home by the visiting nurse.

The interview portion of the assessment guide can actually be a part of the questionnaire and demonstration. The questionnaire should always be followed by a review, at which time the educator reinforces correct knowledge and gains further information about incorrect knowledge; for example, the educator may find out whether the patient has misunderstood the question. This is also the time to correct misconceptions. In addition, an interview gives the educator the opportunity to assess emotional status and gain further information about the patient's family, work, and activities.

ASSESSMENT GUIDE FOR USE IN HOME, HOSPITAL, CLINIC AND OFFICE*

Patient's name _____ Interview date _____

Nurse's name _____

Doctor's orders: _____

_____

_____

Date of order: _____ Ordered by: _____

1. Tell me what the doctor wants you to do about your urine (get name of tests, times). _____

_____

_____

What has been possible for you to do?

For sugar:

Patient says he tests _____ times a day / week

at _____ and _____ AM

at _____ and _____ PM

For acetone:

Does not test _____; or patient says: _____

_____

Observe when possible:

2. What do you use to test your urine for sugar?

Uses _____

(check color of tablets; expiration date of tape)

For acetone?

Uses _____

3. Show me how you test your urine.

Tested correctly according to method used	Yes	No
Compared results with appropriate color chart	Yes	No
Read results correctly	Yes	No

Where indicated:

Show me how you test your urine for acetone.

Tested correctly	Yes	No
Read correctly	Yes	No

4. How do you collect the urine for testing?

Uses double voiding technique	Yes	No

5. Do you ever change the times you test your urine?

Knows when to test more frequently	Yes	No

Observe when possible:

6. Do you keep a written record?   Yes   No

What do you include? _____

_____

Shows record to doctor   Yes   No

GUIDELINES FOR INSTRUCTOR*

Below are statements numbered to correspond with each question on the [preceding] assessment guide. Each statement indicates what "the patient should know" about the various aspects of urine testing.

The patient should know:

1. The doctor's orders regarding the test to be used and when to test.
2. That he should use only the test ordered by his doctor because the meaning of the test results varies according to the test used.

    That discolored tablets and outdated tape should never be used because they will not give accurate results.

    That test supplies (tablets, tape, etc.) should be kept in tightly covered containers to keep them from absorbing moisture.

    That the test ends of the "stix" should never be touched because this will affect the chemical reaction.
3. That he should follow the test directions exactly because *any* deviation will influence results.

    That color charts for the various tests are different and cannot be interchanged.
4. That freshly voided urine will give a more accurate indication of the blood sugar level at that time. (If the doctor agrees, the patient should use the "double-voiding technique," which means he should void and discard the first specimen, then void again within one-half hour, testing the second specimen.)
5. That high urine sugar content usually means high blood sugar content and for this reason, he should test more often when:
    a. He feels ill or has an infection.
    b. The test shows large amounts of sugar and/or acetone.

    That he should contact his doctor when:
    a. His urine contains acetone.
    b. His urine contains much more sugar and/or acetone than usual.
    c. His urine becomes negative for sugar when it has usually been positive.
6. That he should keep a written record of his urine test results and show it to the doctor because the doctor will find it helpful in deciding whether the regimen prescribed is appropriate.

*Reproduced with the permission of The American Diabetes Association North Carolina Affiliate, Inc.

PURPOSE OF ASSESSMENT

The information the assessment gives to the educator can also be used to individualize the patient teaching materials. It may be obvious from the initial assessment that certain materials would be too complex for the patient and more simplified ones should be used. Certain information, such as adjustment of insulin dosage, may be inappropriate for some patients and should be deleted from their teaching.

The information the assessment gives to the patients may help motivate them toward the end result. Morreau states, "In many cases, clients will be able to proceed independently if provided with clear statements of what they need to be able to do and how they can learn to do it."[4] The idea of actually listing the goals and objectives of the teaching program in an initial assessment and telling the patient how to reach the goals may be quite foreign to the usual way of proceeding. However, it may save much time and money in the long run and is certainly worthy of consideration.

Having greater knowledge of the patients may also cut down on the frustration experienced by the staff when there are teaching problems. When the problems are anticipated, greater efficiency and motivation often develop.

Finally, the diabetic's family needs to be involved in the teaching program. Early assessment will reveal what form the involvement should take, and appropriate steps can then be taken to ensure their participation. Family members will usually be responsible for assisting the patient in the home, and their monitoring of the patient's progress will often motivate the individual toward increased self-care.

FOLLOW-UP REASSESSMENT

Assessment should never end with discharge from the hospital. Because it is in the home where patients will be managing their diabetes, it is in the home where assessment should continue. It would be ideal if every person with diabetes could be visited in the home by a health professional within the first month after discharge and periodically thereafter. In practice, home visits are difficult because of lack of personnel. However, there are many patients who do receive home visits, and many times astonishing facts are discovered. Watkins and others[5] did a 24-hour recall diet study in 1967, making home visits to 60 patients who regularly attended two university metabolic clinics. An attempt was made to discover how closely these patients followed their diet plans at home, regarding both food intake and regularity of meals. Their findings showed that only 12% received the maximum score on food intake, indicating at least some adherence to the diet plan, while 32% were following the diet very little. The meal regularity scores showed that only 27% had acceptable spacing of meals.

Because of weaknesses in the 24-hour recall method, a second study was performed.[5] This time 17 patients were asked to keep food records for 7 days. They were visited in their homes each day by a nutritionist or public health nurse to "insure completeness insofar as possible." The findings of this study showed that "over three-fourths of the patients were not eating the foods prescribed with the frequency prescribed."[5]

Other studies by Watkins disclosed serious errors in insulin administration and urine testing.[6,7] While further studies are needed with patients in other settings, the studies in this setting indicate the difficulty in achieving patient compliance in the home, even while under close medical supervision. It can be guessed that the percentage of noncompliance with other groups of diabetic patients would also be quite high. In order to change these ratios, it would appear that some changes need to be made in the treatment and education of diabetic patients. Perhaps early assessment is one way to identify needs and problems at the outset so that patients would have the full benefit of our knowledge of them and educational programs could be better tailored to the needs of each individual. Reassessment of false notions and the need for reeducation and new education must be a part of each clinic visit.

ASSESSMENT TOOLS

While not intended to serve as a model, the format evolved by the Diabetes Treatment and Education Center at Good Samaritan Hospital in Portland has been helpful in identifying and meeting assessment and educational needs. An abbreviated interview form is used on admission to the hospital (see p. 222). This form identifies specific information quickly and easily. During the second day of teaching an interdisciplinary conference is held with the nurses, dietitians, physicians, instructors, public health coordinator, and social worker to review and share information each has about the patients. Are they learning at the ex-

PATIENT INTERVIEW*
Diabetic ambulatory unit

I.   A. Color _____

GENERAL   B. Mobility _____

APPEARANCE   C. Communication _____

D. Deformities _____

E. Affect _____

F. Obesity _____

II.   A. "Why are you here?" _____

CONCEPT   _____

OF ILLNESS   "What are you expecting from hospitalization?" _____

B. Concept of diabetes

1. Length of disease _____

2. Do you recognize your reactions—treatment? _____

3. Do you know when your blood sugars are high—treatment? _____

4. Urine testing—method used and frequency _____

5. Previous class instruction _____

III.   Temp _____ Pulse _____ Resp _____

PHYSICAL   B/P _____ Height _____ Weight _____

HISTORY   A. Systems review

1. Respiratory (smoker, SOB, etc.) _____

2. Circulatory (legs, edema, blood pressure problems) _____

3. Sensory (blurry vision, ears, touch) _____

4. GI (bowels, stomach, ulcers, elimination needs) _____

5. GU (urinary, reproductive) _____

6. Skin (feet, leg ulcers) _____

7. Neuro-skeletal (arthritis, neuritis, Parkinson's, CVA, Fx, etc.) _____

8. Metabolic (thyroid, diabetes) _____

B. Past hospitalizations and surgeries _____

*Reproduced with permission from Diabetes Treatment and Education Center, Samaritan Hospital and Medical Center, Portland, Oregon.

PATIENT INTERVIEW —cont'd
Diabetic ambulatory unit —cont'd

III.
PHYSICAL
HISTORY
—cont'd

C. Allergies (drug, food, cosmetics, tape, etc.) _____
_____

D. Medications (current); insulin (kinds and times) _____
_____

E. Diet (C-P-F, calculation/exchange); special needs; snacks _____
_____

F. Prosthesis
   1. Dentures (upper-lower, partial bridge) _____
   _____

   2. Glasses or contacts _____

   3. Other (limb, eyes, special equipment—walker, cane, etc.) _____
   _____

IV.
PERSONAL
DATA

A. Home life—who does patient live with or near? _____
_____

B. Social assistance (VNA, social welfare) _____
_____
_____
_____

C. Spiritual needs (chaplain, pastor, priest or rabbi to be notified?)
   yes ☐   no ☐

V.
EMOTIONAL
STATE

Circle appropriate descriptive terms:

Alert	Confused	Fearful
Angry	Critical	Hostile
Answers questions readily	Demanding	Hyperactive
Answers questions reluctantly	Disoriented	Tearful
Anxious	Embarrassed	Withdrawn
Belligerent	Euphoric	

VI.
INTERVIEWER'S
COMMENTS

Comments: _____
_____
_____
_____
_____

VII.

Do you have any concerns not included in this interview? _____
_____
_____

Signature _____

Date _____

TEACHING FLOW SHEET FOR DIABETIC PATIENTS*

Name: _____ Admitting date: _____

A. **Initial evaluation**
   of patient's understanding of diabetes.

B. **Urine testing**
   1. Notation that patient understands reasons for testing, correct method and times for him specifically.

---

   2. Demonstrates proper care of testing equipment.

C. **Insulin administration**
   1. Notation of patient's insulin sites and current rotation pattern.

---

   2. Instruct and/or review insulin technique.

---

   3. Preparation of syringe (mixed and/or single dose).

---

   4. Review needle length.
   5. Instructed on U-100 insulin.

---

   6. Family members assist with insulin.

D. **Oral hypoglycemic agent**
   1. Verbalized knowledge of uses, action, and appropriate admin. time.

E. **Diet management**
   1. Notation that patient has received information on: free foods, foods to avoid, and achieving and maintaining a desirable weight.

---

   2. Attended exchange and/or calculated diet class.

---

   3. Demonstrates knowledge of his diet by doing practice menus.

---

   4. Patient received going home diet plan.

---

   5. Patient instructed and understands when to take snacks.

---

   6. Patient can explain effects of alcohol on blood sugar.

F. **Concept of diabetes regulation**
   1. Explains causes, treatment, and prevention of hypoglycemia. Recognizes symptoms.

---

   2. Explains causes, symptoms, treatment and prevention of hyperglycemia.

---

*Reproduced with permission from Diabetes Treatment and Education Center, Good Samaritan Hospital and Medical Center, Portland, Oregon.

TEACHING FLOW SHEET FOR DIABETIC PATIENTS—cont'd

F. **Concept of diabetes regulation**—cont'd
    3. Review metabolic sheet
        a. Explains action of insulin
        b. Knows insulin dose
        c. Understands insulin adjustment
        d. Understands need for an exercise program

G. **Complications**
    1. Notation that patient can list complications of diabetes.

H. **Foot care**
    1. Notation that patient explains foot care technique.

I. **Illness**
    1. Notation that patient has understanding of diabetic routine during illness.

    2. Explains signs and symptoms of ketoacidosis.

    3. Notation that patient indicates that illness, esp infection, vomiting, diarrhea, etc. may precipitate ketoacidosis.

J. **Discharge note**
    1. Verbalizes confidence regarding his independence in self-management

Visiting nurse follow-up and reason:

Nurses discharge evaluation:

pected rate? Are there certain limitations, either physical, intellectual, or emotional? Will they need discharge follow-up by the visiting nurse or social worker? It is found that a clearer picture of the diabetic person is revealed by the group than by any one member of the team.

During the first week of teaching, a flow sheet is used (see p. 224). It identifies skills the patient should possess, has a place for indicating the data or dates when these skills were practiced or learned, and space for any relevant remarks. This flow sheet can be filled out by the nurse on the unit or the instructor in the classroom. By the end of the first week of teaching it should be quite complete.

SUMMARY

Whatever form the evaluation takes, the instructor should feel free to update in it from time to time. No method is perfect, and any method should be adjusted as situations change. There are, however, some guidelines that can be helpful to anyone setting up criteria for assessment:

1. Begin the assessment during the initial contact with the patient. (It is very discouraging to find out on the day of discharge that the patient's vision is so poor she cannot see the markings on the syringe and that her poor vision may be the reason for the poor control that brought her to the hospital in the first place.)

2. Assess physical, social, and emotional needs as well as the current diabetic orientation. (The patient's wife does the cooking; thus she should be involved in the education process, too. Or, the patient recently had a death in the family. Feelings about the death may prevent him from learning.)

3. Use more than one method of assessment —questionnaire, demonstration, interview. (The patient may be able to verbalize exactly how to do the Clinitest, but may be too shaky to drop the urine into the test tube.)

4. Continually assess throughout the education process, including after the patient's discharge. (Each time the patient returns to the physician's office or clinic, someone needs to review some things with him. Further teaching or reinforcement of earlier teaching will help to remind the patient of his responsibilities in self-management.)

5. A copy of the assessment should be available for the physician's office, visiting nurse, or public health nurse. This will greatly assist and enhance the follow-up process.

Assessment of patient knowledge, understanding ability, and needs is an important part of patient education and management. Assessment should be performed initially and repeatedly during the education process.

Reassessment should be performed on some aspect of patient knowledge and compliance at each office or clinic visit for optimal diabetic management and the optimal conservation of patient health.

REFERENCES

1. Lawrence, P.: Diabetes mellitus. *In* Kay, Corman, and Kintzel, editors: Advanced concepts in clinical nursing, Philadelphia, 1972, J. B. Lippincott Co., pp. 105-129.
2. Nickerson, D.: Teaching the hospitalized diabetic, Am. J. Nurs. **5**:935,1972.
3. North Carolina Regional Medical Program: Assessment guides for use in home, hospital, clinic and office, Chapel Hill, North Carolina.
4. Morreau, L. E.: Developing a systems approach to patient education, Diabetes Educator **1**(1):6, 1975.
5. Watkins, J., Williams, T., Anderson, E., and Coyle, V.: Dietary errors made at home by patients with diabetes, J. Am. Diet. Assoc. **51**:19, 1967.
6. Watkins, J., Williams, T. F., and Martin, D. A.: A study of diabetic patients at home, Am. J. Public Health **57**:452, 1967.
7. Watkins, J., Williams, T. F., and Roberts, D. E.: Observation of medication errors made by diabetic patients in the home, Diabetes **16**:882, 1967.

19

Research developments

Diana W. and Richard A. Guthrie

Research in diabetes has secured no major breakthroughs since the discovery of insulin in 1921. However, the slow but steady accumulation of knowledge continues and, in the last 10 years, at an ever increasing pace. Major impetus to basic biomedical research has come from the development of new tools with which to carry out the investigations. Such major tools as the radioimmunoassay and new space age technologies have greatly enhanced the pace of these investigations. Research funds however have not kept pace with technology, and much needed research, now technically feasible, remains undone because funds and trained manpower are lacking. The American Diabetes Association, the Juvenile Diabetes Foundation, other similar private foundations, and the federal government, through the National Diabetes Act of 1974, are beginning to address these problems. It is therefore anticipated that the pace of biomedical research aimed at a prevention and a cure of diabetes will accelerate more rapidly in the near future.

A cure and a prevention remain elusive. Though they remain the only ultimately acceptable solutions to the diabetes problem and though we are more optimistic for a cure in the foreseeable future than at any time since 1921, they still are the wave of the future. In the meantime, treatment must be carried out and the search for better methods of treatment (including health care delivery and education) must also con-

tinue. Though some treatment programs seem to achieve better results than others, those involved in the health care of diabetic individuals must be innovative and willing to submit all ideas, treatments, delivery systems, and educational approaches to careful clinical investigation to validate their effectiveness and establish their possible effect on complications.

The current status of biomedical and clinical research is discussed in this chapter, as are the major controversies in the field, in order to introduce some of the questions that remain to be answered. It should be pointed out that present and future health professionals, for whom this volume has been developed, as well as physicians can and should be involved in both biomedical and clinical research. Much is needed and much is and will be demanded by the population with diabetes. In addition, basic information about research should be communicated to the diabetic person and/or the family. One of the most frequently asked questions by diabetic persons and by the public is "What's being done?" The question is constantly reasked and must be reanswered. The information should be incorporated in the basic education programs for those with diabetes and must be constantly updated. The editors are aware of the fact that this chapter may well be obsolete by the time of publication, and we sincerely hope that the pace of the accumulation of new knowledge is such that it is. However, we include it as the latest available knowledge, which the health care team should know and impart to the diabetic population.

INSULIN

With the development of the radioimmunoassay in the early 1960's by Berson and Yalow,[1] it became possible for the first time to measure circulating insulin levels directly. This led to a whole new understanding of insulin secretion and action and made possible many additional steps. A prevention or a cure will be possible only after there is an understanding of all of the steps in insulin synthesis, secretion, transport, action, and degradation. The radioimmunoassay for insulin, and now for other protein hormones as well, has made research to understand each of these steps in the insulin story possible. Once these steps are fully understood, we can then begin to see where these steps go wrong in the diabetic individual, outside factors that affect them, why the beta cell fails, and perhaps what can be done to prevent the cell from failing or to rejuvenate the failing cell.

Major steps have been taken recently to promote an understanding of the mechanisms of insulin synthesis and release. Using the electron microscope, radioimmunoassay, and radioactive labeling techniques, Lacy[2] and Milner and Hales[3] have added greatly to our understanding of the synthetic steps in insulin production. More recently Orci and others[4] using freeze etching and the scanning electron microscope have greatly enhanced our knowledge of insulin release. The studies of Steiner, Rubenstein, and associates[5] and Chance and others[6] have supplemented the work of Lacy and Orci with the development of the biochemical concepts of synthesis. These authors[5,6] developed the concept of proinsulin, a precursor of insulin, and the need for degradation of proinsulin before secretion. A spin-off of their research has been the development of an assay for the connecting or C-peptide, the fragment broken off from proinsulin, to make the finished insulin molecule.

The assay for C-peptide now makes possible the study of beta cell function in the individual receiving insulin. C-peptide, the breakdown product of proinsulin, is secreted in a molar relationship to insulin. The levels of C-peptide in the blood then give a measure of the insulin-secreting ability of the beta cell in an individual in whom insulin cannot be measured directly because of interfering antibodies or because the assay cannot distinguish between endogenous and exogenous insulin. As a result of this development, we have learned that after initial treatment, the beta cell may temporarily recover some insulin-secreting ability. The declining insulin requirements and stability of the so-called honeymoon period (often seen in children with juvenile diabetes soon after treatment) are accompanied by rising C-peptide levels. This indicates recovery of endogenous insulin secretion. The obvious implication of this remarkable finding is that we should be attempting to design a therapeutic regimen to preserve and protect this beta cell function. More research in this area is urgently needed now that the tools are available.

CELL MEMBRANES

One of the newest and most promising areas of basic biomedical research is in the area of membrane physiology. Insulin acts at the cell membrane level, activating some secondary messenger within the cell membrane that carries out the desired function within the cell. It is entirely possible that some types of diabetes may not result from a primary failure of the beta cell but from a resistance to insulin action at the cell membrane level or within the secondary messenger system. This may well be true of those individuals with chemical diabetes who are insulin hypersecreters. Tools are now available to study this important area and research is in progress. It is possible that methods may be developed to enhance insulin action at the cell membrane or reduce its resistance to insulin action.

GLUCAGON AND SOMATOSTATIN

For many years after its initial discovery, glucagon was the forgotten hormone. Pediatricians used it to treat hypoglycemia, but it received little other attention. Radioimmunoassay for glucagon has now been developed, and glucagon is now beginning to emerge as an important biologic entity. Unger and Orci[7] have carried this important research to the point of discovering that diabetes is a bihormonal, or two-hormone, disease, at least in certain individuals. This concept is supported by the finding that in many diabetic persons the glucagon levels are high even in the presence of marked hyperglycemia and seem to be nonsuppressible by glucose. In the nondiabetic person, glucose will suppress glucagon levels. It has also been shown recently that ketosis is more a function of glucagon excess than of insulin lack and that the marked variability in glucose levels observed in the person with brittle diabetes can be markedly minimized by suppression of glucagon. This finding has lead to the search for agents that will suppress glucagon secretion and to the discovery of somatostatin, a potent hormonal substance (produced in the hypothalamus and perhaps elsewhere) that will suppress glucagon and other hormones, including growth hormone and insulin. Therapy with somatostatin is not at present practical because of its short duration of action (3 to 5 minutes) and its toxicity (somatostatin is toxic to the liver and other organs when given exogenously). Its discovery has opened whole new avenues of research into the regulatory mechanism (insulin), counterregulatory mechanisms (glucagon, growth hormone, and epinephrine), and now the counter-counterregulatory mechanism (somatostatin) for glucose. What should emerge is not only a better understanding of the interrelationship of these regulatory mechanisms but also an understanding of why they fail in the person with diabetes and, if not a prevention, at least improved methods of treatment that will minimize ketosis and the wide variability in blood glucose levels in the person with brittle diabetes.

ETIOLOGY OF DIABETES

The cause of diabetes remains unknown. New research however is leading us to the concept that there may be many causes of diabetes. Diabetes may not be one disease but the common pathway for many diseases that ultimately cause beta cell failure. Diabetes therefore may be more logically classified as a syndrome of multiple etiologies rather than a disease.

Diabetes has always been thought of as a genetic or inherited disease, although the mode of inheritance has not been characterized. This is largely true because a genetic marker for the disease in nondiabetic relatives of diabetic persons has not been found. Data are now beginning to emerge to indicate that diabetes is in fact an inherited disease but that there are many modes of inheritance. These modes of inheritance are different in different families; moreover, the different environmental factors that determine (at least partially) the manifestations of the inheritance may be different for the different inheritance patterns.

Genetic markers that are being developed with the human lymphocyte antigen (HLA) system used in tissue typing for transplants indicate that certain people with diabetes and perhaps their families have certain HLA antigens. For example, though no consistant HLA patterns have been found in adult maturity-onset diabetics, two HLA antigens have been found consistently in juvenile-onset diabetes. The HLA-B8 and B-15 antigens appear to be genetic markers for this type of diabetes. With this information, it should be possible now to identify people who are potential diabetics and study various environmental factors that determine the expression of the genes. If these environmental factors can be identified, it might become possible to eliminate them and prevent diabetes.

Recent virus research indicates that some diabetes may be caused by viruses. New research indicates that persons with the specific HLA types may also be susceptible to certain viruses. Thus, it may be that both the appropriate HLA gene and the virus infection (or other environmental insult) may be necessary for the development of diabetes. If the hypothesis is true, as Tattersall and Fajans[8] and others believe, it could explain the fact that occasionally only one in a pair of identical twins develops diabetes. The nonaffected twin may have the same genetic makeup but may have escaped the environmental or viral insult. In any event, the advent of genetic markers has opened whole new fields for genetic research as well as research aimed at identifying and eliminating or preventing environmental insults to the genetically susceptible individual.

VIRUSES

More study into the relationship between infectious agents and diabetes is needed. Some groups have studied the parallelism of infection with diabetes by time[9-15] and others by serologic techniques.[16] Studies of the association of certain viruses, such as coxsackie virus B (type 4),[17] with diabetes continue but without conclusive data in man. An association between diabetes and the mumps virus[9] seems strongest in man, while other "diabetes-causing" viruses are stronger in animals. In studies at the University of Missouri, it has been noted that infection increases glucose intolerance in children.[18]

An "autoimmune" diabetes mellitus might also be a result of these viruses. The virus may modify islet tissue, creating foreign antigens that might cause the formation of antibodies that cross-react with the person's own insulin-making ability. This type of situation would be analogous to the relationship between the streptococcus and rheumatic fever.

The importance of this research is that if viruses are involved in the etiology of all or some diabetes and they can be identified and grown, it should be possible to develop a vaccine that would prevent these infections and some cases of diabetes.

COMPLICATIONS OF DIABETES AND NEW MODES OF THERAPY

Perhaps no area of diabetes is more controversial or more important to the diabetic person than the area of complications. Because a cure is not going to be available tomorrow or next year, persons with diabetes must be concerned about the possibility of vascular and neurologic complications and must be concerned about treatment and control until a cure is possible. The controversy centers around conflicting data. Depending on how one selects the data to be analyzed, one can support the concept that vascular and neurologic disease in diabetics is either (1) a concomitant of diabetes, genetically predetermined and unaffected by treatment or control or (2) a complication of diabetes and preventable by proper treatment and control. The data regarding macrovascular disease, most often observed in adults with maturity-onset diabetes, are very inadequate at present and do not as yet present any conclusive evidence that treatment alters outcome. Nonetheless, therapy still remains the best and only hope for a good patient outcome, and until the data are more conclusive, the diabetic person must be given the benefit of the doubt, or at least the choice.

The data for microvascular disease and neuropathy and their relationship to control are much better, though the case is by no means proved and much research is still needed.

Biophysical and chemical studies are increasingly supporting the need for a closely controlled disease in order to prevent or delay vascular complications. The goals for control are: blood glucose levels within normal limits a majority of the time without significant insulin reactions, normal blood lipid levels, adequate weight for height, and normal growth and development in the child.

Basement membrane biochemistry

In 1968, Siperstein and associates[19] published data on vascular disease in diabetes using a new technique that has opened a whole new area of research. Siperstein developed the technique of muscle biopsy, using a small needle in the quadriceps muscle and studying the muscle tissue under the electron microscope. When the electron microscope is used, the capillaries can be studied in detail and the thickness of the various layers measured. The significant lesion of blood vessels observed in the diabetic person is a thickening of the basement membrane surrounding the capillaries. The thickness of these basement membranes can be easily measured in a muscle biopsy specimen, and the degree and course of the vascular disease studied. Kilo and others[20] found that the basement membrane surrounding the capillary does not become thickened prior to the development of carbohydrate intolerance. These findings contradicted the previous studies on an older population by the Siperstein group. Osterby,[21] Jackson,[22] Fajans,[23] and their associates found capillary membranes to be of normal thickness in the majority of newly diagnosed children with overt or chemically abnormal diabetes. The Osterby study[21] was especially important because kidney (the important target organ) biopsies were used. Children with juvenile diabetes had normal kidney biopsies at onset of diabetes. After 3 to 5 years of poorly controlled diabetes, however, the membranes were markedly and progressively thickened. Lundbaek,[24] in the same clinic, studied a group of similar patients who had diabetes of up to 5 years' duration and were kept aglycosuric. These children had essentially normal capillary basement membranes. Jackson, Guthrie, and others[22] observed that a high level of metabolic control in diabetic persons with a duration of the disease up to 17 years

resulted in normal basement membrane thickness (see Tables 19-1 to 19-4).

In one study, four newly diagnosed children with diabetes had mildly thickened basement membranes; after 9 months of treatment with insulin, the thickness decreased to normal. Basement membrane studies by several groups continue on a longitudinal basis and promise new understanding of this important area. Work on the basic biochemical mechanisms of the development of microvascular and neurologic disease continues and should be expanded and accelerated.

Spiro and Spiro[25] studying basement membrane biochemistry have found in the basement membranes of the kidneys (and probably other vascular tissue as well) en-

Table 19-1. Capillary basement membrane thickness of nondiabetic boys and girls

Age	Value*	Standard deviation†	Age	Value	Standard deviation
9	696	±171	14	704	±178
9	735	±128	14	905	±167
10	679	±79	14	924	±160
10	724	±148	14	933	±306
10	778	±113	14	910	±180
10	854	±280	14	1004	±334
11	750	±185	14	1005	±334
11	859	±183	15	860	±104
11	869	±159	15	742	±157
11	1002	±164	15	743	±282
12	738	±123	15	880	±104
12	754	±215	15	651	±148
12	787	±103	15	820	±153
12	867	±92	15	833	±202
12	794	±101	15	836	±126
12	871	±273	15	860	±101
12	940	±218	16	641	±211
12	947	±146	16	1006	±433
12	948	±308	16	1010	±306
12	1005	±313	16	1042	±399
13	735	±259	17	854	±96
13	994	±265	17	884	±276
13	1033	±168	18	738	±68
14	664	±134	19	902	±191
14	766	±254	20	1067	±403
14	841	±156	21	754	±130

*Mean 847.3; coefficient of variance 0.1245.
†Standard deviation of values 101.2.

Table 19-2. Capillary basement membrane thickness in girls and boys with chemical diabetics

Age	Value*	Standard deviation	Years' duration of diabetes
10	886	±213	5
12	651	±197	3
13	691	±165	5
13	914	±249	3
14	872	±184	5

*Mean 780.835.

Table 19-3. Capillary basement membrane thickness in girls and boys with recent-onset overt diabetes

Age	Value*	Standard deviation
8	715	±191
9	642	±134
11	751	±107
12	724	±132
13	1047	±318
13	818	±183
14	758	±92
14	844	±146
14	1044	±312
5	1017	±323

*Mean 814.5; coefficient of variance 0.1318.

Table 19-4. Relationship of duration of diabetes and degree of control to capillary basement membrane thickness

	5 years' duration			5-10 years' duration			10-15 years' duration			Over 15 years' duration	
Age	Value	Standard deviation	Age	Value	Standard deviation	Age	Value	Standard deviation	Age	Value	Standard deviation
Girls and boys with good control											
14	882	±186	9	973	±227	13	511	±124	16	982	±286
16	1064	±154	9	778	±203	15	706	±171			
			9	857	±142	15	783	±203			
			11	710	±85	15	842	±212			
			12	677	±121	18	702	±156			
			14	734	±210	18	783	±294			
			14	677	±121	21	902	±193			
			16	641	±186						
			17	827	±224						
			18	837	±213						
			18	642	±127						
				764	±180						
	Mean 973			*Mean* 759			*Mean* 733.3				
Girls and boys with fair control											
5	624	±102	9	636	±173	12	860	±248	21	1812	±418
7	736	±177	12	760	±146						
9	803	±216	12	729	±216						
14	1146	±224	15	807	±204						
			15	867	±236						
			17	997	±211						
			17	993	±251						
			18	1417	±494						
			18	1223	±556						
			22	1091	±460						
	Mean 759.5			*Mean* 951							

Table 19-4. Relationship of duration of diabetes and degree of control to capillary basement membrane thickness—cont'd

5 years' duration			5-10 years' duration			10-15 years' duration			Over 15 years' duration		
Age	Value	Standard deviation	Age	Value	Standard deviation	Age	Value	Standard deviation	Age	Value	Standard deviation
Girls and boys with fair to poor control											
12	829	±223	12	1161	±371	18	1146	±273			
13	933	±270	14	1178	±337						
			15	1302	±165						
			18	982	±305						
	Mean 882			*Mean* 1097.5								
Girls and boys with poor control											
13	1094	±262	16	1591	±507	21	1906	±937			
13	1058	±334	17	1423	±641		906	±437			
13	1283	±373	18	1492	±182						
14	1206	±237									
14	981	±225									
16	1171	±285									
16	883	±167									
	Mean 1047			*Mean* 1502			*Mean* 1406				

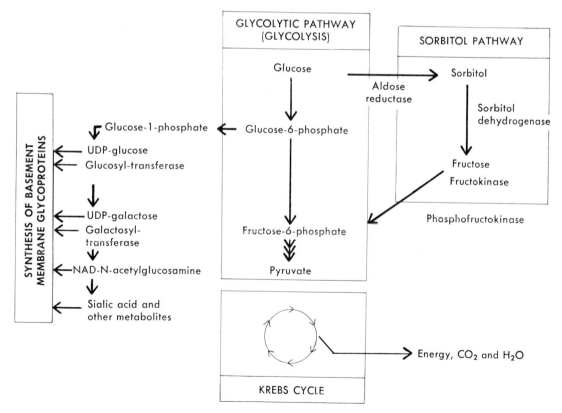

Fig. 19-1. Metabolic pathway: synthesis of basement membrane glycoproteins. (Reproduced with permission of The Upjohn Co.)

zymes called transferases (glucosyltransferase and galactosyltransferase), which are responsible for the conjugation of glucose and galactose, as a disaccharide unit, onto the amino acids of the protein structure of the basement membrane. This conjugation of disaccharide units onto the basement membrane results in thickening of the membrane at that point. The disaccharide content of the basement membrane is increased in diabetic persons and appears to increase with duration of diabetes and with lesser degrees of its control. Spiro and Spiro found that the enzymes (transferases) responsible for this reaction are elevated in poorly controlled diabetic animals and can be suppressed by insulin therapy. It appears that when the insulin level is low, the transferase enzymes are active and the substrates for the transferases are also high. When an enzyme is active and the substrate is present in large amounts, the enzyme can be expected to carry out its intended action

—in this case, the thickening of the capillary basement membrane. Spiro has stated, "It appears that insulin administration must be conducted in a meticulous manner in order to restore to normal the machinery of basement membrane synthesis."* An alternate explanation for basement membrane thickening has been proposed by Maurer,[26] who feels that the initial lesion is the accumulation of material in the mesangium area of the kidney. The function of the mesangium is to remove basement membrane material. Maurer feels that the defect is an altered ability of mesangium to remove basement membrane material. Maurer finds however that the function of the mesangical cells is adversely affected by elevated glucose levels; thus this mechanism of basement

---

*Spiro, R. G., and Spiro, M. J.: Effect of diabetes in the brosynthesis of the renal glomerular basement membranes, Studies on the glycosyltransferase, Diabetes **20**:641, 1971.

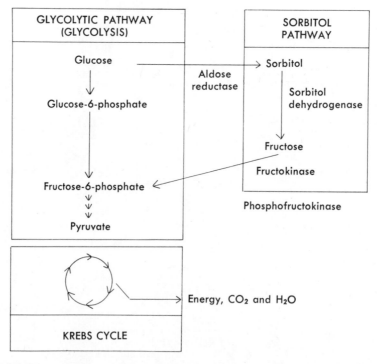

Fig. 19-2. Metabolic pathway: sorbitol pathway, a section of Fig. 19-1. (Reproduced with permission of The Upjohn Co.)

membrane thickening may also be caused by high blood glucose levels or poor control. Maurer has found that he can reverse these changes by improving control in experimental animals.

Polyol pathways of glucose metabolism

Another promising avenue of research has been research into the polyol pathways of glucose metabolism. The polyols are sugar alcohols and represent an alternate pathway of glucose metabolism when insulin-dependent pathways are blocked. Morrison and Winegrad[27] have demonstrated the presence of enzymes of the polyol pathway (aldose reductase and sorbitol dehydrogenase) in various tissues of the body, including capillaries, large vessels, nerves, and the lens of the eye. When glucose levels are high and the normal insulin-dependent glycolytic pathways are blocked by low insulin levels (poor control), the polyol products are formed and accumulate in the respective tissues. The accumulation of polyols increases the osmotic gradient in the tissue, resulting in an influx of water and tissue edema. Tissue edema results in decreased oxygen diffusion and tissue damage.

The polyol accumulation is almost certainly the mechanism of diabetic cataract formation, especially in the young diabetic person, and may be the basic mechanism of diabetic neuropathy.[28] The relationship between the polyol pathway and vascular disease is less well established, but there is some evidence that it may be involved in large vessel, or macrovascular, disease. The polyol pathway in eye, nerve, or vascular tissue is a function of the blood glucose level. If the mechanism is involved in disease of these tissues, then it is imperative that blood glucose levels be kept as nearly normal as possible at all times.

PANCREATIC REPLACEMENT

The attempt to replace or simulate pancreatic action has been studied for many years. Progress is now being made in both the replacement (transplantation) of the pancreas, pancreatic islet cells, and even beta cells and in the simulation of pancreatic action (the artificial pancreas). Actual transplant of all or parts of the pancreas has been tired in various settings. Although tissue transplants involving the pancreas have all the problems associated with heart, lung, or kidney transplants, because of the necessary introduction of immunosuppressant drugs, many feel this is the type of procedure that holds the most promise in long-term control of the disease. The donor pancreas corrects the diabetic condition with heartening results. The recipient pancreas is left in place, while the donor pancreas is either anastomosed to the ureter or connected to the jejunum.[29,30] The basic failure to retain whole pancreas transplants has been a result of either autolysis (self-destruction) or fistula formation secondary to exocrine secretions.[31,32] Tissue rejection and infection resulting from immunosuppression have also been problems.

Islet cell transplant

Islet cell transplantation has opened up new avenues of study. The major centers, such as the University of Minnesota, Washington University, the University of Texas, and Montefiori Hospital, have experimented with whole islet cell transplants and with transplant of the beta cells alone. These transplants have been placed in various parts of animals bodies to ascertain areas of most positive growth and least rejection. The cells have been introduced into the liver through the portal vein as well as into the peritoneal cavity and into the muscle.[33,34]

In a number of studies,[33,34] animals were made diabetic by the introduction of streptozotocin. After injection of islet cells into the liver tissue through the portal vein, the responses of a group of rats favorably paralleled the responses of the nondiabetic control group. The researchers[33] concluded that the liver would be an ideal place for transplantation. However, one large problem has been noted. The beta cells have

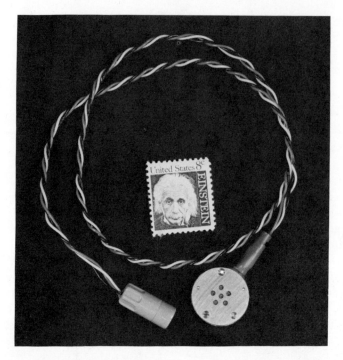

Fig. 19-3. Glucose sensor. (From Soeldner, J. S., and Spiro, R.: Special report: Current status of the artificial beta cell and implantations of islets, Forecast **26**(4):2, July-Aug. 1973. (Used with permission of the American Diabetes Association, Inc.)

been found to undergo fibroblastic formation, such as that observed in the early stages of cancer cell development. Ongoing observation over a period of time will determine whether this formation in the liver will develop into a life-threatening situation.

Artificial pancreas

The artificial pancreas is making notable headway. This mechanical development involves everything from a glucose sensor to an insulin-filled reservoir. When perfected, the mechanism will closely resemble the functioning pancreas. The glucose sensor recently perfected by Soeldner and associates[35] is the size of a dime with a sensitivity of 99%, and in controlled conditions, it is being used to monitor the blood glucose levels of research subjects. To match the physical release of insulin and replace the present system of injection, the artificial pancreas will need a glucose sensor, a computer, a power supply, pump, and a reservoir of insulin. In order to have a fail-safe device, a glucagon or glucose reservoir and release mechanism have also been introduced as part of the unit. The sensor is closest to use in human experimentation. Much research needs to be done before the total device is perfected and miniaturized.

Another device consisting of the sensor and a transmitting device has been used to measure blood or tissue glucose levels in animals. This device may have practical application in warning of a falling or low blood glucose level during the treatment of ketoacidosis, during surgery, or at night. This device will soon undergo human trial in Germany. A large, external, artificial pancreas has been successfully used in Canada and Europe as a research tool and to control therapy in ketoacidosis, delivery, and during surgery.

The artificial pancreas, in order to be practical, must be miniaturized to the size of a cardiac pacemaker, will need to cost about $1000 or less, will need to be replaced no more than every two years and will need to be refilled with insulin no more than every one to four weeks by syringe through the skin into the reservoir.

The first step in the artificial pancreas, the internal glucose sensor and transmitter and the external receiver will help monitor food, exercise and medication. It may replace the need for testing urine. It would also signal an alarm for the occurrence of hypoglycemia. Space technology helped in the miniaturization and functioning in this research project. Soeldner and Bessman[36] have been the pioneers in this field. Engineers from the Space Sciences Division at the Whittaker Corporation have been working closely with Dr. Soeldner at the Joslin laboratory especially in the development of the glucose sensor and appropriate miniaturization of the artificial pancreas components.

Summary

The artificial pancreas and beta cell transplants are often referred to as cures for diabetes. It should be pointed out however that neither of these important projects are cures. Both beta cell transplants and the artificial pancreas are highly sophisticated forms of improved treatment. Neither the families with diabetes nor the public should be told that these are cures because this raises false hopes and gives false impressions. Diabetics should be kept informed of progress in these and other areas but should not be given false hopes.

PREVENTION

The most important but least heralded aspect of research in diabetes is the prevention of the occurrence of diabetes mellitus. Scientific investigation of the functioning of the pancreas, of the associated metabolism of glucagon, and of the hypothalmic-pituitary axis are parts of the puzzle under study. The influence of nutrition on the body and the place of diet in diabetic control need further elucidation. Even

though much is known about insulin, such as its molecular structure and its chemical structure, there still are many gaps of information yet to be unearthed. In the recognition of the role of glucagon, much more information has been analyzed, which has, in fact, opened the door to even newer questions. Although the cure of diabetes may be closer at hand and prevention is becoming a reality as researchers increase knowledge about the general function of the body and its systems, much research remains to be done. Informing the person with diabetes about the ongoing research supports the individual with motivating hope.

A variety of areas of basic research, such as the mechanisms of insulin secretion and action and the role of various treatment regimens in preventing vascular disease, still need further study. Areas of applied research requiring further study are the beta cell transplantation, the artificial pancreas, genetics, and viruses and their applications in prevention of diabetes.

Finally, much research is needed into better methods of treatment and better methods of securing compliance with prescribed treatment. Research into better methods of education of persons with diabetes and the psychosocial aspects of compliance are vital areas of research that should be undertaken by the health care team.

REFERENCES

1. Berson, S. A., and Yalow, R. S.: Diagnosis, radioimmunoassay of plasma insulin. *In* Diabetes mellitus: diagnosis and treatment, vol. 1, American Diabetes Association, Inc., 1964, pp. 47-54.
2. Lacy, P. E.: Beta cell secretion from the standpoint of a pathobiologist, Banting Memorial Lecture, Diabetes 19(12):895, 1970.
3. Milner, R. D. C., and Hales, G. W.: The role of calcium and magnesium in insulin secretion from rabbit pancreas studied in vitro, Diabetologia 3:47, 1967.
4. Malaisse-Lagae, F., Ravazzola, M., and Orci, L.: Electron microscope cytochemical demonstration of the external coat of islet

cells, Excepta Medica, 7th Congress of the International Diabetic Federation, 1973, p. 4.

5. Steiner, D. F., Hollan, O., Rubenstein, A., and others: Isolation and properties of proinsulin, intermediate forms and other minor components from crystalline bovine insulin, Diabetes 17:725, 1968.

6. Chance, R. E., Ellis, R. M., and Bromer, W. W.: Porcine proinsulin characterization and amino acid sequence, Science 161:165, 1968.

7. Unger, R. H., and Orci, L.: The essential role of glucagon in the pathogenesis of diabetes mellitus, Lancet 1:14, 1975.

8. Tattersall, R. B., and Fajans, S. S.: A difference between the inheritance of classical juvenile-onset and maturity-onset type of diabetes of young people, Diabetes 24:1, 1975.

9. Hinden, R.: Mumps followed by diabetes, Lancet 1:1381, 1962.

10. McCraw, W. M.: Diabetes following mumps, Lancet 1:1300, 1963.

11. Gamble, D. R., Kinsley, M. L.; and others: Viral antibodies in diabetes mellitus, Br. Med. J. 3:627, 1969.

12. Craighead, J. E., and Steinke, J.: Diabetes mellitus–like syndrome in mice infected with encephalomycarditis virus, Am. J. Pathol. 63:119, 1971.

13. Johnson, G. M., and Tudor, R. B.: Diabetes mellitus and congenital rubella infection, Am. J. Dis. Child. 120:453, 1970.

14. Forrest, J. M., Menser, M. A., and Burgess, J. A.: High frequency of diabetes mellitus in young with congenital rubella, Lancet 2:332, 1971.

15. Bunnell, C. E., and Monif, C. R. G.: Interstitial pancreatitis in the congenital rubella syndrome, J. Pediatr. 80:465, 1972.

16. Karam, J. H., Grodsky, G. M., and Forsham, P. H.: Coxsackie virus and diabetes, Lancet 2:1209, 1971.

17. Burch, G. E., Tsui, C. Y., Harb, J. M., and Colcolongli, H. L.: Pathologic findings in the pancreas of mice infected with coxackie virus B4, Arch. Intern. Med. 128:40, 1971.

18. Jackson, R. L., and Guthrie, R. A.: The child with diabetes, Kalamazoo, Mich., 1975, The UpJohn Co., p. 15.

19. Siperstein, M. D., Unger, R. H., and Madison, L. L.: Studies of muscle capillary base-

ment membranes in normal subjects, diabetic and prediabetic patients, J. Clin. Invest. 47:1973, 1968.

20. Kilo, C., Vogler, N., and Williamson, J. R.: Muscle capillary basement membrane changes related to aging and diabetes mellitus, Diabetes 21:881, 1972.

21. Osterby, R.: Morphometric studies of the peripheral glomerular basement membrane in early juvenile diabetes. I. Development of initial basement membrane thickening Diabetologia 8:84, 1972.

22. Jackson, R. L., Guthrie, R. A., Esterly, J., and others: Muscle capillary basement membrane changes in normal and diabetic children, Diabetes 24 (Suppl. 2):400, 1975.

23. Fajans, S. S., Williamson, J. R., Weissman, P. N., and others: Basement membrane thickening in latent diabetes. *In* Basement membrane thickening in latent diabetes. Camerini-Davalos, K. A., and editors: Cole, H. F., Early diabetes advances in metabolic disorders (Suppl. 2), New York, 1973, Academic Press, p. 393.

24. Lundbaek, K.: Diabetic angiopathy, Acter Diabetol. Lat. 10:187, 1973.

25. Spiro, R. G., and Spiro, M. J.: Effect of diabetes in the brosynthesis of the renal glomerular basement membranes, Studies on the glycosyltransferase, Diabetes 20:641, 1971.

26. Maurer, M.: The renal lesions of diabetes—the relation to control, presented at symposium on Diabetes, Grand Rapids, Mich., Oct. 1975.

27. Morrison, A. D., and Winegrad, A. L.: Regulation of polyol pathway activity in aorta, Diabetes 20:329, 1971.

28. Gabbay, K. H.: The sorbitol pathway and the complications of diabetes, N. Engl. J. Med. 288:831, 1973.

29. Goetz, F. C.: Organ transplantation in diabetes mellitus, Diabetes mellitus: diagnosis and treatment, vol. 3, New York, 1971. American Diabetes Association, Inc., pp. 363-367.

30. Lillehei, R. C, Simmons, R. L., Najarian, J. S., and others: Pancreatico-duodenal allotransplantation: experimental and clinical experience, Ann. Surg. 172:405, 1970.

31. Gliedman, M. L.; Gold, M., Whittaker, J., and others: Clinical segmented pancreatic transplantation with ureter-pancreatic duct

anastomosis for exocrine drainage, Surgery **74:**171, 1973.

32. Connolly, J. E., Martin, D. C., Steinberg, T., and others: Clinical experience with pancreaticoduodenal transplantation, Arch. Surg. **106:**489, 1973.

33. Ballenger, W. F., and Lacy, P. E.: Transplantation of intact pancreatic islets in rats, Surgery **72:**175, 1972.

34. Amamoo, D. E., Woods, J. E., and Donovan, J. L.: Preliminary Experience with Pancreatic islet-cell implantation, Mayo Clin. Proc. **49:**289, 1974.

35. Soeldner, J. S., Chang, K. W., Hiebert, J. M., and Arnsenberg, S.: The development of a glucose sensor suitable for implantation, Exerpta Medica, 7th Congress of the International Diabetes Federation, 1973. p. 218.

36. Bessman, S. P., and Schultz, R. D.: Glucose sensor for the artificial pancreas, Exerpta Medica, 7th Congress of the International Diabetes Federation, 1973, p. 217.

Appendices

APPENDIX A

Glossary of terms

AADE American Association of Diabetes Educators. A national voluntary organization of professionals interested in education of the person and/or family with diabetes.

acetone A ketone body formed in greater abundance in the liver from fatty acids when glucose is not available to the cells to burn. Acetone is found in the blood and urine of people with uncontrolled diabetes, causing their breath to have a fruity odor.

acidosis An acid condition of the body resulting from abnormal amounts of acid such as ketones. Acidosis occurs in people who do not have enough insulin.

ADA American Diabetes Association, Inc. is a national voluntary health organization in the field of diabetes.

adrenal glands Two tent-shaped organs whose medulla (center part) secretes epinephrine (see *epinephrine*) and cortex (outside part) secretes glucocorticoids (see *glucocorticoids*) and aldosterone.

adult diabetes A type of diabetes that is usually found in adults over 40 years of age. The onset is gradual. The symptoms are often minimal. The patients are often overweight and are less prone to acute complications such as acidosis and coma. Adult diabetes is treated by diet alone or by diet plus oral hypoglycemic agent. Insulin injections are not usually required. Also called non-insulin-dependent diabetes, non-ketosis-prone, or maturity-onset diabetes.

alpha cells Cells that produce glucagon; found in the islets of Langerhans of the pancreas.

atrophy A decrease in the amount of fat under the skin. This sometimes occurs at the sites of insulin injection and results in hollowed-out areas that are cosmetically undesirable.

basement membrane Layers of concentric circles, or chains, of glycoproteins with infrequent glucose and galactose molecules, protectively surrounding capillaries of kidney, muscle, retina of the eye, etc.

beta cells Cells that produce insulin; found in the islets of Langerhans of the pancreas.

biguanides Drugs such as phenformin (DBI and DBI-TD, Metrol) that are used in treating diabetes. They do not stimulate the pancreas to produce more insulin; they prevent glucose uptake from the intestine, prevent gluconeogenesis, and promotes anaerobic glycolysis, to name a few actions.

blood glucose level The concentration of glucose in the blood. It is commonly called blood sugar and is usually measured in milligrams per deciliters (100 milliliters), mg/dl.

brittle diabetes A type of diabetes in which the blood glucose level fluctuates widely from high to low. Brittle diabetes may be caused by the complete loss of ability to produce any insulin, too high an insulin dose, or other factors and can often be improved by a good treatment program. Also called unstable diabetes.

callus A thickening of the skin caused by friction or pressure.

calorie A unit for the measurement of heat. The heat-producing or energy-producing value of foods is measured in calories (called *kilocalories*).

carbohydrate One of the three main constituents of foods. Carbohydrates are composed mainly of sugars and starches.

cardiovascular disease Disease of the heart and large blood vessels; tends to occur more often and at a younger age in people with diabetes and may be related to how well the diabetes is controlled.

cell membrane The material that surrounds all cells and acts to retain helpful substances, exclude harmful substances, and allow glucose, with the help of insulin, to pass into the cells.

cesarean section An operation that delivers an infant by removing it from the mother's womb through an incision in the abdomen. Infants of diabetic mothers (IDM) are frequently delivered before term by this means.

chemical diabetes A type of diabetes in which there

243

are no symptoms and normal results from a fasting blood glucose test but abnormal results from the rest of an oral glucose tolerance test.

Charcot's joint Chronic progressive degeneration of the stress bearing action of a joint.

corns Hard, thickened areas of the skin caused by friction or pressure. They usually occur on the feet and may result in foot ulcers in people who have a loss of pain sensation in their feet.

diabetes mellitus A disease in which the body is unable to use and store glucose normally because of a decrease or lack of insulin production or ineffective insulin production by the pancreas. Diabetes mellitus is usually inherited but may be caused by any process that destroys the pancreas (mainly beta cells).

diabetic coma Unconsciousness occurring during ketoacidosis. Associated symptoms include dry skin and mouth, fruity odor of the breath, very deep and rapid respirations, rapid pulse, and low blood pressure. Diabetic coma is caused by a deficiency of insulin.

diabetic ketoacidosis (DKA) The most severe state of diabetes in which there are markedly elevated glucose levels in blood and urine, elevated ketones in blood and urine, dehydration, and electrolyte imbalance. (See *ketoacidosis*.)

diabetic ketosis A serious state of diabetes in which there is glucose in blood and urine, ketones in blood and urine, and possibly some dehydration. (See *ketosis*.)

double-void technique The procedure of collecting a urine specimen 30 minutes after first voiding of all the urine. The double-voiding technique is often used in collecting urine to test for glucose and acetone levels. It is a measure of diabetic control at that particular time.

epinephrine A hormone released from medulla of adrenal glands. The main function of epinephrine in diabetes is releasing glucose from the liver, increasing the circulation rate, and preventing release of secreted insulin.

exchange A serving of food that contains a known and relatively constant amount of carbohydrate, fat, and/or protein. The food used in an exchange is usually weighed or measured. The exchanges are divided into several groups called milk exchanges, fruit exchanges, meat exchanges, fat exchanges, bread exchanges, and vegetable exchanges.

fasting blood glucose Blood glucose concentration in the morning before breakfast. Commonly called *FBS,* fasting blood sugar.

fat One of the three main constituents of foods. Fats occur in nearly pure form as liquids or solids, such as oils and margarines, or may be a component of other foods and may be of animal or vegetable origin. Fats have a higher energy content than any other food.

fatty acids Constituents of fat. When there is an insulin deficiency, as in diabetes, fatty acids increase in the blood and are used by the liver to produce ketones.

fractional urine The urine output collected over a period of time and used to test for glucose and acetone levels. Fractions of urine are usually collected from breakfast to lunchtime, from lunchtime to suppertime, from suppertime to bedtime, and bedtime to awakening. These are fractions of a 24-hour urine. Also called *block urine*.

gangrene The death of tissue caused by a very poor blood supply as sometimes occurs in the feet and legs of persons with diabetes. Infection may be a contributing cause.

genes Basic units of hereditary characteristics passed through reproduction (part of chromosomes).

gestational diabetes A period of abnormal glucose tolerance that occurs during pregnancy, usually controlled by diet and possibly insulin.

globin insulin Modified form of insulin produced by attaching a globin molecule to regular insulin, slowing absorption and extending the peak and duration of action. Globin is a clear insulin of acid pH and intermediate action.

glucagon A hormone produced by the alpha cells in the islets of Langerhans of the pancreas. Glucagon causes a rise in the blood glucose level and may therefore be used by injection for the treatment of insulin reactions.

glucocorticoids Hormone released from the cortex of adrenal gland; in relation to diabetes, causes amino acids to be changed into new glucose (gluconeogenesis).

gluconeogenesis The process of converting amino acids and fats to glucose (new glucose) in the liver and kidneys.

glucose The simple sugar, also known as dextrose, that occurs in the blood and is used by the body for energy.

glucose tolerance The ability of the body to use and store glucose. Glucose tolerance is decreased in persons with diabetes mellitus.

glucose tolerance test A test for diabetes mellitus. The person being tested is given a certain amount of glucose to drink; blood glucose levels are measured before ingestion and ½, 1, 2, 3, and sometimes 4 and 5 hours afterward ingestion of the glucose. Also called *oral glucose tolerance test (OGTT)*.

glycogen Glycogen is the storage form of glucose in the liver. It may be broken down to form blood glucose during an insulin reaction or during a fast.

glycogenesis The process whereby the liver converts a portion of glucose to glycogen (beginning of glycogen).

glycogenolysis The breakdown of glycogen to glucose.

glycolysis The breakdown of glucose to carbon dioxide and water.

glycosuria The presence of glucose in the urine. *Glyco* refers to sugar; *uria* to urine.

gram A small unit of weight in the metric system; used in weighing food to determine a specific amount to eat or to burn in kilocalories.

heredity The transmission of a trait, such as blue eyes, from the parents to offspring.

hormone A chemical substance produced by one gland or tissue and carried by the blood to other tissues or organs where it stimulates action resulting in a specific effect. Insulin and glucagon are hormones.

hyperbilirubinemia Condition in which a person has greater than normal value (+12.0 mg/dl in the infant) of bilirubin in the blood. Signs: jaundiced skin and sclera of eyes.

hyperglycemia A greater than normal level of glucose in the blood (high blood glucose). FBS value greater than 120 mg/dl.

hyperinsulinism An excessive amount of insulin, which may be caused by overproduction of insulin by the beta cells of the islets of Langerhans in the pancreas or by an excessive dose of insulin. Hyperinsulinism may cause hypoglycemia (low blood glucose levels).

hypocalcemia Less than normal value (10-12 mg/dl in the infant) of calcium in the blood. Signs: convulsive seizure and irritability of neuromuscular system.

hypoglycemia A less than normal level of glucose in the blood (low blood glucose level). FBS value less than 60 mg/dl.

hypoglycemic agent A drug or substance such as sulfonylureas (Orinase) and biguanides (DBI) used to reduce blood glucose levels.

insulin A hormone secreted by the beta cells of the islets of Langerhans in the pancreas; insulin promotes the utilization of glucose.

insulin reaction A condition with rapidly occurring onset that is the result of low blood glucose levels,

which may be caused by too much insulin, too little food, or by increased exercise without a corresponding increase in food or a decrease in insulin. Symptoms vary from nervousness, shakiness, headaches, and drowsiness to confusion, convulsions, and coma.

islets of Langerhans The small groups of cells in the pancreas that contain alpha and beta cells and produce glucagon and insulin.

isophane insulin NPH (neutral protamine Hagedorn) insulin, a residual pH intermediate-acting insulin.

lente insulin An intermediate-acting insulin that is a mixture of 30% semilente and 70% ultralente insulin.

juvenile diabetes A type of diabetes usually found in people under 40 years of age. The onset is usually rapid. The symptoms are polyuria, (frequent urination), polydipsia (thirst), and polyphagia (increased eating). Other problems such as weight loss, blurring of vision, itching, and slow healing of sores may occur. Controlled by diet and insulin. Also called insulin-dependent diabetes or ketosis-prone diabetes.

ketoacidosis An acid condition of the body resulting from overproduction of ketones. Occurs when there is not enough insulin; thus fat is released to produce ketones in excess. This abnormal production of ketones results in increased acidity of the blood (acidosis), thus *ketoacidosis*. Large amounts of sugar and acetone are found in the urine, electrolytes are imbalanced, and dehydration is present. The onset is usually slow with a loss of appetite, abdominal pain, nausea and vomiting, rapid and deep respiration, and coma. Death may occur.

ketone bodies Substances formed in the liver when a fat is broken down because of insufficient insulin. When insulin is decreased, fats are released as fatty acids and are chemically changed into ketones. Ketones are often found in the blood and urine of persons with uncontrolled diabetes. (See *acetone*.)

ketones Another name for ketone bodies.

ketonuria The presence of ketones in the urine.

ketosis The presence of large amounts of ketones in the body secondary to excessive breakdown of fat caused by insufficient insulin in persons with diabetes mellitus. Ketosis precedes and causes acidosis; the combination (ketosis and acidosis) is called *ketoacidosis*.

kidney threshold The level of a substance (such as glucose) in the blood in the kidney, above which it will be spilled into the urine. Also called *renal threshold*.

Kimmelstiel-Wilson syndrome Nodular lesions of the glomerulus caused by blood vessel degeneration related to poorly controlled diabetes, as described by Drs. Kimmelstiel and Wilson.

Kussmaul's respiration The rapid, deep, and labored respiration observed in patients with diabetic ketoacidosis; an involuntary mechanism to excrete carbon dioxide to reduce carbonic acid level.

labile diabetes A term used for unstable diabetes control. (See *brittle diabetes*.)

latent diabetes An early stage of chemical diabetes in which there is a normal fasting blood glucose level, a sharp rise in glucose level in response to a glucose load, followed by a somewhat rapid drop in blood glucose levels. There are no signs or symptoms other than some hypoglycemic symptoms.

lipolysis The increased fat breakdown in the body tissues that occurs in ketosis (lysis of fat).

maturity-onset diabetes Another name for adult diabetes, mild diabetes, non-insulin-dependent or ketone-resistant diabetes.

Mauriac syndrome A condition observed before puberty in children with prolonged, poorly controlled diabetes. It involves an enlarged, fatty liver, pitting edema, and short stature. The Mauriac syndrome is seen much less as the health team recognizes the need for adequate food and insulin for growth.

meal plan An arrangement whereby the total food allowed daily is expressed in terms of a certain number of points or exchanges to be eaten at specified times.

metabolism All the chemical processes in the body, including those by which foods are broken down and used for tissue or energy production.

microaneurysms Small ballooned-out areas on the capillary blood vessels on the retina of the eye. They may burst and bleed.

nephropathy Disease of the kidneys.

neuritis Inflammation of the nerves.

neuropathy Any disease of the nervous system. Neuropathy may occur in persons with diabetes and be related to poor control. Symptoms such as pain, loss of sensation, loss of reflexes, and/or weakness may occur.

oral glucose tolerance test (OGTT) See *glucose tolerance test*.

oral hypoglycemic agents Another name for blood glucose lowering agents.

pancreas A gland that is positioned near the stomach and secretes at least two hormones—insulin and glucagon—and many digestive juices.

points system A method of quantitating food intake by assigning points to various food components (carbohydrate, fat, protein, calories, sodium, etc.) and correlating the number of each component point needed for a meal or days' intake. This system may be used in place of the less-precise exchange system for diet calculation.

polydipsia Excessive thirst with increased drinking of water.

polyphagia Excessive hunger or appetite resulting in increased food intake.

polyunsaturated fats The type of fats such as corn or other vegetable oils that are liquid at room temperature, unless they are hydrogenated.

polyuria Excessive output of urine.

postprandial Occurring after a meal.

precipitate Particles that settle out of a solution. This may occur in insulin that is used beyond the expiration date, is contaminated, or improperly mixed.

prediabetes The time during the life of a diabetic person before any abnormality in glucose tolerance can be demonstrated. The identical twin of a diabetic or a person whose parents are both diabetic is felt to have prediabetes. Most people do not know they are prediabetic until they develop diabetes.

protein One of the three main constituents of foods. Proteins are made up of amino acids and are found in foods such as milk, meat, fish, and eggs. Proteins are essential constitutents of all living cells and are the nitrogen-containing nutrient.

protamine zinc insulin Protamine zinc insulin is a long-acting insulin prepared with large amounts of protamine combined with regular insulin in the presence of zinc.

regular insulin Short-acting insulin crystallized in the pancreas of animals. Formerly of acid pH, this insulin has now been neutralized and can be pre-mixed with NPH and lente insulins. Also known as clear insulin or crystalline insulin.

renal Pertaining to the kidneys.

renal threshold Another name for kidney threshold.

respiratory distress syndrome (RDS) Difficulty in breathing noted by grunting, respiratory or expiratory wheezing or both, labored respirations, cyanosis, and abnormal rate of respiration.

retina The light-sensitive layer at the back of the inner surface of the eyeball.

retinopathy Disease of the retina. Retinopathy occurs in persons with prolonged, poorly controlled diabetes and involves abnormal growth of and bleeding from the capillary blood vessels in the eye.

saturated fats The type of fat, such as butter, that is usually a solid at room temperature. Saturated fats are usually derived from animal sources.

semilente Insulin prepared by special crystallizing techniques to produce small insulin crystals with a large absorptive surface and a rapid action. Semilente is slower in action than regular insulin but more rapid than the intermediate-acting insulins.

serum glucose The concentration of glucose in the liquid part of the blood after the cells have been removed.

single-void technique The procedure of collecting a urine specimen four times a day before meals and at bedtime. The bladder is not emptied 30 minutes before collecting the specimen.

spot test A urine test performed on a sample collected by the single-void technique.

subclinical diabetes A late stage of chemical diabetes in which the fasting blood glucose level is normal and the response to the glucose load is elevated (blood glucose levels not returning to normal in the prescribed 3 to 4 hour period of time). No signs of symptoms are usually associated with this stage of chemical diabetes.

sulfonylureas Chemical compounds that stimulate production or release of insulin by the beta cells in the pancreas and/or prevent release of glucose from the liver. They are used in the treatment of adult diabetes.

time-action curve A curve that shows the effect of a medicine at various times after it is taken.

twenty-four hour urine Used to measure quantitative glucose levels in urine from a pooled, 24-hour specimen.

ultralente A long-acting insulin produced by special crystallizing techniques that produce large crystals with a small absorptive surface. Equivalent to PZI in action.

unsaturated fats The type of fats such as vegetable oils that are usually liquids at room temperature.

unstable diabetes Another name for *brittle diabetes*.

APPENDIX B

Resources and services

Diabetes related and affiliated associations

American Association of Diabetes Educators
3553 W. Peterson Ave.
Chicago, Ill. 60659

Juvenile Diabetes Foundation
23 E. 26th.
New York, N.Y. 10010

American Diabetes Association
600 Fifth Avenue
New York, N.Y. 10020

ALABAMA

American Diabetes Association
Alabama Affiliate, Inc.
P.O. Box 2022
Huntsville, Ala. 35804
205/534-2515 or 536-4866
Mr. Harry Vincent, Executive Director

ALASKA

Alaska Diabetes Association, Inc.
P.O. Box 4495
Anchorage, Alaska 99509
Mrs. Jocelyn Woodman, President

ARIZONA

Arizona Diabetes Association, Inc.
555 West Catalina Drive #207
Phoenix, Ariz. 85013
602/274-3514
Mrs. Arline Fraser, Executive Director

ARKANSAS

American Diabetes Association
Arkansas Affiliate, Inc.
5422 West Markham
Little Rock, Ark. 72205
Mr. Barrett Lee Brown, Executive Director

CALIFORNIA

American Diabetes Association
Northern California Affiliate, Inc.
255 Hugo Street
San Francisco, Calif. 94122
415/681-9210
Mr. Wesley Franco, Executive Director

American Diabetes Association
Northern California Affiliate, Inc.

Unit
Marin County
First Methodist Church
9 Ross Valley Drive
San Rafael, Calif. 94901
Mrs. Edna Cerruzi, Executive Secretary

American Diabetes Association
Southern California Affiliate, Inc.

Executive office
1801 Century Park East, Suite 2116
Los Angeles, Calif. 90067
213/553-2141 or 879-1534
Mr. D. Rodney Lee, Executive Director

Central office
4849 Van Nuys Boulevard
Sherman Oaks, Calif. 91403
213/872-1385 or 986-6272
Mr. Lawrence Werner, Administrator

Regional offices
1970 Third Avenue
San Diego, Calif. 92101
714/232-7573

17842 Irvine Boulevard, Suite 136
Tustin, Calif. 92690
714/544-9033
Ms. Jean Halliburton, Field Director

COLORADO

American Diabetes Association
Colorado Affiliate, Inc.
1045 Acoma Street
Denver Colo. 80204
303/573-8833
Mr. G. Hayward Shull, Executive Director

CONNECTICUT

Connecticut Diabetes Association, Inc.
17 Oakwood Avenue
West Hartford, Conn. 06119
203/232-8859
Miss Linda Holbrook, Acting Executive Director

DELAWARE

Delaware Diabetes Association, Inc.
1925 Lovering Avenue
Wilmington, Del. 19806
302/656-0030
Mrs. Daphne J. White, Executive Secretary

DISTRICT OF COLUMBIA

American Diabetes Association
Washington, D.C. Area Affiliate, Inc.
P.O. Box 4384, Takoma Park Branch
Washington, D.C. 20012
301/270-8866
Mr. James M. Bruckwick, Executive Director

FLORIDA

American Diabetes Association
Florida Affiliate, Inc.
110 Cesery Blvd., Suite #1
Jacksonville, Fla. 32911
904/743-0822
Mr. Harold E. Aldrich, Jr., Executive Director

GEORGIA

American Diabetes Association
Georgia Affiliate, Inc.
762 Cypress Street, N.E.
Atlanta, Ga. 30308
404/881-1963
Mrs. Elaine Morris, Executive Secretary

Chapter
Diabetes Association of Atlanta
Same address as above
Mrs. J. Ernest Williams, Executive Director

IDAHO

Idaho Diabetes Association, Inc.
Box 7113
Boise, Idaho 83707
208/344-5717
George Baker, M.D., President

ILLINOIS

American Diabetes Association
Greater Chicago and Northern Illinois
 Affiliate, Inc.
620 N. Michigan Avenue
Chicago, Ill. 60611
312/943-8668
Ms. Nike Bradley, Executive Director

American Diabetes Association
Downstate Illinois Affiliate, Inc.
6 Valleyview
Jackson, Ill. 62650
Mrs. Bill Buchanan, President

INDIANA

Indiana Diabetes Association, Inc.
1433 N. Meridian Street
Indianapolis, Ind. 46202
317/634-1719
Mr. Thomas V. Iozzo, Executive Director

Chapter
Diabetes Association of Greater
 Indianapolis, Inc.
Same address as above

IOWA

American Diabetes Association
Iowa Affiliate, Inc.
% Lutheran Hospital
Penn at University
Des Moines, Iowa 50316
515/265-6662
Mrs. Katie Gibson, Executive Secretary

KANSAS

American Diabetes Association
Kansas Affiliate, Inc.
2312 E. Central
Wichita, Kan. 67214
316/265-6671
Mrs. Melva Burt, Executive Director

KENTUCKY

**American Diabetes Association
Kentucky Affiliate, Inc.**
3564 Gloucester Drive
Lexington, Ky. 40504
606/255-6841
Joseph G. Caldwell, M.D., President

LOUISIANA

Diabetes Association of Louisiana, Inc.
1121 Louisiana Avenue
Shreveport, La. 71101
318/422-2158
Arthur A. Herold, Jr., M.D., President

MAINE

See Massachusetts

MARYLAND

**American Diabetes Association
Maryland Affiliate, Inc.**
3701 Old Court Road
Old Court Executive Park, Suite 19
Baltimore, Md. 21208
301/358-7050
Ms. Shyrl Jones, Executive Director

MASSACHUSETTS

**American Diabetes Association
New England Affiliate, Inc.**
377 Elliot Street
Newton Upper Falls, Mass. 02164
617/965-2323
Miss Marjorie Cotton, Executive Director

MICHIGAN

**American Diabetes Association
Michigan Affiliate, Inc.**
6131 West Outer Drive
Detroit, Mich. 48235
313/342-9333
Mr. Hubert H. Baker, Executive Director

MINNESOTA

**American Diabetes Association
Minnesota Affiliate, Inc.**
7601 Bush Lake Road
Minneapolis, Minn. 55435
612/835-2800
Mr. T. Harrison Bryant, Executive Director

Chapter
Twin Cities Diabetes Association
Same address as above
Mrs. Donna Jean Fillmer, Executive
Secretary

MISSOURI

**American Diabetes Association
Greater Kansas City Affiliate, Inc.**
415 East 63rd
Kansas City, Mo. 64110
816/361-3361
Mrs. Mona Marsh, Executive Director

**American Diabetes Association
Missouri Regional Affiliate, Inc.**
Box 11
Columbia, Mo. 65201
Miss Janis Gifford, Coordinator

**American Diabetes Association
Greater St. Louis Affiliate, Inc.**
3839 Lindell Boulevard
St. Louis, Mo. 63108
314/533-4143
Mr. Ernest E. Sellars, Executive Director

MONTANA

Montana Diabetes Association, Inc.
P.O. Box 2088
Great Falls, Mont. 59403
406/761-6794
Ms. Carole Vetsch, Executive Secretary

NEBRASKA

**American Diabetes Association
Nebraska Affiliate, Inc.**
921 Dorcas, Room 221
Omaha, Neb. 68108
402/348-1447
Mrs. Sam DiMauro, Executive Director

NEVADA

**American Diabetes Association
Nevada Affiliate, Inc.**
7784 Wishing Well Road
Las Vegas, Nev. 89119
702/736-3639
Mrs. Nancy Halpin, President

NEW HAMPSHIRE

See Massachusetts

NEW JERSEY

**American Diabetes Association
New Jersey Affiliate, Inc.**
345 Union Street
Hackensack, N.J. 07601
201/487-7228
Mr. William Humphrey Jones, Executive Director

NEW MEXICO

**American Diabetes Association
New Mexico Affiliate, Inc.**
6101 Marble, N.E., Suite 11
Albuquerque, N.M. 87110
505/268-1913
Ms. Eve Land, Executive Director

NEW YORK

**Buffalo Diabetes Association, Inc.
Mercy Hospital**
565 Abbott Road
Buffalo, N.Y. 14220
716/824-3055
Mr. Robert Cochran, Executive Director

**American Diabetes Association
Troy Unit, Inc.**
891 Eighth Avenue
Troy, N.Y. 12182
Mrs. Jean Ryan, President

New York Diabetes Association, Inc.
104 East 40th Street
New York, N.Y. 10016
212/697-7760
Miss Lynne Perry, Acting Executive Director

Chapter
Nassau County
250 Fulton Avenue, Room 502
Hempstead, N.Y. 11550
516/538-6688
Mrs. Geri Brown, Field Coordinator

Rochester Regional Diabetes Association
1351 Mount Hope Avenue
Rochester, N.Y. 14620
716/275-2930
Mrs. William L. Lieberman, Executive Vice-President

NORTH CAROLINA

**American Diabetes Association
North Carolina Affiliate, Inc.**
408 North Tryon Street
Charlotte, N.C. 28202

704/333-1568
Mr. John A. Laurents, Executive Director

Chapter
Mecklenberg Diabetes Association
301 South Brevard Street
Charlotte, N.C. 28202
Mr. Pender R. McElroy, President

NORTH DAKOTA

**American Diabetes Association
North Dakota Affiliate, Inc.**
4919 South Belmont, R.R. #1
Grand Forks, N.D. 58201
701/772-8320
Ms. Mary Ann Keller, Executive Director

OHIO

**American Diabetes Association
Cincinnati Affiliate, Inc.**
2400 Reading Road
Cincinnati, Ohio 45202
513/721-2905
Mrs. Emily H. Robbins, Executive Director

Dayton Area Diabetes Association, Inc.
184 Salem Avenue
Dayton, Ohio 45406
513/228-8166
Mr. Eleanor J. Graham, Executive Secretary

**American Diabetes Association
Akron Area Affiliate, Inc.**
326 Locust Street
Akron, Ohio 44302
216/253-1171
Mr. James Ginther, Executive Director

**American Diabetes Association
Mahoning Valley Chapter, Inc.**
420 Oak Hill Avenue
Youngstown, Ohio 44502
Mrs. Ruthanne Harrison, Secretary

OKLAHOMA

**American Diabetes Association
Eastern Oklahoma Chapter, Inc.**
Kelly Bldg. St. 613
Tulsa, Okla. 74136
918/664-2047
Mrs. Bobette Lang, Executive Director

**American Diabetes Association
Western Oklahoma Chapter, Inc.**
2801 N.W. Expressway, Ste. 146
Oklahoma City, Okla. 73112
Mr. Steve Gann, Executive Director

OREGON

Diabetes Association of Oregon, Inc.
P.O. Box 13510
Portland, Ore. 97213
503/223-6215 or 288-3014
Mrs. Rita Dewart, Executive Director

PENNSYLVANIA

American Diabetes Association
Delaware Valley Affiliate, Inc.
919 Walnut Street, 4th Floor
Philadelphia, Penn. 19107
215/627-7718 and 627-7719
Mr. Jay Reinboth, Executive Director

American Diabetes Association
Pennsylvania Affiliate, Inc.
345 Jefferson Avenue
Scranton, Penn. 18510
Mr. Casmir V. Yanish, Executive Director

RHODE ISLAND

See Massachusetts

SOUTH CAROLINA

South Carolina Diabetes Association, Inc.
P.O. Box 8248, Station A
Greenville, S.C. 29604
803/235-7822
Mr. Adam Fisher, Executive Director

SOUTH DAKOTA

American Diabetes Association
South Dakota Affiliate, Inc.
400 Park Avenue
Yankton, S.D. 57078
William W. Quick, M.D., President

TENNESSEE

Tennessee Diabetes Association, Inc.
% Baptist Hospital
Room 120, West Building
2000 Church Street
Nashville, Tenn. 37236
615/320-0242
Solomon Solomon, M.D. President

American Diabetes Association
Chattanooga Chapter
Tennessee Diabetes Association
921 East 3rd Street
Chattanooga, Tenn. 37402
615/756-8010
Mrs. Julian Katz, Executive Director

Chapters
Middle Tennessee Diabetes Association
Same address as above
Mrs. Janet Hill, Executive Secretary

American Diabetes Association
Memphis-Mid-South Chapter
2805 Lombardy
Memphis, Tenn. 38111
Mr. Bert Ferguson, President

TEXAS

American Diabetes Association
North Texas Affiliate, Inc.
5415 Maple, Suite 210
Dallas, Tex. 75235
214/638-5400
Mr. R. Phillip Davis, Executive Director

American Diabetes Association
South Texas Affiliate, Inc.
1536 E. Anderson Lane, Ste. 36
Austin, Tex. 78711
512/837-1712
Mr. Earl R. Palmer, Executive Director

Chapter
Houston Diabetes Association, Inc.
2706 Richmond, Suite 14
Houston, Tex. 77006
713/524-0377
Mrs. Sylvia Cline, Executive Secretary

UTAH

Utah Diabetes Association, Inc.
5524 Dunbarton Drive
Salt Lake City, Utah 84117
Mr. Charles Hand, Secretary

VERMONT

See Massachusetts

VIRGINIA

American Diabetes Association
Virginia Affiliate, Inc.
P.O. Box 8495
Richmond, Va. 23226
804/285-9819

WASHINGTON

American Diabetes Association
Washington Affiliate, Inc.
1218 Terry Avenue, Suite 209
Seattle, Wash. 98101
206/624-5240
Mr. James Neidigh, Executive Director

WEST VIRGINIA

American Diabetes Association
West Virginia Affiliate, Inc.
P.O. Box 2865
Charleston, W. Va. 25330
304/346-6418
Mrs. Alan J. Arthur, Secretary Treasurer

WISCONSIN

American Diabetes Association
Wisconsin Affiliate, Inc.
5215 North Ironwood Road
Milwaukee, Wis. 53217
414/964-7676
Mr. Richard J. Sandretti, Executive Director

WYOMING

American Diabetes Association
Cheyenne Unit
P.O. Box 2351
Cheyenne, Wyom. 82001
Mrs. Sandra Finch, Chairman

Summer camps for children

ALABAMA

Camp Seale Harris, Scoutshire Woods, Citronelle (near Mobile), Ala. 36522. Sponsored by: American Diabetes Association, Alabama Affiliate, Inc. Contact: Mrs. Donald R. Flack, Director, Camp Seale Harris, P.O. Box 8224, Mobile, Ala, 36608. Telephone: 205/344-3534 (September-June 8 AM to 4 PM 205/342-4355).

ARIZONA

Hidden Valley Ranch, P.O. Box 1431, Prescott, Ariz. 86301. Sponsored by: Arizona Diabetes Association, Inc. Contact: Ms. Arline Fraser. State Secretary, Arizona Diabetes Association, Inc. 555 West Catalina Drive, #207, Phoenix, Ariz. 85013. Telephone: 602/274-3514.

CALIFORNIA

Bearskin Meadow, P.O. Box 55, Kings Canyon National Park, Calif. 93633. Sponsored by: Diabetic Youth Foundation. Contact: M. B. Olney, M.D., Executive Director, Diabetic Youth Foundation, 1128 Irving Street, San Francisco, Calif. 94122. Telephone: 415/731-5113.

Camp Chinnock, Barton Flats in the San Bernardino Mountains, Calif. Sponsored by: American Diabetes Association, Southern California Affiliate, Inc. Contact: Miss Anita Shurack,

Camp Coordinator, American Diabetes Association, Southern California Affiliate, Inc., 4849 Van Nuys Boulevard, Suite 200, Sherman Oaks, Calif. 91403. Telephone: 213/986-6272 or 213/872-1385.

Uni-Betic Camps, University Camps, Angeles Oaks Post Office, Calif. 92305. Sponsored by: Metabolic Foundation of Los Angeles, Inc. Contact: Mrs. Louise O. Simonson, Executive Director, Metabolic Foundation of Los Angeles, Inc., 2525 West Eighth Street, Los Angeles, Calif. 90057. Telephone: 213/285-2917.

COLORADO

Camp Chief Ouray, Granby (100 miles northwest of Denver), Colo. Sponsored by: American Diabetes Association, Colorado Affiliate, Inc. Contact: Mr. G. Hayward Shull, Executive Director, American Diabetes Association, Colorado Affiliate, Inc., 1045 Acoma Street, Denver, Colo. 80204. Telephone: 303/573-8833.

FLORIDA

Florida's Camp for Children and Youth with Diabetes, Camp Swan Lake, State Road 26, Melrose, Fla. 32666. Sponsored by: Florida Diabetes Association, Inc. and other groups. Contact: Mrs. Jack Van Der Beek, Camp Secretary, Florida's Camp for Children and Youth with Diabetes, 1910 Riverside Drive East, Brandenton, Fla. 33505. Telephone: 813/746-7071.

GEORGIA

Ross Stevens Memorial Camp, Camp Waco, Waco, Ga. 30182. Sponsored by: Georgia Diabetes Association, Inc. Contact: Mrs. Elaine Morris, Executive Secretary, Georgia Diabetes Association, Inc., 762 Cypress Street, N.E., Atlanta, Ga. 30308. Telephone: 404/881-1963.

ILLINOIS

Summer Camp for Diabetic Children, Camp Holiday Home, Lake Geneva, Wis. 53147. Sponsored by: American Diabetes Association, Greater Chicago and Northern Illinois Affiliate, Inc. Contact: Ms. Nike Bradley, Executive Director, American Diabetes Association, Greater Chicago and Northern Illinois Affiliate, Inc., 620 North Michigan Avenue, Chicago, Ill. 60611. Telephone: 312/943-8668.

Lake Springfield Camp for Diabetic Children, Springfield, Ill. 62701. Sponsored by: Central

Illinois Diabetes Association. Contact: Mr. Michael J. Baker, Camp Director, Central Illinois Diabetes Association, 424 South Second Street, Springfield, Ill. 62701. Telephone: 217/525-1760.

INDIANA

Camp John Warvel, Bradford Woods, Martinsville, Ind. 46151. Sponsored by: Indiana Diabetes Association, Inc. Contact: Samuel M. Wentworth, M.D., Director, Juvenile Diabetes Services, Riley Hospital, 1100 West Michigan, Indianapolis, Ind. 46202. Telephone: 317/264-3889.

IOWA

Camp Hertko Hollow, YMCA Camp, Boone, Iowa. Sponsored by: American Diabetes Association, Iowa Affiliate, Inc.; Iowa Dietetic Association. Contact: Vivian and Chris Murray, Directors, Camp Hertko Hollow, Route 3, Ames, Iowa 50010. Telephone: 515/292-1785.

KANSAS

Camp Discovery. Sponsored by: American Diabetes Association, Kansas Affiliate, Inc. Contact: Executive Director, American Diabetes Association, Kansas Affiliate, Inc., 2312 E. Central, Wichita, Kan. 67214. Telephone: 316/265-6671.

KENTUCKY

Camp Hendon, % Camp Green Shores, McDaniels, Ky. 40152. Sponsored by: Kentucky Diabetes Association, Inc.; Kentucky Easter Seal Society. Contact: William J. Riley, M.D., Camp Coordinator, Camp Hendon, 1904 Piccadilly Street, Lexington, Ky. 40504. Telephone: 606/233-6370 (after 6:00 PM: 606/255-2595).

LOUISIANA

Camp Singing Waters, YMCA, Holden, La. Sponsored by: Diabetes Association of Greater New Orleans. Contact: Jerome Ryan, M.D., Medical Director, Camp Singing Waters, 1430 Tulane Avenue, New Orleans, La. 70112. Telephone: 504/588-5511.

MARYLAND

Camp Glyndon for Diabetic Children, Route 3, Box 29B, Reisterstown, Maryland 21136. Sponsored by: American Diabetes Association, Maryland Affiliate, Inc. Contact: Ms. Shyrl Jones, Executive Director, American Diabetes Association, Maryland Affiliate, Inc., 3701 Old Court Road, Suite 19, Baltimore, Md. 21208. Telephone: 301/358-7050 or 301/358-2445.

MASSACHUSETTS

Clara Barton Camp for Diabetic Girls, North Oxford, Mass. 01537. Sponsored by: Unitarian Universalist Women's Federation. Contact: Ms. Elizabeth A. Kruczek, Camp Administrator, Unitarian Universalist Women's Federation, 25 Beacon Street, Boston, Mass. 02108. Telephone: 617/742-2100 (Home: 617/757-1211).

Elliot P. Joslin Camp for Diabetic Boys, Charlton, Mass. 01507. Sponsored by: Unitarian Universalist Women's Federation. Contact: Ms. Elizabeth A. Kruczek, Camp Administrator, Unitarian Universalist Women's Federation, 25 Beacon Street, Boston, Mass. 02108. Telephone: 617/742-2100 (Home: 617/757-1211).

MICHIGAN

Camp Midicha, 5125 Klam Road, Columbiaville, Mich. 48421. Sponsored by: Michigan Diabetes Association, Inc. Contact: Mr. Dan Donigan, Director of Youth Activities, Michigan Diabetes Association, 6131 West Outer Drive, Detroit, Mich. 48235. Telephone: 313/342-9333.

MINNESOTA

Camp Needlepoint, Camp St. Croix, Hudson, Wisconsin. Sponsored by: American Diabetes Association, Minnesota Affiliate, Inc. Contact: Mrs. Donna Jean Fillmer, Executive Secretary, American Diabetes Association, Minnesota Affiliate, Inc., 6490 Excelsior Boulevard, Minneapolis, Minn. 55426. Telephone: 612/927-4487.

MISSISSIPPI

Diabetic Youth Camp of Mississippi, Camp Ita Kana (30 miles south of Hattiesburg, Miss.) Sponsored by: Forrest County General Hospital. Contact: W. J. Huddleston, M.D., Medical Director, Diabetic Youth Camp of Mississippi, P.O. Box 1691, Hattiesburg, Miss. 39401. Telephone: 601/544-0511.

MISSOURI

Camp for Children with Diabetes, Camp Lion's Den, Imperial, Mo. Sponsored by: Diabetic Children's Welfare Association. Contact: Mr. Ernest E. Sellars, Executive Director, St. Louis Diabetes Association, Inc., 3839 Lindell Boulevard, St. Louis, Mo. 63108. Telephone: 314/533-4143.

Camp Hope, 5600 East Gregory, Kansas City, Mo. 64132. Sponsored by: American Diabetes Association, Kansas City Affiliate, Inc. Contact: Mr. Jay Hungate, Camp Chairman, American Diabetes Association, Kansas City Affiliate, Inc., 415 East 63rd, #200, Kansas City, Mo. 64110. Telephone: 816/361-3361.

Central Missouri Diabetic Children's Camp, Ron J's Ranch, Northwest of Columbia (just off county route E), Mo. Sponsored by: Central Missouri Diabetic Children's Camp, Inc. Contact: Mr. H. Ralph Franklin, Treasurer, Central Missouri Diabetic Children's Camp, Inc., 2705 Highland Drive, Columbia, Mo. 65201. Telephone: 314/455-4987.

MONTANA

Camp Diamont, Hayalite Lake Camp (10 miles south of Bozeman), Mont. Sponsored by: Montana Diabetes Association, Inc. Contact: Mr. Wilbur D. Visser, Camp Chairman, Camp Diamont, Route 4, Box 48, Bozeman, Mont. 59715. Telephone: 406/586-9305.

NEBRASKA

Camp Floyd Rogers, Bellevue, Neb. Sponsored by: Camp Floyd Rogers, Inc. Contact: Mr. Sherman Poska, Director, Camp Floyd Rogers, 4615 Capitol, Omaha, Neb. 68132. Telephone: 402/551-2662 or 402/556-5161, Ext. 765.

Camp Hope, Nebraska Western College, Pioneer Hall, Scottsbluff, Neb. Sponsored by: Wyo-Braska Diabetes Association, Inc. Contact: Mrs. Jo Ann Crawford, Camp Chairman, Wyo-Braska Diabetes Association, P.O. Box 715, Scottsbluff, Neb. 69361. Telephone: 308/247-3162.

NEW JERSEY

Camp Beta, 345 Union Street, Hackensack, N.J. 07601. Sponsored by: American Diabetes Association, New Jersey Affiliate, Inc. Contact: Mrs. Frances Tasner, Associate Director, American Diabetes Association, New Jersey Affiliate, Inc., 345 Union Street, Hackensack, N.J. 07601. 201/487-7470.

Camp Nejeda, P.O. Box 156, Stillwater, N.J. 07875. Sponsored by: Camp Nejeda Foundation, Inc.; Camp Nejeda Medical Committee. Contact: Mrs. Engel Levison, Executive Director, Camp Nejeda Foundation, Inc., 153 Roseville Avenue, Newark, N.J. 07107. Telephone: 201/483-1122.

NEW MEXICO

Hummingbird Camp, in Jemez Mountains (65 miles northwest of Albuquerque), N.M. Sponsored by: New Mexico Diabetes Association, Inc. Contact: Mrs. Barbara Strome, Camp Committee Chairman, New Mexico Diabetes Association, Inc., 6131 Marble, N.E., Suite 11, Albuquerque, N.M. 87110. Telephone: 505/268-1913.

NEW YORK

Camp Nyda, Burlingham, N.Y. 12722. Sponsored by: New York Diabetes Association, Inc. Contact: Mr. Stanley T. Sajecki, Camp Director, New York Diabetes Association, Inc. 104 East 40th Street, New York, N.Y. 10016. Telephone: 212/697-7760.

NORTH CAROLINA

Carolinas' Camp for Diabetic Children, Eagle's Nest Camp, Pisgah Forest (60 miles east of Brevard and 15 miles west of Hendersonville off U.S. Highway 64), N.C. 28712. Sponsored by: American Diabetes Association, North Carolina Affiliate, Inc.; South Carolina Diabetes Association, Inc. Contact: Mr. John A. Laurents, Executive Director, American Diabetes Association, North Carolina Affiliate, Inc., 408 North Tryon Street, Charlotte, N.C. 28202. Telephone: 704/333-1568. (See also South Carolina.)

NORTH DAKOTA

Camp Sioux, Turtle River State Park, Arvilla, N.D. Sponsored by: American Diabetes Association, North Dakota Affiliate, Inc.; Grand Forks Kiwanis Club. Contact: E. A. Haunz, M.D., Secretary-Treasurer, American Diabetes Association, North Dakota Affiliate, Inc., 221 South Fourth Street, Grand Forks, N.D. 58201. Telephone 701/775-8121, Ext. 214.

OHIO

Camp Ho-Mita-Koda, 14040 Auburn Road, Newbury, Ohio 44065. Sponsored by: Ho Mita Koda, Inc. Contact: Mr. George Cervenka, Camp Director, Camp Ho Mita Koda, 14040 Auburn Road, Newbury, Ohio 44065. Telephone: 216/564-5125.

Camp Ko-Man-She, Lauver Road, Pleasant Hill, Ohio. Sponsored by: Dayton Area Diabetes Association, Inc. Contact: Mrs. Eleanor J. Graham, Executive Secretary, Dayton Area Diabetes Association, Inc., 184 Salem Avenue, Dayton, Ohio 45406. Telephone: 513/228-8166.

Camp Za-Ni-Ka, Camp Stoner, Napoleon, Michigan. Sponsored by: Toledo Diabetes League. Contact: Camp Director, Camp Za-Ni-Ka, % Toledo Diabetes League, 1614 South Byrne Road, Toledo, Ohio 43614. Telephone: 419/385-7517.

Central Ohio Diabetes Association Camp, Loudenville, Ohio. Sponsored by: Central Ohio Diabetes Association, Inc. Contact: Mr. Thomas L. Spitler, Executive Director, Central Ohio Diabetes Association, Inc., 1474 Presidential Drive, Columbus, Ohio 43212. Telephone: 614/486-7344.

OREGON

Gales Creek Camp, Glenwood, Ore. 97120. Sponsored by: Diabetic Children's Camp Foundation. Contact: Mr. C. M. Emeis, President, Diabetic Children's Camp Foundation, 2519 North Mississippi Avenue, Portland, Ore. 97227. Telephone: 503/282-0931.

PENNSYLVANIA

Camp Firefly, Spring Mount, Penn. 19748. Sponsored by: American Diabetes Association, Delaware Valley Affiliate, Inc. Contact: Mr. Joseph C. Hildebrand, Camp Director, American Diabetes Association, Delaware Valley Affiliate, Inc., 919 Walnut Street, Philadelphia, Penn. 19107. Telephone: 215/627-7718.

SOUTH CAROLINA

Carolinas' Camp for Diabetic Children, Eagle's Nest Camp, Pisgah Forest (60 miles east of Brevard and 15 miles west of Hendersonville off U.S. Highway 64), N.C. 28712. Sponsored by: American Diabetes Association, North Carolina Affiliate, Inc.; South Carolina Diabetes Association, Inc. Contact: Mr. Robert A. Bagwell, Chairman, Camp Committee, Carolinas' Camp for Diabetic Children, P.O. Box 8248, Sta. A., Greenville, S.C. 29604. Telephone: 803/235-3395.

SOUTH DAKOTA

Kiwanis Camp Haunz, Black Hills (12 miles from Rapid City), S.D. Sponsored by: Downtown Kiwanis Club, Rapid City, SD. Contact: Mr. Robert R. Calhoon or Mr. John Richards, Co-Chairmen, Kiwanis Camp Haunz, P.O. Box 652, Rapid City, S.D. 57701. Telephone: 605/342-3722.

TENNESSEE

Tennessee Camp for Diabetic Children, Double G Ranch, Soddy, Tenn. 37381. Sponsored by: Tennessee Diabetes Association, Inc. Contact: Mrs. Virginia Eddings, Camp Secretary, Tennessee Camp for Diabetic Children, 519 East Fourth Street, Chattanooga, Tenn. 37403. Telephone: 615/267-7129.

TEXAS

Camp Sweeney Diabetic Educational Training Center, Route 1, Whitesboro, Tex. 76273. Sponsored by: Southwestern Diabetic Foundation, Inc. Contact: Mr. James V. Campbell, Director, Camp Sweeney, P.O. Box 844, Gainesville, Tex. 76240. Telephone: 817/665-9323 or 817/665-9502.

Texas Lions Camps for Diabetic Children (Friendswood and Kerrville) P.O. 247, Kerrville, Tex. 78208. Sponsored by: Texas Lions League, Inc.; American Diabetes Association, South Texas Affiliate, Inc; University of Texas Medical Branch, Galveston, Tex. Contact: Luther B. Travis, M.D., Camp Medical Director and Professor of Pediatrics, Department of Pediatrics, University of Texas Medical Branch, Galveston, Tex. 77550. Telephone: 713/765-2538.

UTAH

Camp Utada, YMCA Camp Roger, Kamas, Utah 84102. Sponsored by: Utah Diabetes Association, Inc. Contact: Mr. Carl Jensen, Committee Chairman, Camp UTADA, 1002 East South Temple, Salt Lake City, Utah 84102. Telephone: 801/355-1452.

VIRGINIA

Camp for Diabetic Boys and Girls, MacKemie Woods Camps (near Williamsburg), Va. Sponsored by: Optimist Club; Medical College of Virginia; Virginia Diabetes Association, Inc; Richmond Area Diabetes Association. Contact: William R. Jordan, M.D., 1631 Monument Avenue, Richmond, Va. 23220.

Camp Holiday Trails, RFD 1, Box 356, Charlottesville, Va. 22901. Sponsored by: Camp Holiday Trails, Inc. Contact: Mr. Alexander Fisher, Executive Director, Camp Holiday Trails, RFD 1, Box 356, Charlottesville, Va. 22901. Telephone: 804/977-3781.

WASHINGTON

Camp Orkila, Orcas Island, Wash. BOYS. Owned by: YMCA. Sponsored by: YMCA. Diabetic Trust Fund; American Diabetes Association, Washington Affiliate, Inc. Contact: Ms. Eloise Schindler, Office Manager, American Diabetes Association, Washington Affiliate, Inc., 1218 Terry Avenue, Room 105, Seattle, Wash. 98101. Telephone: 206/624-5240.

Camp Sealth, Vashon Island, Wash. GIRLS. Owned by: Seattle-King Co. Council of Campfire Girls, Inc. Sponsored by: Camp Fire Girls; Diabetic Trust Fund; American Diabetes Association, Washington Affiliate, Inc. Contact: Ms. Eloise Schindler, Office Manager, American Diabetes Association, Washington Affiliate, Inc., 1218 Terry Avenue, Room 105, Seattle, Wash. 98101. Telephone: 206/624-5240.

WEST VIRGINIA

Camp Kno-Koma, P.O. Box 8184, South Charleston, W.V. 25303. Sponsored by: American Diabetes Association, West Virginia Affiliate, Inc. Contact: Mrs. George Connolly, Secretary, Camp Kno-Koma, P.O. Box 8184, South Charleston, W.V. 25303. Telephone: 304/744-5845.

WISCONSIN

Wisconsin Diabetic Camp, % Camp Sidney Cohen, 2521 North Mill Rd., Delafield, Wisconsin 53018. Sponsored by: Wisconsin Diabetes Association, Inc. Contact: Mr. Richard J. Sandretti, Executive Director, Wisconsin Diabetes Association, Inc., 5215 North Ironwood Road, Milwaukee, Wisc. 53217. Telephone: 414/964-7676.

Camp Needlepoint, YMCA Camp St. Croix, Hudson, Wis. (See Minnesota.)

Summer Camp for Diabetic Children, Camp Holiday Home, Lake Geneva, Wisc. (See Illinois.)

CAMPS IN OTHER COUNTRIES

Information about camps in Canada may be obtained from: The Canadian Diabetic Association, 1491 Yonge Street, Toronto, Ontario M4T 1Z5, Canada.

Information about "children-homes" in other countries may be obtained from: International Diabetes Federation, 3/6 Alfred Place, London WCIE 7E, England.

Drug and supply companies

American Medical Association
535 N. Dearborn St.
Chicago, Ill.
(Diabetes identification)

Ames Company
819 McNaughton Ave.
Elkhart, Ind. 46514
(Urine tests, Dextrostix information)

Becton, Dickinson and Company
P.O. Box 183
Rutherford, N.J. 07070
(Syringes, needles, information)

CIBA-GEIGY
556 Morris Avenue
Summit, N.J. 07901
201/277-5000
(Biguanides, information)

Eli Lilly and Company
Medical Department
307 E. McCarty
P.O. Box 618
Indianapolis, Ind. 46206
(Insulin, Dymelor, urine test, glucagon, information)

Medic Alert Foundation
Turlock, Calif.
(Diabetes identification)

W. A. Morrow Co., Inc.
9633 S.E. 36th St.
P.O. Box 188
Mercer Island, Wash. 98040
(Diabetes identification)

National Identification Co.
3955 Oneida St.
Denver, Colo. 80207
(Diabetes identification)

National Nameplate Co.
Box 40
Greely, Iowa 52050
(Diabetes identification)

Parke Davis & Company
Joseph Campau at the River
Detroit, Mich. 48232
(Syringes, needles, etc.)

Pfizer, Inc.
235 E. 42nd
New York, N.Y. 10017
212/573-2323
(Diabinese, information)

Sherwood Pharmaceutical Co.
62 Madison St.
Hackensack, N.J. 07601
(Needles, syringes, etc.)

E. R. Squibb and Sons
General Office
P.O. Box 4000
Princeton, N.J. 08540
(Insulin, including globin, information)

UpJohn Co.
7000 Portage Rd.
Kalamazoo, Mich. 49001
(Tolbutamide, Tolinase, information)

Other supportive and information services

American Heart Association, Inc.
National Office
44 E. 23rd St.
New York, N.Y. 10010

American Foundation for the Blind
15 W. 16th St.
New York, N.Y. 10011
212/924-0420

Library of Congress
Division for the Blind and Physically
  Handicapped
Washington, D.C. 20524

National Dairy Council
111 N. Canal St.
Chicago, Ill. 60606

**National Easter Seal Society for Crippled
  Children and Adults**
2023 W. Ogden Ave.
Chicago, Ill. 60612

National Kidney Foundation
315 Park Ave. S.
New York, N.Y. 10010
212/982-4450

National Rehabilitation Association
1522 "K" Street, N.W.
Washington, D.C. 20005

Rehabilitation Services Administration
Room 3024
330 C Street, S.W.
Washington, D.C. 20201

U.S. Government Printing Office
Division of Public Documents
Washington, D.C. 20402

APPENDIX C

Suggested course outline

Central objective: This outline is presented to assist the nurse or other health professional in teaching the client to learn as much about the disease, its treatment, methods of communication, and self-care in order to live a useful and productive life.

Subobjectives: On completion of this course, clients should be able to:

1. Relate in simple terms what diabetes is.
2. List action(s) and function(s) of insulin.
3. List action(s) and function(s) of glucagon.
4. Describe the acute complications.
5. Tell what the physician or nurse wishes them to do in regard to acute complications.
6. List the possible chronic complications.
7. Describe early signs and symptoms of chronic complications and report them to physician as soon as they occur.
8. Complete a home record for 3 days.
9. Interpret the outcome of a 3-day record.
10. Demonstrate urine testing procedure(s) and describe an appropriate course of action for continued positive results.
11. Fill out a meal plan for 3 days.
12. List meal plan variations for:
    a. Illness
    b. Travel
    c. Social events
    d. Extra exercise
13. Describe the medication:
    a. Time action
    b. Untoward side effects
    c. Dosage
    d. Method of administration (if insulin—withdrawing, mixing, injecting)
14. Demonstrate care of supplies.
15. Follow through on basics of self-care, which consists of:
    a. Testing urine
    b. Administering medication, as appropriate
    c. Following a meal plan

d. Keeping a record
e. Contacting a health professional, as appropriate

COURSE OUTLINE

I. What is diabetes mellitus

A. Definition of the disease
   Diabetes mellitus is a chronic disease in which there is an inefficient or inadequate supply of insulin or a complete lack of insulin, with the inability of insulin to assist in the body process of metabolizing or burning carbohydrates.

B. Statistics that make diabetes such an important disease
   1. 3rd leading cause of death by disease
   2. 1 out of 20 people; 1 out of 4 families
   3. ½ of heart attacks
   4. ¾ of strokes
   5. ¾ of gangrene

C. Proposed cause of diabetes
   1. Heredity
      a. Genetic theories
      b. Implications of genetics
   2. Infection of pancreas
   3. Tumor of pancreas
   4. Injury to pancreas
   5. Use of stress medications (steroids)
   6. Stress illness (pheochromocytoma, hemochromotosis)

D. Definition of terms
   1. Prediabetes—historical term
   2. Chemical diabetes—normal fasting blood glucose level
      Oral glucose tolerance test—abnormal fasting blood glucose level
   3. Overt diabetes—elevated fasting blood glucose level; abnormal result from oral glucose tolerance test
      a. Non-insulin-dependent diabetes
      b. Insulin-dependent diabetes

259

II. **Complications of diabetes**
  A. Acute complications
    1. Hyperglycemia
    2. Hypoglycemia
  B. Chronic complications
    1. Retinopathy
    2. Microangiopathy
    3. Nephropathy
    4. Neuropathy
    5. Macroangiopathy
III. **Insulin and glucagon**
  A. Action of insulin
    1. Synthesis
    2. Release of insulin
    3. Activity in circulation
    4. Activity with the cell membrane
  B. Action of glucagon
    1. Cause of release
    2. Response to release
    3. Insulin/glucagon ratio
IV. **Medications**
  A. Oral agents—use and action
    1. Types of oral agents
      a. Sulfonylureas
        1. Tolinase
        2. Orinase
        3. Dymelor
        4. Diabinese
      b. Biguanides
        1. DBI
        2. DBI-TD
        3. Metrol
    2. Untoward effects
    3. Use in the body
    4. Research on oral agents
  B. Insulin—use and action
    1. Types of insulin
      a. Short-acting insulin
        1. Regular
        2. Semilente
      b. Intermediate-acting insulin
        1. Lente
        2. NPH
        3. Globin
      c. Long-acting insulin
        1. PZI
        2. Ultralente
    2. Use in the body
    3. Untoward effects
    4. U-40, U-80, U-100
    5. Single-peak insulin
    6. Single-component insulin
    7. Research on insulin

V. **Urine testing procedures**
  A. What tests are available
    1. To test for glucose
      a. Glucose oxidase tests
        1. Clinistix
        2. Testape
        3. Diastix
      b. Reducing substance test: Clinitest
        1. 5-drop test
        2. 2-drop test
        3. 1-drop test
    2. To test for ketones
      a. Ketostix
      b. Acetest
  B. Methods of testing
    1. Single-void technique (or first-voided specimen)
    2. Double-void technique (or second-voided specimen)
  C. Advantages of tests
  D. Disadvantages of tests
  E. Problems associated with tests
  F. Test supplies and their care
VI. **Insulin injection procedures**
  A. Supplies needed
  B. Withdrawing insulin
    1. Needles
      a. Gauge 25, 26, 27
      b. 1 inch, ⅝ inch, ½ inch
    2. Syringes
      a. U-40
      b. U-80
      c. U-100
      d. U-100/50 unit
      e. Tuberculin syringe
    3. Alcohol wipes
  C. Withdrawing insulin
  D. Mixing insulin (as appropriate)
    1. Mixing in a syringe
    2. Mixing in a sterile vial
    3. Diluting insulin
      a. U-50
      b. U-25
      c. U-10
      d. U-1
  E. Injecting of insulin
  F. Rotating injection sites
    1. Where to rotate
    2. Why rotate
  G. Untoward effects
    1. Hypertrophy
    2. Atrophy
    3. Allergy effects
    4. Insulin resistance

H. How to care for supplies
1. Reusable syringes
2. Disposable syringes
3. Injections
4. Hypo-sprays (jet injectors)

VII. **Hypoglycemia**
A. Causes
1. Glucose levels below 60 mg/dl
2. Blood glucose below accustomed levels
B. Treatment
1. Mild hypoglycemia: food
2. Moderate hypoglycemia: simple sugar (20 to 40 calories)
   a. Prepared products—Reactose, tube glucose, other
   b. Household products—juice, table sugar, honey, other
3. Severe hypoglycemia (seizure possibilities): simple sugar, glucagon
C. Identification
1. Bracelets   3. Cards
2. Necklaces   4. School cards
D. Prevention of hypoglycemia

VIII. **Meal planning**
A. Normal nutrition
1. Carbohydrate
2. Proteins
3. Fats
4. Vitamins and minerals
5. Calories
B. The meal plan (choice of one)
1. Exchange system
2. Points system
3. Total available glucose
C. Keeping of food records
1. Following a system
2. Variations of a system
3. System during illness
D. Food and exercise
1. Increased exercise
2. Decreased exercise
3. Somogyi effect
E. Social events and travel
1. Dining out
2. Parties
3. Travel, including driving
4. Back packing
5. Cultural differences
6. School

IX. **Exercise**
A. Action of exercise
1. Decreased exercise
2. Increased exercise

B. Food versus exercise
C. Somogyi effect

X. **Record keeping**
A. What to record
B. Why to record it
C. Interpretation of recording—what to do for:
1. Sugar-free urine
   a. Increased activity
   b. Decreased food
   c. Increased hypoglycemia
2. 75% to 80% sugar-free urine
   a. No change in insulin. When insulin is increased to make urine more than 80% sugar free, also causes hypoglycemia
   b. Increased insulin or decreased food
3. Patterned spill—before same time of glucose spilled in urine
   a. Decrease previous snack (or meal)
   b. Decrease previous snack and meal
   c. Return food and increase insulin
   d. Expect to see decrease of glucose in urine if exercise increased or if food decreased.
4. Increased spill
   a. Increase of insulin
   b. Decrease of food
   c. Increase of exercise
5. When to call the physician, nurse, dietitian, or other health professional

XI. **General hygiene**
A. Eye care (include routine check up as well as check for retinopathy)
B. Care of teeth
C. Skin care
1. General care
2. Cuts and scratches
3. Foot care
   a. Observation—what to look for
   b. Procedures—what to care for, equipment needed

XII. **Illness**
A. Review of diet during illness
B. Insulin and illness
1. Variations management
2. Use of regular insulin
C. When to notify the health professional

XIII. **Research**
A. Pancreatic replacement
1. Islet/beta cell transplants
2. Artificial pancreas
B. Microangiopathy

1. Basement membrane thickening
2. Insulin action
3. Control

C. Other
   1. Medications
   2. Physiology
   3. Genetic markers

XIV. Review
A. Return demonstration
   1. Insulin procedure
   2. Urine test procedures
   3. Meal planning
   4. Record keeping
B. Description and treatment of
   1. Hyperglycemia
   2. Hypoglycemia
   3. General hygiene
C. Evaluation
   1. Testing
   2. General discussion
      a. Methods of communication
         1. Clinic
         2. Phone
         3. Letter
         4. Record
      b. Follow-up
         1. Clinic
         2. American Diabetes Association
         3. Continuing education

MET levels of activities*

Definitions

MET: Work metabolic rate = oxygen consumption
  Resting metabolic rate = oxygen consumption at sitting rest
  (Note: Values do not refer to duration of effort or total expenditure over some period of time.)

Static tension (+): Static or isometric component of an activity that *increases* the work required of the heart.

Points to consider before initiating specific tasks:
1. MET level at which you are functioning.
2. Environment: temperature, clothing, emotional stress, position.
3. Duration: you should have full recovery without fatigue within one hour of activity.

ACTIVITIES LISTED BY MET LEVELS

Self-care

	METs
Sit in chair as tolerated, fully supported	1
Care for fingernails	1.2
Brush teeth	1.2
Feed self in bed, back supported	1.3
Wash hands and face, back supported	1.5
Wash upper body (except back) with back supported	1.5
Feed self sitting on edge of bed	1.5
Baths in tub (excluding transfer)	1.5
Comb hair, male and female	1.5
Sit on edge of bed	1.5
Sit on bedside commode with assisted transfer	1.5+
Shaving, electric and safety razor	1.6
Washing hair, male and female	1.5+

Self-care—cont'd

	METs
Setting hair	1.6+
Wash entire body at bedside	1.7+
Wash entire body sitting in bathroom (excluding transfer)	1.7+
Showering, sitting (excluding transfer)	1.8+
Dressing and undressing bedclothes	2+
Dressing and undressing street clothes	2+
Showering, standing	3.8
Use bedpan	4.8

Housework

	METs
Machine sewing, household	2.3
Washing small clothes	2.5
Mix batter	2.5+
Peeling potatoes	3.2
Fix simple meal (breakfast or lunch)	2-3+
Fold clothes	2-3+
Wash clothes (by machine)	2-3+
Fix complex meal (dinner)	3+
Wash dishes	3+
Ironing, house, standing	3++
Scrubbing at counter height, standing	3++
Making bed	2-3++
Bending and stooping (pick up newspaper)	3++
Cleaning stove (inside)	3-4++
Scrub pots and pans	3-4++
Dusting/polishing (reaching with arms)	3-4++
Changing bed	3-4++
Wringing by hand	4.5
Hanging wash	4.6
Mopping floors (hands and knees)	3-5++

*From Gordon, Edward E.: The use of energy costs in regulating physical activity in chronic disease, AMA Arch. Indus. Health **16**:437, 1957. Copyright 1957, American Medical Association.

Housework—cont'd	METs	*Avocational/recreational*—cont'd	METs
Vacuuming (bare floor to pile rugs)	4-5++	Chip carving, back supported	2.1
		Copper tooling	2.2
Sweeping floor	4-5++	Weaving, table loom	2.2
Mopping (standing)	4-5++	Leather carving, sitting	2.3
Grocery shopping	4-5++++	Painting, sitting	2.5
Scrubbing, polishing, waxing, floors, walls, cars, windows while standing	5-6+++	Chisel carving with mallet, sitting	2.5
		Printing (hand composition)	2.6
		Horseshoes	3
Turning mattress	7+++++	Horseback riding, walk	3.3
Vocational		Playing organ, sitting	3.5
Sitting at desk, writing, calculating	1.5	Playing piano	2-3++
		Hammering	3++++
Lying down under a car as by service mechanic	1.5	Walking, 2.5 mph	3+
		Lift 20 lb maximum; frequently lift 10 lb	3.5±±±
Use hand tools	1.8		
Light assembly work	1.8	Volleyball	3.8
Radio repair	1.8	Planting	3-4
Driving a truck	1.8	Riding motorcycle	3-4+++
Working heavy levers	2	Paint wall	3-4++
Dredge	2	Cycling, 5.5 mph	3-4++
Watch repairing	2.1	Sexual activity	3-4+++
Bookbinding, light	2.3	Playing drums	4.3
Typing rapidly	2.3	Bowling	4.5
Power sanding or sawing	2.6	Gardening	4.7
Armature winding	2.6	Badminton	4-5
Bricklaying	3-5+++	Ping-Pong	4-5
Plastering	3-5+++	Archery	4-5
Carpentry	4-6++++	Walking downstairs	4.5
Lift maximum 50 lb; frequently lift or carry 25 lb	4-6++++	Swimming, breast stroke, 20 yd/min	5
Wheeling barrow, 50 lb.	4++++	Weeding	3-5+
Shoveling	5-7++++	Sailing	2-5+
Digging holes	5-7++++	Walking, 3.5 mph	5.5+
Chopping wood	5-7++++	Hoeing	4-6++
Light/heavy farming	5-7+++	Planing	4-6+++
Light/heavy industrial	5-7+++	Canoeing, 2-5 mph	3-6+++
Lift maximum 100 lb; frequently lift/carry 50 lb	6-8+++++	Golfing	4-7
		Hunting	4-6
Avocational/recreational		Sawing wood	5-7
Phoning, conversation	1.0	Ice skating	5-7
Leather punching, lacing, back supported	1.8	Horseback riding, trotting	7.5
		Mowing lawn by hand or power	8
Leather tooling, back supported	1.8	Dancing, fox-trot	5-7±±±
Making link belt, back supported	1.9	Spading	3-8
Rug hooking, sitting	1.9	Cycling, 13 mph	7-9
Hand sewing	2	Skiing (snow or water)	9
Knitting, 23 st/min	2	Squash	9
Embroidery	2	Tennis	5-15+
Playing cards or any sitting competitive game	2		

Some calorie/exercise expenditures*

The following are lists of various classifications of work and recreation in relation to calories expended per minute.

	kcal/min		kcal/min
Work		*Self-care*—cont'd	
Light	2.5	Stand, relaxed	1.4
Moderate	5.0	Eating	1.4
Heavy	7.5	Conversation	1.4
Very heavy	10.0	Dressing, undressing	2.3
Extremely heavy	12.5	Washing hands, face,	2.5
Rest	1.25	brushing hair	
Locomotion		Washing and shaving	2.6
Wheelchair, 1.2 mph	2.4	Washing and dressing	2.6
Walking, 2.5 mph	3.6	Using bedside commode	3.6
Walking, 2.75 mph	5.6	Showering	4.2
Walking downstairs	5.2	Using a bed pan	4.7
Walk, crutches and braces,	8.0	Bathing in tub	
1.2 mph		*Household tasks*	
Walking upstairs (17-lb load,	9.0	Hand sewing	1.4
27 ft/min)		Knitting	1.5
Walking upstairs (no load)	—	Sweeping	1.7
Exercises		Ironing, standing	1.7
Bending at waist (sideways),	2.2	Machine sewing	1.8
13/min		Simple work, sitting	1.7
Sitting on floor, touching toes,	2.4	Brushing boots	2.2
16/min		Polishing	2.4
Balancing exercises	2.5	Peeling potatoes	2.9
Abdominal exercises	3.0	Scrubbing, standing	2.9
Lying on floor, leg raising,	3.5	Washing small clothes	3.0
10/min		Bringing in wash	3.3
Trunk bending	3.5	Kneading dough	3.3
Arm swinging, hopping	6.5	Getting coal	3.5
Deep knee bends, 16/min	6.7	Scrubbing floors	3.6
Push ups, 16/min	7.5	Making beds	3.9
Self-care		Cleaning windows	3.7
Rest supine	1.0	Mopping	4.2
Sitting	1.2	Wringing by hand	4.4
		Hanging wash	4.5
		Polishing floors	4.8
		Beating carpets	4.9

*Data from Berg, R. H.: One sensible way to diet, Look **33:**84-90, Dec. 16, 1969.

265

Household tasks—cont'd	kcal/min	*Occupations*	kcal/min
		CLERICAL WORK	
Breaking firewood	4.9	Electric typewriter, 30 w/min	1.16
Bed making and stripping	5.4	Electric typewriter, 40 w/min	1.31
Clearing floors, kneeling, bending	6.0	Mechanical typewriter, 30 w/min	1.39
Vacuum cleaning	—	Mechanical typewriter, 40 w/min	1.48
Dusting	—	Misc. office work, sitting	1.6
Children's recreation		Misc. office work, standing	1.8
Sitting, listening to radio	1.0	LIGHT ENGINEERING WORK	
Sitting, playing at puzzle	1.2	Watch and clock repair	1.6
Sitting, singing	1.4	Light assembly line	1.8
Standing, drawing	1.5-1.9	Draftsman	1.8
Cycling	2.4-3.1	Armature winding	2.2
Carpentry	3.0	Light machine work	2.4
Recreation		Radio assembly	2.7
Sitting, listening to radio	2.0-2.5	PRINTING INDUSTRY	
Painting	2.0	Hand composition	2.2
Sitting, writing	1.9-2.2	Printing	2.2
Playing cards	2.2	Paper laying	2.5
Playing piano	2.5	LEATHER TRADE	
Playing violin	2.7	Polishing shoes	1.8
Car driving	2.8	Filing soles	2.3
Canoeing	3.0-2.5 mph	Fixing soles	2.4
Horseback riding, slow	3.0	Shoe repairing	2.7
Playing volleyball	3.5	Shoe manufacturing	3.0
Playing with children	3.5	PRESS GOODS INDUSTRY	
Playing drums	4.0-4.2	Pressing, household utensils	3.8
Sculling, 51 m/min, 12 mph	4.1	LOCKSMITH	
Bowling	4.4	Filing with large file	3.3-3.7
Cycling, 5.5 mph	4.5	Five other processes	2.1-2.9
Golf	5.0	TAILOR	
Swimming	5.0-20 yd/min	Hand sewing	2.0-1.9
Archery	5.2	Cutting	2.4-2.7
Dancing	5.5	Machine sewing	2.8-2.9
Gardening, weeding	5.6	Pressing	3.5-4.3
Recreational swimming	6-7.0	Ironing	4.2
Tennis	7.1	POSTMAN CLIMBING STAIRS	
Trotting on a horse	8.0	Postal load, 11 kg	9.8
Spading	8.6	Postal load, 16 kg	9.8-13.8
Gardening, digging	8.6	PICK, SHOVEL, AND WHEELBARROW	
Playing football	8.9	Shoveling, 8-kg load, less than 1-m lift, 12 throws/min	7.5
Skiing	9.9	Shoveling, 8-kg load, from 2-m lift, 12 throws/min	9.5
Playing squash	10.2		
Climbing slope, 1 inch 5.75 kg lead	10.7	Shoveling, 16 lb	8.5
Cycling, 13 mph	11.0	Wheelbarrow, 115 lb, 2.5 mph	5.0
Swimming, breast stroke, 40 yd/min	10.0	Hoeing with pick	7.0
Swimming, side stroke, 40 yd/min	11.0	BUILDING INDUSTRY	
Swimming, back stroke, 40 yd/min	11.5	Measuring wood	2.4
Swimming, crawl, 45 yd/min	11.5	Machine sawing	2.4

Occupations—cont'd	**kcal/min**	*Occupations*—cont'd	**kcal/min**
Light work in laying stones or bricks	3.4	Drilling hardwood	7.0
		Sawing hardwood	6.3
Measuring and sawing	3.5	Planing softwood	8.1
Misc. work, carrying	3.6	Planing hardwood	9.1
Shaping stones with mason's hammer	3.8	Using heavy hammer	6.3-9.8
		MISCELLANEOUS	
Making wall with bricks and mortar	4.0	Tractor	4.2
		Plowing	5.9
Plastering	4.1	Haying	7.3
Joining floor boards	4.4	Mowing lawn by hand	7.3
Mixing cement	4.7	Felling tree	8.0
Chiseling	5.7	Tending furnace	10.2
Sawing softwood	6.3	Ascending, 22-lb load, 54 ft/min	16.2

Revised exchange list, 1976*

LIST 1: NONFAT MILK EXCHANGES

One exchange of nonfat milk contains 12 gm of carbohydrate, 8 gm of protein, a trace of fat, and 80 calories.

Milk is a basic food for your Meal Plan for very good reasons. Milk is the leading source of calcium. It is a good source of phosphorus, protein, some of the B-complex vitamins, including folacin and vitamin B_{12}, and vitamins A and D. Magnesium is also found in milk.

Since it is a basic ingredient in many recipes you will not find it difficult to include milk in your Meal Plan. Milk can be used not only to drink but can be added to cereal, coffee, tea, and other foods.

This list shows the kinds and amounts of milk or milk products to use for one Milk Exchange. Those that appear in CAPS are nonfat. Low-fat and whole milk contain saturated fat.

	Weight† (gm)	Amount to use
Nonfat fortified milks		
SKIM OR NONFAT MILK	240	1 cup
POWDERED (NONFAT DRY, BEFORE ADDING LIQUID)	60	⅓ cup
CANNED, EVAPORATED SKIM MILK	120	½ cup
BUTTERMILK MADE FROM SKIM MILK	240	1 cup
YOGURT MADE FROM SKIM MILK (PLAIN, UNFLAVORED)		1 cup
Low-fat fortified milk		
1% fat fortified milk (omit ½ Fat Exchange)		1 cup

	Weight (gm)	Amount to use
2% fat fortified milk (omit 1 Fat Exchange)	240	1 cup
Yogurt made from 2% fortified milk (plain, unflavored) (omit 1 Fat Exchange)	240	1 cup
Whole milk (omit 2 Fat Exchanges)		
Whole milk	240	1 cup
Canned, evaporated whole milk	120	½ cup
Buttermilk made from whole milk	240	1 cup
Yogurt made from whole milk (plain, unflavored)	240	1 cup

LIST 2: VEGETABLE EXCHANGES

One exchange of vegetables contains about 5 gm of carbohydrate, 2 gm of protein and 25 calories.

The generous use of many vegetables, served either alone or in other foods such as casseroles, soups or salads, contributes to sound health and vitality.

Dark green and deep yellow vegetables are among the leading sources of vitamin A. Many of the vegetables in this group are notable sources of vitamin C— asparagus, broccoli, brussels sprouts, cabbage, cauliflower, collard greens, kale, dandelion, mustard and turnip greens, spinach, rutabagas, tomatoes, and turnips. A number are particularly good sources of potassium—broccoli, brussels sprouts, beet greens, chard, and tomato juice. High folacin values are found in asparagus, beets, broccoli, brussels sprouts, cauliflower, collards, kale, and lettuce. Moderate amounts of vitamin B_6 are supplied by broccoli, brussels sprouts, cauliflower, collards, spinach, sauerkraut, and tomatoes and tomato juice. Fiber is present in all vegetables.

Whether you serve them cooked or raw, wash all vegetables even though they look clean. If fat is added

---

*From Meal planning with exchange lists, New York, June 1976, The American Diabetes Association Inc.
†Weights obtained from Church, F., C., and Church, H. N.: Food values, ed. 12, Philadelphia, 1975, J. B. Lippincott Co.; Adam, C. F.: Nutritive values of American foods, Handbook No. 456, U.S. Department of Agriculture, Washington, D.C., 1975, U.S. Government Printing Office.

in the preparation, omit the equivalent number of Fat Exchanges. The average amount of fat contained in a Vegetable Exchange that is cooked with fat meat or other fats is one Fat Exchange.

This list shows the kinds of *vegetables* to use for one Vegetable Exchange. One exchange is ½ cup.

Asparagus	Mustard
Bean sprouts	Spinach
Beets	Turnip
Broccoli	Mushrooms
Brussels sprouts	Okra
Cabbage	Onions
Carrots	Rhubarb
Cauliflower	Rutabaga
Celery	Sauerkraut
Cucumbers	String beans, green or
Eggplant	yellow
Green pepper	Summer squash
Greens	Tomatoes
Beet	Tomato juice
Chards	Turnips
Collards	Vegetable juice cocktail
Dandelion	Zucchini
Kale	

The following *raw vegetables* may be used as desired:

Chicory	Lettuce
Chinese cabbage	Parsley
Endive	Radishes
Escarole	Watercress

Starchy vegetables are found in the Bread Exchange List.

LIST 3: FRUIT EXCHANGES

One exchange of fruit contains 10 grams of carbohydrate and 40 calories.

Everyone likes to buy fresh fruits when they are in the height of their season. However, you can also buy fresh fruits and can or freeze them for off-season use. For variety, serve fruit as a salad or in combination with other foods for dessert.

Fruits are valuable for vitamins, minerals, and fiber. Vitamin C is abundant in citrus fruits and fruit juices and is found in raspberries, strawberries, mangoes, cantaloupes, honeydew melons, and papayas. The better sources of vitamin A among these fruits include fresh or dried apricots, mangoes, cantaloupes, nectarines, yellow peaches, and persimmons. Oranges, orange juice, and cantaloupe provide more folacin than most of the other fruits in this listing. Many fruits are a valuable source of potassium, especially apricots, bananas, several of the berries, grapefruit, grapefruit juice, mangoes, canta-

loupes, honeydew melons, nectarines, oranges, orange juice, and peaches.

Fruit may be used fresh, dried, canned or frozen, cooked or raw, as long as no sugar is added.

This list shows the kinds and amounts of *fruits* to use for one Fruit Exchange.

	Weight (gm)	Amount to use
Apple	80	1 small
Apple juice	80	⅓ cup
Applesauce (unsweetened)	100	½ cup
Apricots, fresh	80	2 medium
Apricots, dried	15	4 halves
Banana	50	½ small
Berries	50	
Blackberries	150	½ cup
Blueberries	100	½ cup
Raspberries	150	½ cup
Strawberries	150	¾ cup
Cherries	75	10 large
Cider	80	⅓ cup
Dates	15	2
Figs, fresh	50	1
Figs, dried	15	1
Grapefruit	125	½
Grapefruit juice	100	½ cup
Grapes	75	12
Grape juice	60	¼ cup
Mango	70	½ small
Melon		
Cantaloupe	200	¼ small
Honeydew	150	⅛ medium
Watermelon	150	1 cup
Nectarine	50	1 small
Orange	100	1 small
Orange juice	100	½ cup
Papaya	90	¾ cup
Peach	100	1 medium
Pear	75	1 small
Persimmon, native	50	1 medium
Pineapple	80	½ cup
Pineapple juice	80	⅓ cup
Plums	100	2 medium
Prunes	25	2 medium
Prune juice	65	¼ cup
Raisins	15	2 tbsp
Tangerine	100	1 medium

Cranberries may also be used as desired if no sugar is added.

LIST 4: BREAD EXCHANGES (includes bread, cereal, and starchy vegetables)

One exchange of bread contains 15 grams of carbohydrate, 2 grams of protein and 70 calories.

In this list, whole-grain and enriched breads and cereals, germ and bran products, and dried beans and peas are good sources of iron and among the better sources of thiamin. The whole-grain, bran, and germ products have more fiber than products made from refined flours. Dried beans and peas are also good sources of fiber. Wheat germ, bran, fried beans, potatoes, lima beans, parsnips, pumpkin, and winter squash are particularly good sources of potassium. The better sources of folacin in this listing include whole-wheat bread, wheat germ, dried beans, corn, lima beans, parsnips, green peas, pumpkin, and sweet potato. Starchy vegetables are included in this list because they contain the same amount of carbohydrate and protein as one slice of bread.

This list shows the kinds and amounts of *breads, cereals, starchy vegetables,* and *prepared foods* to use for one Bread Exchange. Those that appear in CAPS are low fat.

	Weight (gm)	Amount to use
Bread		
WHITE (INCLUDING FRENCH AND ITALIAN)	25	1 slice
WHOLE WHEAT	25	1 slice
RYE OR PUMPERNICKEL	25	1 slice
RAISIN	25	1 slice
BAGEL, SMALL	25	½
ENGLISH MUFFIN, SMALL	25	½
PLAIN ROLL, BREAD	35	1
FRANKFURTER, ROLL	20	½
HAMBURGER BUN	40	½
DRIED BREAD CRUMBS	100	¼ cup
TORTILLAS, 6 inch	30	1
Cereal		
BRAN FLAKES	25	½ cup
OTHER READY-TO-EAT UNSWEETENED CEREAL	20	¾ cup
PUFFED CEREAL (UNFROSTED)	20	¾ cup
CEREAL (COOKED)	20	½ cup
GRITS (COOKED)	20	½ cup
RICE OR BARLEY (COOKED)	100	½ cup
PASTA (COOKED), SPAGHETTI, NOODLES, MACARONI	100	½ cup
POPCORN (POPPED, NO FAT ADDED)	20	3 cups
CORNMEAL (DRY)	17	2 Tbs

Cereal—cont'd		
FLOUR	20	2½ Tbs
WHEAT GERM	50	⅓ cup
Crackers		
ARROWROOT	15	3
GRAHAM, 2½-inch square	20	2
MATZOTH, 4 × 6 inch	10	½
OYSTER	45	5 small
PRETZELS, 3⅛ inches long, ⅛ inch d	25	15
RYE WAFERS, 2 × 3½ inches	20	3
SALTINES	20	6
SODA, 2½-inch square	30	4
Dried beans, peas, and lentils		
BEANS, PEAS, LENTILS (DRIED AND COOKED)	90	½ cup
BAKED BEANS, NO PORK (CANNED)	50	¼ cup
Starchy vegetables		
CORN	80	⅓ cup
CORN ON COB	140	1 small
LIMA BEANS	50	½ cup
PARSNIPS	125	⅔ cup
PEAS, GREEN (CANNED OR FROZEN)	100	½ cup
POTATO, WHITE	100	1 small
POTATO (MASHED)	100	½ cup
PUMPKIN	170	¾ cup
WINTER, ACORN, OR BUTTERNUT SQUASH	100	½ cup
YAM OR SWEET POTATO	50	¼ cup
Prepared foods		
Biscuit, 2-inch d (omit 1 Fat Exchange)	35	1
Corn bread, 2 × 2 × 1 inch (omit 1 Fat Exchange)	35	1
Corn muffin, 2-inch d (omit 1 Fat Exchange)	35	1
Crackers, round butter type (omit 1 Fat Exchange)	20	5
Muffin, plain small (omit 1 Fat Exchange)	35	1
Potatoes, french fried, 2 to 3½ inches long (omit 1 Fat Exchange)	30	5
Potato or corn chips (omit 2 Fat Exchanges)	30	15
Pancake, ½ × 5 inches (omit 1 Fat Exchange)	55	1
Waffle, ½ × 5 inches (omit 1 Fat Exchange)	75	1

LIST 5: MEAT EXCHANGES (Lean Meat)

One exchange of lean meat (1 oz) contains 7 gm of protein, 3 gm of fat and 55 calories.

All of the foods in the Meat Exchange Lists are good sources of protein, and many are also good sources of iron, zinc, vitamin B_{12} (present only in foods of animal origin), and other vitamins of the B-complex.

Cholesterol is of animal origin. Foods of plant origin have no cholesterol.

Oysters are outstanding for their high content of zinc. Crab, liver, trimmed lean meats, the dark muscle meat of turkey, dried beans, peas, and peanut butter all have much less zinc than oysters but are still good sources.

Dried beans, peas, and peanut butter are particularly good sources of magnesium and potassium.

Your choice of meat groups through the week will depend on your blood lipid values. Consult with your diet counselor and your physician regarding your selection.

You may use the meat, fish, or other meat exchanges that are prepared for the family when no fat or flour has been added. If meat is fried, use the fat included in the Meal Plan. Meat juices with the fat removed may be used with your meat or vegetables for added flavor. Be certain to trim off all visible fat and measure meat after it has been cooked. A 3-ounce serving of cooked meat is about equal to 4 ounces of raw meat.

To plan a diet low in saturated fat and cholesterol, choose only those exchanges in CAPS. This list shows the kinds and amounts of *lean meat* and other *protein-rich foods* to use for one Low-Fat Meat Exchange.

	Weight (gm)	Amount to use
Beef: BABY BEEF (VERY LEAN), CHIPPED BEEF, CHUCK, FLANK STEAK, TENDERLOIN, PLATE RIBS, PLATE SKIRT STEAK, ROUND (BOTTOM, TOP), ALL CUTS RUMP, SPARE RIBS, TRIPE	30	1 oz
Lamb: LEG, RIB, SIRLOIN, LOIN (ROAST AND CHOPS), SHANK, SHOULDER	30	1 oz
Pork: LEG (WHOLE RUMP, CENTER SHANK), HAM, SMOKED (CENTER SLICES)	30	1 oz

	Weight (gm)	Amount to use
Veal: LEG, LOIN, RIB, SHANK, SHOULDER, CUTLETS	30	1 oz
Poultry: MEAT WITHOUT SKIN OF CHICKEN, TURKEY, CORNISH HEN, GUINEA HEN, PHEASANT	30	1 oz
Fish		
ANY FRESH OR FROZEN	30	1 oz
CANNED SALMON, TUNA, MACKEREL, CRAB, AND LOBSTER		¼ cup
CLAMS, OYSTERS, SCALLOPS, AND SHRIMP	30	5 or 1 oz
SARDINES, DRAINED	30	3
CHEESES CONTAINING LESS THAN 5% BUTTERFAT	30	1 oz
COTTAGE CHEESE, DRY AND 2% BUTTERFAT	30	¼ cup
DRIED BEANS AND PEA (omit 1 Bread Exchange)	90	½ cup

LIST 5: MEAT EXCHANGES (Medium-Fat Meat)

For each exchange of medium-fat meat omit ½ Fat Exchange (7 gm protein, 5 gm fat, and 75 calories).

This list shows the kinds and amounts of *medium-fat meat* and other *protein-rich foods* to use for one Medium-Fat Meat Exchange.

	Weight (gm)	Amount to use
Beef: ground (15% fat), corned beef (canned), rib eye, round (ground commercial)	30	1 oz
Pork: loin (all cuts tenderloin), shoulder arm (picnic), shoulder blade, Boston butt, Canadian bacon, boiled ham	30	1 oz
Liver, heart, kidney and sweetbreads (these are high in cholesterol), and creamed cottage cheese	30	1 oz
Cheese: mozzarella, ricotta, farmer's cheese, Neufchatel, Parmesan	60	¼ cup 3 Tbs
Egg (high in cholesterol)	50	1
PEANUT BUTTER (omit 2 additional Fat Exchanges)	30	2 Tbs

LIST 5: MEAT EXCHANGES (High-Fat Meat)

For each exchange of high-fat meat omit 1 Fat Exchange (7 gm protein, 7 gm fat, and 95 calories).

This list shows the kinds and amounts of *high-fat meat* and other *protein-rich foods* to use for one High-Fat Meat Exchange.

	Weight (gm)	Amount to use
Beef: brisket, corned beef (brisket), ground beef (more than 20% fat), hamburger (commercial), chuck (ground commercial), roasts (rib), steaks (club and rib)	30	1 oz
Lamb: breast	30	1 oz
Pork: spare ribs, loin (back ribs), pork (ground), country style ham, deviled ham	30	1 oz
Veal: breast	30	1 oz
Poultry: capon, duck (domestic), goose	30	1 oz
Cheese: cheddar types	30	1 oz
Cold cuts	45	4½ × ⅛ inch
Frankfurter	50	1

LIST 6: FAT EXCHANGES

One exchange of fat contains 5 grams of fat and 45 calories.

Fats are of both animal and vegetable origin and range from liquid oils to hard fats. Oils are fats that remain liquid at room temperature and are usually of vegetable origin. Common fats obtained from vegetables are corn oil, olive oil, and peanut oil. Some of the common animal fats are butter and bacon fat.

Since all fats are concentrated sources of calories, foods on this list should be measured carefully to control weight. Margarine, butter, cream, and cream cheese contain Vitamin A. Use the fats on this list in the amounts on the Meal Plan.

This list shows the kinds and amounts of *fat-containing foods* to use for one Fat Exchange. To plan a diet low in saturated fat select only those exchanges that appear in CAPS. They are polyunsaturated.

	Weight (gm)	Amount to use
MARGARINE, SOFT, TUB OR STICK*	5	1 tsp
AVOCADO, 4-inch d†	25	⅛
OIL, CORN, COTTONSEED, SAFFLOWER, SOY SUNFLOWER	5	1 tsp
OIL, OLIVE†	5	1 tsp
OIL, PEANUT†	5	1 tsp
OLIVES†	50	5 small
ALMONDS†	10	10 whole
PECANS†	5	2 large whole
PEANUTS†		
SPANISH	10	20 whole
VIRGINIA	10	10 whole
WALNUTS	15	6 small
NUTS, OTHER†	15	6 small
Margarine, regular stick	5	1 tsp
Butter	5	1 tsp
Bacon fat	5	1 tsp
Bacon, crisp	10	1 strip
Cream, light	30	2 Tbs
Cream, sour	30	2 Tbs
Cream, heavy	15	1 Tbs
Cream cheese	15	1 Tbs
French dressing‡	15	1 Tbs
Italian dressing‡	15	1 Tbs
Lard	5	1 tsp
Mayonnaise‡	5	1 tsp
Salad dressing, mayonnaise type‡	10	2 tsp
Salt pork	5	¾-inch cube

---

*Made with corn, cottonseed, safflower, soy or sunflower oil only.

†Fat content is primarily monounsaturated.

‡If made with corn, cottonseed, safflower, soy, or sunflower oil, can be used on fat modified diet.

Index